A superior work of scholarship that blends cross-sectoral dimensions needed for building the art of public health at the grassroots, at tables of governance, and also for academic understanding. Practitioners of the global health trade must get their hands on this book for resolving bottlenecks and building resilient societies.

Edmond Fernandes, *Director, Edward & Cynthia Institute of Public Health, India*

This book gives research-based insights into the impact of agricultural diversity on the nutritional status of children, issues in capturing child nutrition challenges and the journey to sustainable food production, and the role of fortification and nutrigenomics in India. It also highlights the benefits and challenges of promoting millets and pathways to sustainable food choices, women's empowerment for nutritional well-being, and harnessing artificial intelligence for enhanced nutritional outcomes. This book will be useful for prospective and future researchers in the field of public health, food and nutrition, and gender and women's studies.

Neerja Sood, *Associate Professor, School of Health Sciences, IGNOU, New Delhi, India*

Agriculture, Nutrition, and Resilience

This book aims to provide a comprehensive analysis of food security by exploring the interconnections between agricultural practices, nutritional status, socioeconomic factors, and technological advancements. It addresses the challenges posed by population growth, climate change, and socioeconomic disparities, focusing on sustainable agriculture, equitable access to food, and community resilience. The book integrates insights from multilevel modeling, structural equation modeling, and case studies to highlight effective strategies for combating malnutrition, promoting gender equality, and enhancing food systems. It also emphasizes the importance of policy interventions, community engagement, and innovative technologies in fostering a sustainable, resilient, and equitable global food landscape.

Key features

- **Multidisciplinary Approach:** Integrates nutrition, agriculture, economics, and gender studies to offer a comprehensive view of food security challenges and solutions.
- **Advanced Analytical Methods:** Employs multilevel modeling and structural equation modeling to identify key factors affecting child nutrition and the impact of agricultural productivity.
- **Focus on Gender Equality:** Highlights the critical role of women's health and empowerment in improving food systems and achieving sustainable development goals.
- **Practical Solutions:** Proposes actionable strategies such as rice fortification and millet promotion, tailored to diverse socioeconomic and climatic conditions.
- **Holistic Framework:** Combines theoretical insights with real-world applications to create a sustainable, resilient, and equitable global food system.

The target audience for this book includes researchers, policymakers, public health professionals, agricultural and environmental scientists, NGOs, community leaders, students, educators, and development agencies. It provides insights into food security, sustainable agriculture, nutrition, gender equality, and community engagement, making it valuable for those involved in related fields and initiatives.

Agriculture, Nutrition, and Resilience

Recent Insights and Innovations

Edited by
Shikha Saxena and Chhavi Taliwal

CRC Press
Taylor & Francis Group
Boca Raton London New York

CRC Press is an imprint of the
Taylor & Francis Group, an **informa** business

Designed cover image: Shikha Saxena

First edition published 2025
by CRC Press
2385 NW Executive Center Drive, Suite 320, Boca Raton FL 33431

and by CRC Press
4 Park Square, Milton Park, Abingdon, Oxon, OX14 4RN

CRC Press is an imprint of Taylor & Francis Group, LLC

Library of Congress Cataloging-in-Publication Data
Names: Saxena, Shikha, editor. | Taliwal, Chhavi, editor.
Title: Agriculture, nutrition, and resilience : recent insights and innovations /
Shikha Saxena and Chhavi Taliwal.
Description: First edition | Boca Raton, FL : CRC Press, 2025. |
Includes bibliographical references and index.
Identifiers: LCCN 2024051008 (print) | LCCN 2024051009 (ebook) |
ISBN 9781032782409 (hardback) | ISBN 9781032782966 (paperback) |
ISBN 9781003487227 (ebook)
Subjects: LCSH: Nutrition. | Food security. | Nutrition policy.
Classification: LCC QP141 .A43 2025 (print) | LCC QP141 (ebook) |
DDC 363.8–dc23/eng/20250102
LC record available at https://lccn.loc.gov/2024051008
LC ebook record available at https://lccn.loc.gov/2024051009

ISBN: 978-1-032-78240-9 (hbk)
ISBN: 978-1-032-78296-6 (pbk)
ISBN: 978-1-003-48722-7 (ebk)

DOI: 10.1201/9781003487227

Typeset in Times
by Newgen Publishing UK

Contents

Preface

Food security is shaped by a myriad of factors, including population growth, urbanization, climate change, and socioeconomic disparities. Addressing these challenges requires integrated approaches that encompass policy interventions, technological innovations, and community-based solutions. Governments play a crucial role in supporting sustainable agriculture and ensuring equitable access to food, while technological advancements and community engagement enhance resilience. A holistic strategy is essential for developing a more equitable and resilient food system.

Understanding the nutritional status of children is a complex process influenced by maternal health, education, local health facilities, and agricultural productivity. This book employs multilevel modeling to identify key factors affecting child stunting and underweight, revealing significant associations with agricultural production and infrastructure access. Structural equation modeling further indicates that maternal BMI mediates these impacts, with crop production indirectly influencing child nutrition through economic and consumption changes.

Addressing food security also involves tackling issues like poverty, hunger, and climate change, improving food distribution systems, and advancing agricultural technologies. Sustainable practices such as crop diversification and soil management are vital components of these efforts. Collaboration among stakeholders, continuous policy implementation, and the promotion of inclusive policies and innovation are crucial for ensuring a resilient and food-secure future.

This book explores the intricate relationship between nutritional security, women's health, and empowerment. Using a blend of literature, databases, and state-led models, it highlights the positive impact of gender equality on food systems. Improvements in food consumption and women's anthropometric profiles are noted, despite persistent malnutrition and anemia. Empowering women beyond traditional societal norms can significantly enhance national and global development indices. International frameworks should adopt gender-neutral, equity-oriented approaches, with strategic interventions to address vulnerabilities and ensure community food security.

Focusing on child malnutrition in India, this book emphasizes the importance of village-level data for understanding and addressing this issue. Despite economic growth, high rates of child malnutrition persist. The need for early-stage nutrition interventions, detailed data for planning, and consideration of socioeconomic factors is underscored, with regional differences showcased through case studies. Effective, targeted treatments and evidence-based policymaking rely on comprehensive village-level data collection, as highlighted by programs like the National Nutrition Mission.

Rice fortification emerges as an effective strategy to enhance food security and combat malnutrition, aligning with United Nations Sustainable Development Goal 2. Adding essential nutrients to rice, a staple food, addresses hidden hunger and nutrient deficiencies while preserving cultural diets. This scalable solution supports public health initiatives, ensuring long-term sustainability and a healthier global food landscape.

Genetic variability significantly affects nutrient bioavailability and metabolism, making nutrigenomics crucial for personalized nutrition and medicine. This approach, similar to pharmacogenomics, tailors dietary recommendations and medication efficacy by targeting genes related to diseases like cancer and diabetes. Successful implementation requires biomarker trials, global collaboration, and robust databases for effective health improvement.

Promoting millets can significantly enhance food and nutrition security, especially in climate-vulnerable regions. This requires consumer education, market expansion, farmer training, and supportive policies. Successful initiatives in Karnataka and Odisha demonstrate the benefits of millets, supporting sustainable agriculture, better nutrition, and a healthier, more equitable food system.

The carbon footprint of food consumption has a significant impact on the environment, contributing to greenhouse gas emissions. Strategies to reduce this impact include consuming locally grown food, reducing meat consumption, and choosing sustainable food products. Emphasizing nutritional value and life cycle impact is crucial. Sustainable farming practices, efficient resource use, and individual actions like promoting local foods and home gardening can mitigate climate change and promote sustainability. Everyone has a responsibility to adopt low-carbon footprint diets for a sustainable future.

Food security is further compromised by adverse weather, political instability, and economic issues, leading to decreased well-being, particularly among the poor. Sustainable food systems aim to meet current needs while preserving ecosystems and promoting fairness. Precision agriculture driven by artificial intelligence (AI) optimizes resource use, improves productivity, and mitigates environmental impact, addressing food insecurity and hunger challenges. AI enhances crop yield prediction, pest management, and food safety. However, it brings challenges such as unemployment and the digital divide, which must be addressed through proactive strategies like job creation, digital training, and cybersecurity measures.

This book delves into these multifaceted aspects of food security, offering insights and strategies to build a more sustainable, resilient, and equitable food system for the future.

About the Editors

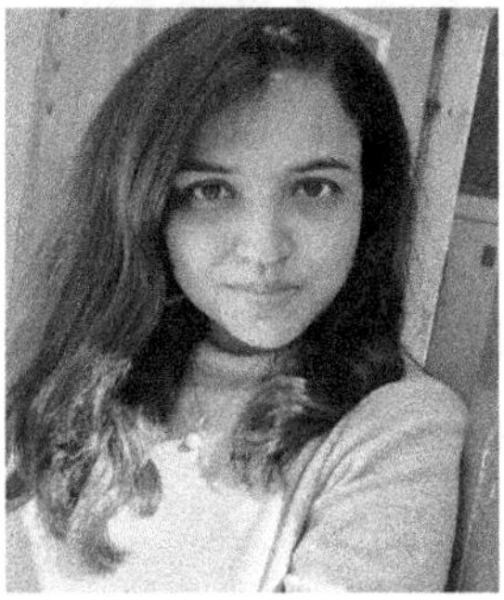

Shikha Saxena holds a PhD in Public Health Nutrition from the Centre for Social Medicine and Community Health, Jawaharlal Nehru University, New Delhi (2019). Specializing in household food security and women's nutrition, and mixed method research, she investigates the determinants of household food security and their impact on the nutritional status of women in slums in India. She was awarded a DAAD fellowship in Germany during her PhD studies. She concluded her NIHR-funded postdoctoral research at the National Institute for Cancer Prevention and Research, ICMR, in 2022. She has over 13 years of experience as a faculty member, nutritionist, and consultant for India's reputed education, healthcare, and research institutions. She has been actively engaged in community-based projects, demonstrating proficiency in quantitative and qualitative analysis. She has worked as a consultant on interim projects for WHO and Jhpiego. Additionally, she has worked for the Centre for Policy Research and Public Health Foundation of India. She has authored a book titled *Women Nutrition in Developing Countries: A Mixed Method Study*. She has also presented her research at national and international conferences. She is a member of the Nutrition Society of India, the Indian Dietetic Association, the Canadian Obesity Network, and the Nutrition Society of the United Kingdom. She has also served as an Online Academic Expert at Australia's Victoria University. At present, she is working as an Associate Professor at the School of Health Sciences and Technology, UPES, in Dehradun, Uttarakhand, India.

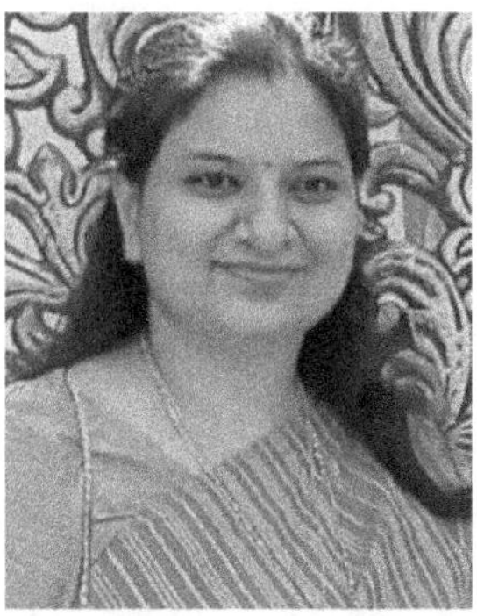

Chhavi Taliwal is a distinguished nutritionist and academician with over 15 years of experience in food and nutrition. She has made significant contributions to nutritional analysis, meal planning, food product development, and public health. Dr. Taliwal holds an MSc in Foods & Nutrition from Chaudhary Charan Singh University, an MPhil in Home Science from Devi Ahilya Vishwavidyalaya University, Indore, MP and a PhD from Amity University, Noida, UP, where she researched supplementary food for lactating mothers. Currently, Dr. Taliwal serves as a Project Assistant Professor at the National Institute of Nutrition (NIN), ICMR, in Hyderabad. Her role involves mentoring students in Applied and Sports Nutrition, coordinating courses, and developing innovative food products. Prior to this, she worked as a dietician at Shivam Clinic in Delhi and held academic positions at Amity University, Gurgaon, Haryana and Ginni Devi Modi Girls Post Graduate College in Modinagar, UP. Dr. Taliwal's research focuses on optimizing nutritional products for vulnerable populations. She has published extensively in Scopus-indexed journals and presented her work at national and international conferences, earning several awards. Additionally, she has been an invited speaker for the POSHAN Program, contributing to government efforts to improve nutrition in schools and colleges. Her commitment to research, education, and public health has made a lasting impact, benefiting students, professionals, and the broader community. Dr. Taliwal is a respected figure in the field, actively contributing to the advancement of nutrition science.

Contributors

Naga Jyothi Ala
MYAS, ICMR-National Institute of Nutrition, Hyderabad, Telangana, India-500007

Prachi Bhasin
School of Health Sciences and Technology, UPES, Dehradun, Uttarakhand, 248007, India

Aparna Chaudhary
Independent researcher

Neha Goyal
IMS Unison University, Dehradun

Jagriti Jaiswal
School of Management, IILM University, Gurgaon

Rati Kapoor
International Food Policy Research Institute (IFPRI), New Delhi

Maheshwar Mekam
MYAS, ICMR-National Institute of Nutrition, Hyderabad, Telangana, India-500007

Shambhavi Mishra
Department of Statistics, University of Lucknow, Lucknow, Uttar Pradesh

Shireesha Mukka
MYAS, ICMR-National Institute of Nutrition, Hyderabad, Telangana, India-500007

Jharna Puppala
MYAS, ICMR-National Institute of Nutrition, Hyderabad, Telangana, India-500007

Shikha Saxena
School of Health Sciences and Technology, UPES, Dehradun, Uttarakhand, 248007, India

Lochan Sharma
National Centre for Promotion of Employment for Disabled People (NCPEDP), New Delhi-110065

Arpit Singh
International Center for Research on Women (ICRW-Asia), New Delhi

Chhavi Taliwal
MYAS, ICMR-National Institute of Nutrition, Hyderabad, Telangana, India-500007

Harika Vasa
MYAS, ICMR-National Institute of Nutrition, Hyderabad, Telangana, India-500007

Abbreviations

3D	Three-dimensional
AFSC	Agri-food supply chain
AI	Artificial Intelligence
AICRP-PM	All India Coordinated Research Project on Pearl Millet
ANFIS	Adaptive neuro-fuzzy inference system
ANN	Artificial neural network
AWW	Anganwadi worker
BMI	Body mass index
BNN	Biological neural network
CED	Chronic energy deficiency
CNN	Convolutional neural networks
COVID-19	Coronavirus disease 2019
DCNN	Deep convolutional neural networks
DEM	Digital elevation model
DL	Deep learning
DSS	Decision support systems
ET	Evapotranspiration
FAO	Food and Agriculture Organization
FAO-AMIS	FAO's agricultural market information system
FDR	Frequency domain reflectometry
GC	Ground coverage
GDI	Gender Development Index
GGGI	Global Gender Gap Index
GHG	Greenhouse gas
GII	Gender Inequality Index
GIS	Geographic information system
ICDS	Integrated Child Development Scheme
ICMR	Indian Council of Medical Research
ICRISAT	International Crops Research Institute for the Semi-Arid Tropics
IFAD	International Fund for Agricultural Development
IFPRI	International Food Policy Research Institute
IIMR	Indian Institute of Millets Research
INSIMP	Initiative for Nutritional Security through Intensive Millets Promotion
IoT	Internet of Things
IP	Image processing
KNN	K-nearest neighbors algorithm
ML	Machine learning
MPI	Multidimensional Poverty Index
NDVI	Normalized difference vegetation index
NFSM	National Food Security Mission
NFHS	National Family Health Survey

OPHI	Oxford Poverty and Human Development Initiative
PA	Precision agriculture
POSHAN	Partnerships and Opportunities to Strengthen and Harmonize Actions for Nutrition in India
RF	Radiofrequency
RNN	Recurrent neural network
RSM	Response surface methodology
SDG	Sustainable Development Goals
SVM	Support vector machine
SVR	Support vector regression
TDR	Time domain reflectometry
UAV	Unmanned aerial vehicle
UNCTD	United Nations Conference on Trade and Development
UNDP	United Nations Development Programme
UNICEF	United Nations Children's Fund
USAID	United States Agency for International Development
WEAI	Women's Empowerment in Agriculture Index
WEF	World Economic Forum
WENI	Women's Empowerment and Nutrition Index
WFP	World Food Programme
WHO	World Health Organization
WSN	Wireless sensor network

1 Delving into Food Security

A Multidimensional Exploration Through Scholarly Research and Contemporary Advancements

Shikha Saxena

1.1 INTRODUCTION: THE EVOLUTION OF FOOD SECURITY CONCEPTS

Food security research has evolved significantly, expanding from specific topics to include food availability, diversification, sustainability, and effectiveness. This interdisciplinary field now intersects with environmental science, demography, and sociology, emphasizing the need for comprehensive, field-based research. The theoretical framework should be enhanced by integrating ecological, economic, and social perspectives. The focus should shift from fundamental science to technical applications, prioritizing sustainable development through the coordination of economic, environmental, and social factors, supported by technological advancements and policy management (Xie et al., 2021). Food security, crucial for human well-being, now encompasses availability, access, utilization, and stability of food sources, addressing not just calorie sufficiency but also nutrition, sustainability, and resilience to shocks like climate change and economic fluctuations.

Availability

Food availability refers to the supply of food through production, distribution, and exchange. Recent trends indicate a significant shift towards enhancing agricultural productivity through technological innovations and sustainable farming practices. The advent of precision agriculture, biotechnology, and digital farming tools has revolutionized food production. Precision agriculture revolutionizes farming with technologies like GPS, sensors, drones, and data analytics, enabling data-driven decisions, increased efficiency, reduced resource waste, and improved yields. It supports real-time monitoring and variable rate technology, enhancing sustainability and productivity. Future advancements in AI and automation promise further

DOI: 10.1201/9781003487227-1

efficiency and sustainability (Maurya et al., 2024). These technologies have enabled farmers to optimize resource use, increase crop yields, and reduce environmental impact. However, challenges such as land degradation, water scarcity, and climate change continue to threaten food availability. According to the Food and Agriculture Organization (FAO), global food production must increase by 70% by 2050 to meet the demands of a growing population (FAO, 2009).

Modern industrial farms and advanced agricultural methods are essential to addressing the global food security crisis. Data-driven solutions to enhance yields, reduce costs, and minimize waste have been already introduced by the industries. This review examines the current state of digital technologies in agriculture, noting that many, including big data, analytics, and blockchain, are still in development. Challenges and opportunities are highlighted, with an emphasis on the value of these technologies. Despite some limitations in the literature search, the overall conclusions remain robust (Abiri et al., 2023)

Access

Food access involves the economic and physical means to obtain food. Socioeconomic disparities significantly affect food access, with poverty, inequality, and economic instability being major barriers. Recent trends show an increasing focus on social protection programs and policies aimed at improving food access for vulnerable populations (Hidrobo et al., 2018). Initiatives such as food subsidies, cash transfers, and school feeding programs have proven effective in enhancing food security. Additionally, the COVID-19 pandemic highlighted the importance of resilient food supply chains and the need for policies that ensure continuous food access during crises (Laborde et al., 2020).

Utilization

Food utilization refers to the nutritional value of food and its impact on health. Beyond calorie sufficiency, contemporary concerns include micronutrient deficiencies, dietary diversity, and the rising prevalence of non-communicable diseases linked to poor diets. Recent trends emphasize the importance of nutrition-sensitive interventions and the promotion of healthy eating habits (Hawkes et al., 2020). The double burden of malnutrition, where undernutrition and obesity coexist, is a growing concern globally. Efforts to address this issue include fortification of staple foods, diversification of diets, and public health campaigns to promote balanced nutrition.

Stability

Stability encompasses the reliability of food access over time, addressing factors such as economic shocks, climate change, and political instability. The increasing frequency of extreme weather events, driven by climate change, poses significant threats to food security. Recent trends highlight the importance of building resilience in food systems to withstand and recover from such shocks (Owino et al., 2022). Strategies include the development of climate-smart agriculture practices, improvement of disaster risk management, and investment in infrastructure to enhance the stability of food supplies.

1.2 FROM FOOD TO NUTRITION SECURITY

The concept of food security has evolved from a focus on calorie intake to a more holistic approach that includes nutrition, sustainability, and resilience. This shift reflects a growing recognition that food security is not just about quantity but also about quality and equity.

Nutritional security is now a critical component of food security. Ensuring access to diverse, nutrient-rich foods is essential for preventing malnutrition and promoting overall health. Recent trends in nutrition policy emphasize the integration of nutrition objectives into broader food security and agricultural strategies (Hawkes et al., 2020). This approach aims to address the root causes of malnutrition, such as poor dietary diversity and lack of access to nutritious foods. Sustainability is increasingly recognized as a cornerstone of food security. Sustainable food systems aim to provide food in a way that is environmentally sound, socially and economically viable, and in line with the adoption of circular economy principles (FAO, 2009). These efforts seek to balance the need for increased food production with the imperative to protect natural resources and reduce greenhouse gas emissions.

Building resilience in food systems is crucial for ensuring long-term food security. Resilience involves the capacity to anticipate, prepare for, and respond to various shocks and stresses. Recent trends highlight the importance of diversifying livelihoods, improving risk management, and fostering adaptive capacity in communities (Bene, 2020). Investment in infrastructure, early warning systems, and social safety nets are key components of building resilience in food systems.

1.3 GLOBAL CHALLENGES

Despite advancements, significant global challenges continue to impact food security. These challenges are multifaceted and interconnected, requiring coordinated efforts at local, national, and international levels.

Evidence demonstrates that micro studies on food safety and nutrition poverty should be linked to macro food security developments including climate change's influence on agricultural productivity and global food crises. Although extensive and multidisciplinary food safety research has potential, it is difficult to theoretically and empirically connect global and regional dimensions of change (crisis) with meso (policy) and micro (individual behavior) dimensions.

Food security as a multidimensional topic is depicted in Figure 1.1, which shows the thematic clusters in the food security literature (2000–20) (Righettini & Bordin, 2023).

Climate change and economic inequality

Climate change poses one of the most significant threats to global food security. Changes in temperature, precipitation patterns, and the frequency of extreme weather events affect crop yields, livestock productivity, and fisheries. Adaptation and mitigation strategies are essential to address the impacts of climate change on food security (Wheeler & von Braun, 2013). Climate-smart agriculture, which includes crop diversification, conservation agriculture, and integrated pest management, is a promising

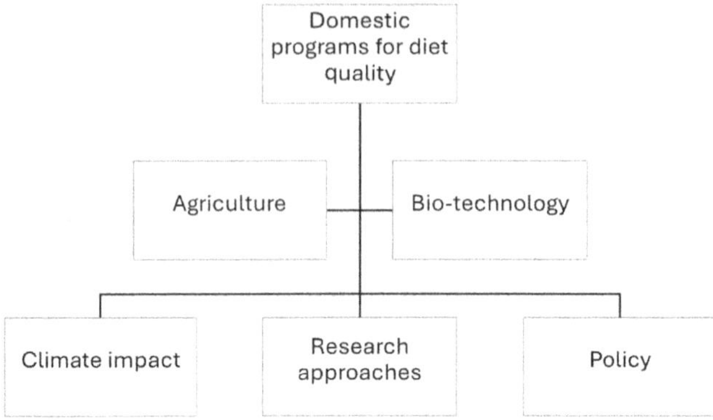

FIGURE 1.1 Descending the hierarchy of thematic clusters in food security (2000–20). (Adapted from Righettini & Bordin, 2023.)

approach to enhancing resilience to climate change. Economic inequality remains a major barrier to food access. Income disparities, lack of employment opportunities, and inadequate social protection exacerbate food insecurity, particularly in low- and middle-income countries. Addressing economic inequality requires comprehensive policies that promote inclusive economic growth, social protection, and access to education and healthcare (FAO, 2009).

Political instability

Political instability and conflict disrupt food production and distribution, leading to acute food insecurity. Regions affected by conflict often experience displacement, loss of livelihoods, and destruction of infrastructure. Efforts to address food insecurity in conflict-affected areas include humanitarian assistance, peacebuilding initiatives, and support for rebuilding agricultural systems (FAO, 2009).

Global pandemic

The COVID-19 pandemic underscored the vulnerability of global food systems to health crises. The pandemic disrupted supply chains, reduced incomes, and increased food prices, exacerbating food insecurity for millions of people. Lessons learned from the pandemic highlight the need for resilient food systems that can adapt to and recover from such shocks (Laborde et al., 2020).

1.4 FACTORS INFLUENCING FOOD SECURITY AND STRATEGIES FOR IMPROVEMENT

The landscape of food security is influenced by multiple factors such as population growth, urbanization, climate change, and socioeconomic disparities. Each of these factors poses unique challenges to ensuring a stable and accessible food supply. Addressing these challenges requires a multifaceted approach that integrates social, economic, and environmental strategies. This chapter explores the impact of these factors on food security, drawing on recent academic research and data to highlight the urgency and complexity of the issue.

Population growth

Population growth remains a fundamental challenge to food security. The global population is projected to reach 9.7 billion by 2050, which necessitates a substantial increase in food production (United Nations, 2019). However, the capacity to expand food production is constrained by limited natural resources, including arable land and freshwater. The growing population increases the demand for food, leading to intensified agricultural practices that can deplete soil quality and reduce biodiversity (Godfray et al., 2010).

The strain on food production is particularly acute in developing countries where population growth rates are highest. These regions often lack the infrastructure and technology necessary to increase agricultural productivity sustainably. As a result, they are more susceptible to food shortages and malnutrition. Enhancing agricultural productivity through technological innovations, improved farming practices, and investment in agricultural research is essential to meet the growing food demand (Ray et al., 2013).

Urbanization

Urbanization is another critical factor affecting food security. By 2050, it is expected that 68% of the world's population will live in urban areas (United Nations, 2018). This shift from rural to urban living creates significant challenges for food production and distribution. Urban areas typically have limited space for agriculture, leading to a reliance on food transported from rural regions or imported from other countries. The dependence on complex supply chains makes urban food systems vulnerable to disruptions. For instance, during the COVID-19 pandemic, lockdown measures and transportation restrictions caused significant delays and shortages in urban food supplies (FAO, 2020). Furthermore, urbanization often changes dietary patterns, with increased consumption of processed foods that are high in calories but low in nutritional value, contributing to rising rates of obesity and diet-related diseases (Casari et al., 2022).

Improving urban food security requires innovative solutions such as urban agriculture, vertical farming, and improved logistics and supply chain management. These strategies can help cities become more self-sufficient and resilient to external shocks

Urban agriculture (UA) faces economic challenges but offers significant socio-environmental benefits. This review examines UA's value in social, health, disaster risk reduction, and environmental aspects. It highlights the need for adaptive policies and technological advancements to bridge gaps, enhance profitability, and integrate UA into sustainable urban development (Yuan et al., 2023). UA can enhance city resilience against environmental and socioeconomic disturbances but is underappreciated. The success factors include scale, integration, inclusiveness, production efficiency, and safety. These depend on institutional support, knowledge, collaboration, and resourcefulness. Increasing UA's resilience benefits requires more research, collaboration, and innovative, context-specific solutions (Gulyas & Edmondson, 2021). Vertical farming faces challenges such as high initial costs, expertise shortage, and the need for controlled environments. Despite this, its potential for sustainable and reliable food production is promising. Benefits include reduced water use, less land degradation, lower pesticide use, and shorter supply chains. More research and collaboration are needed to enhance sustainability and optimize product quality in agriculture and horticulture (Oh & Lu, 2023).

Climate change

Climate change poses a severe threat to agricultural productivity and food security. Changes in temperature, precipitation patterns, and the frequency of extreme weather events such as droughts and floods directly impact crop yields. The Intergovernmental Panel on Climate Change (IPCC) projects that climate change could reduce global crop yields by up to 25% by 2050 (IPCC, 2019). The effects of climate change are particularly devastating in vulnerable regions where agriculture is a primary source of livelihood. For example, in sub-Saharan Africa and South Asia, changing climate conditions are expected to exacerbate food insecurity by reducing agricultural productivity and increasing food prices. Climate change destabilizes global food systems, decreasing food security and diet quality, and exacerbating malnutrition, especially in vulnerable populations. Pandemics like COVID-19 compound these issues. Sustainable, resilient food systems and climate-smart agriculture are needed to ensure diverse, nutritious diets and environmental conservation (Owino et al., 2022). Smallholder farmers in these regions often lack the resources and technology to adapt to changing conditions, making them more susceptible to crop failures and income loss. Adaptation strategies are crucial to mitigate the impact of climate change on food security. These include developing drought-resistant crop varieties, improving water management practices, and adopting sustainable agricultural practices. However, the success of these strategies depends on the availability of resources, technology, and supportive policies. The disparity between food security and climate adaptation in the Global North and South, not least in rural India and the USA during COVID-19, highlights the unique challenges and solutions, policy differences, and their impacts on food security (Raj et al., 2022).

Socioeconomic disparities

Socioeconomic disparities significantly influence food security, particularly among marginalized communities. Economic instability, poverty, and lack of access to resources create barriers to obtaining nutritious food. According to the FAO, more than 820 million people were hungry in 2018, with the highest prevalence in low-income countries (FAO, 2019). Marginalized communities often face multiple layers of disadvantage. Economic instability can lead to job loss and reduced income, making it difficult for families to afford sufficient and nutritious food. These communities may also lack access to markets, healthcare, and education, all of which are critical for maintaining food security. Furthermore, socioeconomic disparities often influence dietary choices, with low-income households relying on cheaper, energy-dense foods that are low in nutritional value, leading to higher rates of malnutrition and diet-related diseases (Darmon & Drewnowski, 2015).

The double burden of malnutrition (DBM) includes stunting, overweight, and obesity, leading to health issues like impaired development, infectious diseases, and non-communicable diseases. This results in economic costs through lost wages, productivity, and higher medical expenses (Nugent et al., 2020). Addressing food security disparities requires targeted interventions like food assistance, cash transfers, and nutrition programs, alongside policies promoting inclusive economic growth, education, and healthcare to reduce poverty and enhance resilience.

1.5 INTEGRATED APPROACHES TO FOOD SECURITY

Addressing the multifaceted challenges of food security necessitates integrated approaches that consider the interconnected nature of population growth, urbanization, climate change, and socioeconomic disparities. Policy interventions, technological innovations, and community-based solutions all play a role in improving food security.

Policy interventions
Governments can implement policies that support sustainable agricultural practices, provide financial assistance to farmers, and ensure equitable access to food. For example, subsidies for smallholder farmers can help them invest in better seeds and technology, increasing their productivity. Additionally, social safety nets can provide immediate relief to vulnerable populations during crises (Barrett, 2021).

Technological innovations
Advances in agricultural technology can significantly enhance food production and resilience. Precision agriculture, for instance, uses data and technology to optimize farming practices, increasing efficiency and yields. Biotechnology can also contribute by developing crops that are more resistant to pests, diseases, and climate change. A systematic review and meta-analysis of 57 studies assessed global food security projections to 2050, showing a 35%–56% increase in food demand and varied hunger risk changes. Climate change impacts these projections slightly but with no significant differences (van Dijk et al., 2021)

Community-based solutions
Empowering local communities to develop their food security strategies is crucial. Community gardens, cooperatives, and local markets can improve access to fresh food and create economic opportunities. Education and awareness campaigns can also promote healthy eating habits and sustainable food practices.

Adopting integrated soil and agronomic management practices to improve fertilizer efficiency requires understanding diverse conditions and resource constraints. Increased investment in localized, adaptive farm-level research and extension systems is essential for sustainable intensification in Africa (Jayne et al., 2019).

Impact of the COVID-19 pandemic on food systems
Global events such as the COVID-19 pandemic have starkly revealed the vulnerabilities within food systems, leading to significant disruptions in supply chains and worsening food insecurity. The pandemic has demonstrated how quickly crisis can impact food availability and accessibility, emphasizing the need for resilient and sustainable food systems. Addressing these challenges necessitates holistic approaches that integrate social, economic, and environmental factors. Effective strategies

include enhancing agricultural productivity, promoting sustainable farming practices, improving market access for smallholder farmers, and investing in social safety nets.

The COVID-19 pandemic disrupted global food supply chains on an unprecedented scale, affecting every stage from production to consumption. Lockdowns, travel restrictions, and social distancing measures hindered the movement of labor and goods, causing delays and shortages. According to the FAO, these disruptions have been particularly severe for perishable goods, which depend on timely transportation and processing (FAO, 2020). Agricultural production suffered as farmers faced difficulties in accessing essential inputs like seeds, fertilizers, and machinery. The restriction on movement also meant that many seasonal laborers could not travel to farms, resulting in labor shortages and reduced harvests. Additionally, the closure of food processing plants and markets, especially in urban areas, led to significant post-harvest losses and decreased incomes for farmers (World Bank, 2021).

1.6 SOCIOECONOMIC AND ENVIRONMENTAL FACTORS

Addressing the vulnerabilities exposed by the pandemic requires a comprehensive approach that considers the interconnectedness of social, economic, and environmental factors. Socioeconomic disparities significantly influence food security, with marginalized communities often bearing the brunt of food system disruptions. These communities typically have less access to resources, making it harder to cope with shocks such as those caused by the pandemic. In early 2020, COVID-19 prompted India to implement strict measures. Phone-based surveys with 1515 smallholder farmers in Haryana and Odisha revealed significant differences in lockdown impacts, influenced by market infrastructure and state policies, affecting labor costs, procurement, and food availability (Ceballos et al., 2020).

Environmental factors also play a crucial role. Climate change, land degradation, and biodiversity loss continue to threaten agricultural productivity and food security. Sustainable farming practices are essential to mitigate these environmental impacts and build more resilient food systems (Altieri et al., 2015).

Enhancing agricultural productivity

Increasing agricultural productivity is vital for improving food security. This can be achieved through various means, including the adoption of modern farming techniques, improved crop varieties, and better resource management. Research and development (R&D) in agriculture are critical for innovation and the dissemination of new technologies that can help farmers increase yields and reduce losses (FAO, 2020). Precision agriculture, which utilizes data and technology to optimize farming practices, is one such innovation. Farmers can monitor crop health, soil conditions, and weather patterns using sensors, drones, and satellite imagery in real time, allowing for more precise and efficient use of inputs such as water and fertilizers (Barrett & Bevis, 2015).

Promoting sustainable farming practices

Sustainable farming practices are essential for ensuring long-term food security and environmental health. These practices include crop rotation, agroforestry, conservation tillage, and integrated pest management. Such methods help maintain soil fertility, reduce erosion, and enhance biodiversity, making agricultural systems more resilient to climate change and other stresses (Altieri et al., 2015).

Agroecology, which emphasizes the ecological principles of farming, offers a holistic approach to sustainable agriculture. By integrating ecological practices into farming systems, agroecology aims to create more diverse and productive agricultural landscapes that are better equipped to withstand environmental and economic shocks (Altieri et al., 2015).

Improving market access for smallholder farmers

Smallholder farmers, who produce a significant portion of the world's food, often face challenges in accessing markets. Improving market access for these farmers is crucial for enhancing their livelihoods and ensuring food security. This can be achieved through investments in rural infrastructure, such as roads and storage facilities, which help reduce post-harvest losses and transportation costs (FAO, 2009). Moreover, strengthening farmer cooperatives and organizations can enhance collective bargaining power, giving smallholder farmers better access to markets and fair prices for their products. Digital platforms and mobile technology can also play a role in connecting farmers to markets, providing real-time information on prices, demand, and best practices. Food systems worldwide are part of a global network dominated by large exporters and corporations, focusing on high production of key products. The unequal structure and risks of this network, propose "next best transition steps" to empower and improve resilience for peripheral food systems (Lahde et al., 2023).

Investing in social safety nets

Social safety nets are critical for protecting vulnerable populations from food insecurity, especially during crises like the COVID-19 pandemic. These safety nets include food assistance programs, cash transfers, and nutrition programs that provide immediate relief and support long-term resilience (World Bank, 2021). During the pandemic, many countries expanded their social safety nets to help those affected by lockdowns and economic downturns. For example, the World Food Programme (WFP) scaled up its efforts to provide food and cash assistance to millions of people facing hunger due to the pandemic (WFP, 2020). Investing in robust social safety nets can help cushion the impact of future shocks and ensure that vulnerable populations have access to sufficient and nutritious food.

1.7 HOLISTIC APPROACHES TO FOOD SECURITY

A holistic approach to food security requires integrating social, economic, and environmental strategies. This involves collaboration among governments, international organizations, the private sector, and civil society to create inclusive and sustainable food systems.

Achieving food security in the 21st century is a multifaceted challenge that requires comprehensive strategies addressing the diverse dimensions of food access, availability, utilization, and stability. Technological innovations such as precision agriculture and biotechnology offer promising solutions to enhance food production and sustainability. However, these innovations must be accompanied by equitable distribution mechanisms and inclusive policies to ensure that the benefits are accessible to all segments of society. This chapter explores the potential of these technological advancements and the importance of integrating them into broader, inclusive strategies to achieve food security.

Policy interventions

Governments play a crucial role in creating an enabling environment for food security through policies that support sustainable agriculture, market access, and social protection. Policies should focus on providing incentives for sustainable farming practices, investing in agricultural R&D, and ensuring that safety nets reach the most vulnerable populations (FAO, 2020).

International cooperation

Global challenges such as food insecurity require international cooperation. Organizations like the FAO, WFP, and the International Fund for Agricultural Development (IFAD) work to address food security through various programs and initiatives. International cooperation is also essential for sharing knowledge, technologies, and best practices across countries and regions (FAO, 2009).

Community engagement

Engaging local communities in food security initiatives is critical for their success. Community-based approaches can empower people to take ownership of their food systems, ensuring that solutions are tailored to local needs and contexts. Education and capacity-building programs can also help communities adopt sustainable practices and improve their resilience to shocks. Community-based programs play a very important role in tackling food insecurity. Involving local farmers, administrators, and community advocates in planning and implementing solutions helps guide and improve food availability and access (Hasnat Milton et al., 2022).

1.8 PRECISION AGRICULTURE

Precision agriculture is a farming management concept that uses technology to monitor and optimize agricultural processes. It involves the use of sensors, GPS, data analytics, and IoT devices to collect real-time data on crop health, soil conditions, weather patterns, and pest activity. This data-driven approach allows farmers to make more informed decisions, enhancing productivity and reducing waste. The benefits of precision agriculture are listed below.

Increased efficiency

Precision agriculture enables farmers to apply inputs such as water, fertilizers, and pesticides more precisely, reducing waste and enhancing crop yields. Precision agriculture technologies optimize crop production and minimize environmental impacts. Innovations include crop sensing with hyperspectral imaging, variable rate technologies to reduce waste, data analytics for site-specific interventions, robotics for field operations, and advanced breeding techniques (Naresh et al., 2024).

Cost savings

By optimizing resource use, precision agriculture can reduce costs associated with inputs and labor. Precision farming uses information and technology to identify, evaluate, and manage local and temporal variability in fields to improve productivity, profitability, sustainability, and land resource protection while minimizing production costs. We must adapt agricultural management to preserve water, air, and soil while remaining lucrative as public environmental consciousness rises. Chemical fertilizers and insecticides at the right amounts, times, and places (site-specific management). In recent decades, irrigation projects have produced almost a third of the world's food. Market-based global competition in agricultural commodities is jeopardizing established agricultural systems and requiring new, dynamic production methods (Hakkim et al., 2016).

Environmental sustainability

Targeted application of inputs minimizes environmental impact, reducing runoff and soil degradation (Gebbers & Adamchuk, 2010).

Challenges and considerations regarding precision agriculture

Smallholder and resource-poor farmers may lack access to the necessary technology and infrastructure, exacerbating existing inequalities (Lowenberg-DeBoer & Erickson, 2019). The extensive use of data in precision agriculture raises concerns about data privacy and security (Wolfert et al., 2017).

1.9 BIOTECHNOLOGY IN AGRICULTURE

This involves the use of genetic engineering, molecular markers, tissue culture, and other technologies to improve crop yields, enhance nutritional quality, and develop resistance to pests and diseases. The benefits of biotechnology are listed below.

Improved crop varieties

Genetically modified (GM) crops can be engineered to exhibit desirable traits such as drought tolerance, pest resistance, and enhanced nutritional content (ISAAA, 2018).

Enhanced food security

Biotechnology can contribute to food security by increasing agricultural productivity and resilience to climate change (Qaim, 2020).

Sustainability

Biotechnology can reduce the need for chemical inputs, promoting more sustainable agricultural practices. Agricultural science involves a commitment to humanitarian and environmental ethics. Historically focused on maximizing production, it now needs to address urgent issues like environmental degradation, climate change, and social inequality. Modern agricultural science should prioritize multidimensional food systems over mere productivism to better solve these problems (Haring et al., 2023).

Regulatory and ethical issues regarding GM crops

The adoption of GM crops is often hindered by regulatory hurdles and ethical concerns about genetic modification. Many GM food and non-food crops exhibit distinctive traits and are commercially grown. The most extensively farmed crops for pest resistance and herbicide tolerance include soybean, maize, canola, and cotton. More GM crops are being developed and not yet sold. The FAO's 2017 State of Food Security and Nutrition in the World report highlights food insecurity and malnutrition in most Asian and developing nations. GM crops might solve malnutrition and food security by improving crop nutrition and output. India has made considerable progress in GM crop research, evaluation, and monitoring over the past two decades, but the regulatory system has been impeded by a lack of coordination and unified attitude on GM technology across administrations, and ministries GMOs cause food safety, environmental, and social issues (Shukla et al., 2018).

Public perception

Public skepticism and opposition to GM crops can limit their acceptance and adoption. Understanding what influences consumer acceptance of novel functional foods has been deemed crucial for successful product launches. A review of 75 global studies has identified five key determinants: product, sociodemographic, psychological, behavioral, and physical characteristics, providing insights for product developers and marketers (Baker et al., 2022).

1.10 EQUITABLE DISTRIBUTION MECHANISMS

Technological innovations alone are not sufficient to achieve food security. Equitable distribution mechanisms are essential to ensure that the benefits of these technologies reach all farmers, particularly smallholders and marginalized communities.

Strategies for equitable distribution include the following:

- *Subsidies and financial support:* Governments and organizations can provide subsidies, grants, and low-interest loans to help smallholder farmers access modern technologies (Pingali, 2012).
- *Training and education:* Extension services and training programs can equip farmers with the knowledge and skills needed to adopt and effectively use new technologies (Anderson, 2007).
- *Infrastructure development:* Investments in rural infrastructure such as roads, storage facilities, and irrigation systems can enhance access to markets and reduce post-harvest losses (FAO, 2014).
- *Inclusive policies:* Inclusive policies are critical for creating an enabling environment that supports technological adoption and ensures food security for all.

These policies should address social, economic, and environmental dimensions, promoting equity and sustainability.

- *Key policy areas*
    - *Research and development:* Governments should invest in agricultural R&D to develop and disseminate innovative technologies tailored to local contexts and needs. Governments and development organizations promote agricultural technologies to increase productivity and reduce poverty, but adoption rates remain low. This study analyzes 367 regression models, finding that farmer education, household size, land size, credit access, land tenure, extension services, and organization membership positively influence technology adoption. Recommendations emphasize adapting promotion efforts to local contexts (Ruzzante et al., 2021).
    - *Market access:* Policies should facilitate market access for smallholder farmers, including fair trade practices and support for local markets (Barrett et al., 2012).
    - *Social protection:* Social protection programs such as food assistance, cash transfers, and nutrition interventions can help vulnerable populations access sufficient and nutritious food (HLPE, 2012).
    - *Climate-smart agriculture:* Policies promoting climate-smart agriculture can enhance resilience to climate change while improving agricultural productivity and sustainability (Lipper et al., 2014).

1.11 COMPREHENSIVE STRATEGIES FOR FOOD SECURITY

Achieving food security requires a holistic approach that integrates technological innovations, equitable distribution mechanisms, and inclusive policies. This comprehensive strategy should address the four dimensions of food security: access, availability, utilization, and stability.

- *Access:* Ensuring that all individuals have physical and economic access to sufficient, safe, and nutritious food.
- *Availability:* Enhancing food production and supply through sustainable agricultural practices and technological innovations.
- *Utilization:* Promoting proper food utilization through education, healthcare, and nutrition programs.
- *Stability:* Ensuring the stability of food supply and access over time, particularly in the face of economic, environmental, and social shocks.

Innovation in food systems

Innovation is critical in addressing the myriad challenges facing global food systems. Technological advancements and new methodologies can enhance productivity, efficiency, and resilience in agriculture. Precision agriculture, for example, uses data analytics, sensors, and automation to optimize farming practices, thereby increasing crop yields and reducing resource waste (Lajoie-O'Malley et al., 2020).

Ensuring food security for all requires a multifaceted approach that encompasses innovation, sustainability, and inclusivity. The goal is to create a food system where every individual has access to safe, nutritious, and culturally appropriate food. Achieving this vision necessitates the collective effort of stakeholders including governments, private sector players, non-governmental organizations (NGOs), and local communities. This essay explores how embracing these key principles can contribute to a more equitable and resilient food system.

Biotechnology also holds promise, with GM crops offering improved resistance to pests and diseases, and enhanced nutritional profiles. These advancements can be particularly beneficial in regions prone to agricultural instability (Fischer et al., 2014). Additionally, innovative food processing and preservation techniques can reduce post-harvest losses and extend the shelf life of food products, thereby improving food availability and reducing waste (Aulakh & Regmi, 2013).

Moreover, digital platforms can revolutionize market access for smallholder farmers by providing real-time information on prices, demand, and weather conditions. These platforms can also facilitate direct sales to consumers, thus bypassing intermediaries and improving farmers' income (Reardon et al., 2019). Mobile technology is increasingly being used to disseminate agricultural knowledge and best practices, empowering farmers with the information they need to enhance productivity and sustainability (Tripathi et al., 2016).

Sustainability in food systems

Sustainability is at the heart of creating a resilient and long-lasting food system. Sustainable agriculture practices not only protect the environment but also ensure the longevity of food production systems. Agroecology, which integrates ecological principles into agricultural practices, promotes biodiversity, enhances soil health, and reduces dependency on chemical inputs (Altieri et al., 2015).

Conservation agriculture, which includes minimal soil disturbance, crop rotation, and cover cropping, helps maintain soil fertility and reduce erosion. These practices are crucial in mitigating the impacts of climate change, which poses a significant threat to global food security (Pretty et al., 2018). Additionally, water-efficient practices such as drip irrigation and rainwater harvesting are essential in regions facing water scarcity, ensuring that crops receive adequate hydration without wasting precious resources (Zhang et al., 2021). Sustainable livestock practices, such as rotational grazing and integrated crop-livestock systems, can also contribute to environmental health. These methods enhance soil fertility, reduce greenhouse gas emissions, and improve animal welfare (Herrero et al., 2016). Moreover, promoting plant-based diets and reducing meat consumption can alleviate pressure on natural resources and decrease the carbon footprint associated with food production (Willett et al., 2019).

Inclusivity in food systems

Inclusivity ensures that all stakeholders, particularly marginalized and vulnerable groups, are considered in food security strategies. Social equity in food systems addresses disparities in access to resources, opportunities, and decision-making processes. This involves empowering women, smallholder farmers, indigenous communities, and other marginalized groups who play a crucial role in food production and distribution (FAO, 2020). Women, for example, are integral to agricultural activities in many regions, yet they often face barriers such as limited access to land, credit, and education. Empowering women through targeted policies and programs can significantly enhance food security. Studies have shown that when women have equal access to resources, agricultural productivity increases, and food insecurity decreases (Essilfie et al., 2024)

Similarly, supporting smallholder farmers is vital for global food security. These farmers produce a large portion of the world's food, yet they often struggle with limited access to markets, finance, and technology. Providing training, financial services, and infrastructure can help smallholder farmers increase their productivity and resilience (IFAD, 2021). Initiatives such as farmer cooperatives and community-supported agriculture can also enhance market access and bargaining power for smallholders (Kassam et al., 2020). Indigenous communities possess traditional knowledge and practices that are invaluable for sustainable agriculture and biodiversity conservation. Recognizing and integrating this knowledge into broader agricultural policies can contribute to more resilient and sustainable food systems (FAO, 2020).

1.12 STRATEGIES FOR FUTURE FOOD SECURITY

To ensure a future where all individuals have access to safe, nutritious, and culturally appropriate food, stakeholders must adopt holistic and integrated strategies.

- *Policy and governance:* Effective policies and governance structures are crucial for supporting innovation, sustainability, and inclusivity. Governments should implement policies that promote sustainable agricultural practices, protect smallholder farmers, and ensure equitable access to resources. International cooperation is also essential to address global food security challenges, share knowledge, and develop common strategies (Pingali, 2015).
- *Investment in R&D:* Continued investment in agricultural R&D is necessary to drive innovation and find new solutions to emerging challenges. This includes funding for public research institutions, partnerships with the private sector, and support for local research initiatives. Innovations in biotechnology, climate-resilient crops, and sustainable farming practices should be prioritized (Fischer et al., 2020).
- *Education and capacity building:* Education and capacity-building programs are essential for empowering farmers and communities with the knowledge and skills they need to adopt new technologies and practices. Extension services, vocational training, and community-based education initiatives can help disseminate best practices and support sustainable development (Tripathi et al., 2016).
- *Public-private partnerships:* Collaboration between the public and private sectors can drive innovation and scale up successful initiatives. Public-private

partnerships can facilitate the development and dissemination of new technologies, improve market access, and leverage private sector investment in sustainable agriculture (AIF, Policy brief, 2023).

- *Social safety nets:* Investing in social safety nets is critical to protect vulnerable populations from food insecurity. These safety nets should include food assistance programs, cash transfers, and nutrition programs that provide immediate relief and support long-term resilience. Ensuring that these programs reach the most vulnerable populations is essential for building a more inclusive food system (World Bank, 2021).

The food security understandings have evolved via research, practice, and worldwide events. Increasing usage of the four pillars of food security highlights the need for a clear way to express its complexities. This method has shown policymakers that its root causes are complex and that strengthening food security policies requires multifaceted efforts. The food policy authorities, including the CFS, should update existing food security policy frameworks to account for new research, notably on agency and sustainability. International food rights legislation would be formalized. These other qualities should be incorporated in food security policy and research, however hard to evaluate. Agency and sustainability indicators may be used to analyze both aspects and their relationships (Clapp et al., 2022).

1.13 CONCLUSION

Food security is a complex and dynamic issue that extends beyond mere calorie sufficiency to encompass nutrition, sustainability, and resilience. Recent trends highlight the importance of technological innovations, social protection programs, nutrition-sensitive interventions, and climate-smart practices in addressing food security challenges. However, significant global challenges such as climate change, economic inequality, political instability, and pandemics continue to threaten food security. Addressing these challenges requires coordinated efforts and comprehensive policies that promote inclusive, sustainable, and resilient food systems.

The COVID-19 pandemic has highlighted the vulnerabilities in global food systems, emphasizing the need for holistic approaches to address food insecurity. Enhancing agricultural productivity, promoting sustainable farming practices, improving market access for smallholder farmers, and investing in social safety nets are crucial strategies. By integrating social, economic, and environmental factors, we can build more resilient and equitable food systems that can withstand future shocks and ensure food security for all.

Technological innovations such as precision agriculture and biotechnology offer significant potential to enhance food security in the 21st century. However, the benefits of these technologies must be equitably distributed, and inclusive policies are essential to ensure that all populations, particularly marginalized communities, can access and benefit from these advancements. Comprehensive strategies that integrate social, economic, and environmental dimensions are crucial to addressing the complex challenges of food security. By fostering collaboration among governments, international organizations, the private sector, and civil society, we can build resilient, equitable, and sustainable food systems that ensure food security for all.

By embracing innovation, sustainability, and inclusivity, stakeholders can work towards a future where all individuals have access to safe, nutritious, and culturally appropriate food. This vision requires collective effort and collaboration across sectors and borders. By integrating these principles into food security strategies, we can ensure the well-being of present and future generations, creating a more equitable and resilient food system.

The landscape of food security is shaped by a complex interplay of factors including population growth, urbanization, climate change, and socioeconomic disparities. Addressing these challenges requires a comprehensive approach that includes policy interventions, technological innovations, and community-based solutions. By understanding and addressing the root causes of food insecurity, we can work towards a future where all individuals have access to sufficient, safe, and nutritious food.

REFERENCES

Abiri, R., Rizan, N., Balasundram, S. K., Shahbazi, A. B., & Abdul-Hamid, H. (2023). Application of digital technologies for ensuring agricultural productivity. *Heliyon*, *9*, 22601. https://doi.org/10.1016/j.heliyon.2023.e22601

AIF, Policy Brief. (2023). *Food, Agriculture and Forestry (FAFD) ASEAN Economic Community Leveraging Investments through Public-Private Partnerships: Agrinnovation Fund in ASEAN (AIF). AIF Policy Brief.* Jakarta: ASEAN. https://asean.org/wp-content/uploads/2023/10/19.-Policy-Brief-on-Leveraging-Investment-through-Public-Private-Partnerships-AIF.pdf

Altieri, M., Nicholls, C., Henao, A., & Lana, M. (2015). Agroecology and the design of climate change-resilient farming systems. *Agronomy for Sustainable Development*, *35*. https://doi.org/10.1007/s13593-015-0285-2

Anderson, J. R., & Feder, G. (2007). Agricultural extension. In R. Evenson & P. Pingali (Eds.), Handbook of Agricultural Economics (Vol. 3, pp. 2343–2378). Elsevier. ISSN 1574-0072, ISBN 9780444518736. https://doi.org/10.1016/S1574-0072(06)03044-1

Aulakh, J., & Regmi, A. (2013). Post-harvest food losses estimation-development of consistent methodology. In *Selected Poster Prepared for Presentation at the Agricultural & Applied Economics Association's 2013 AAEA & CAES Joint Annual Meeting*. Washington, DC, August 4–6. www.fao.org/fileadmin/templates/ess/documents/meetings_and_workshops/GS_SAC_2013/Improving_methods_for_estimating_post_harvest_losses/Final_PHLs_Estimation_6-13-13.pdf

Baker, M. T., Lu, P., Parrella, J. A., & Leggette, H. R. (2022). Consumer acceptance toward functional foods: A scoping review. *Public Health*, *19*, 1217. https://doi.org/10.3390/ijerph19031217

Barrett, C. B., Bachke, M. E., Bellemare, M. F., Michelson, H. C., Narayanan, S., & Walker, T. F. (2012). Smallholder participation in contract farming: Comparative evidence from five countries. *World Development*, *40*(4), 715–730. https://doi.org/10.1016/j.worlddev.2011.09.006

Barrett, C. B., & Bevis, L. E. M. (2015). The self-reinforcing feedback between low soil fertility and chronic poverty. *Nature Geoscience*, *8*(12), 907-912.

Barrett, C. B., Ghezzi-Kopel, K., Hoddinott, J., Homami, N., Tennant, E., Upton, J., & Wu, T. (Eds.) (2021). *Methods and Evidence, AEP WP*. Applied Economics and Policy Working Paper No. 2021-03. Ithaca: Cornell SC Johnson School of Business. https://doi.org/10.22004/ag.econ.309952.

Bene, C. (2020). Resilience of local food systems and links to food security – A review of some important concepts in the context of COVID-19 and other shocks. *Food Security*, *12*, 805–822. https://doi.org/10.1007/s12571-020-01076-1

Casari, S., Di Paola, M., Banci, E., Diallo, S., Scarallo, L., Renzo, S., Gori, A., Renzi. S., Paci, M., de Mast, Q., Pecht, T., Derra, K., Kaboré, B., Tinto, H., Cavalieri, D., & Lionetti, P. (2022). Changing dietary habits: The impact of urbanization and rising socio-economic status in families from Burkina Faso in Sub-Saharan Africa. *Nutrients*, *14*(9), 1782. PMID: 35565752; PMCID: PMC9104313. https://doi.org/10.3390/nu14091782

Ceballos, F., Kannan, S., & Kramer, B. (2020). Impacts of a national lockdown on smallholder farmers' income and food security: Empirical evidence from two states in India. *World Development*, *136*, 105069. https://doi.org/10.1016/j.worlddev.2020.105069

Clapp, J., Moseley, W. G., Burlingame, B., & Termine, P. (2022). Viewpoint: The case for a six-dimensional food security framework. *Food Policy*, *106*, 102164. https://doi.org/10.1016/J.FOODPOL.2021.102164

Darmon, N., & Drewnowski, A. (2015). Contribution of food prices and diet cost to socio-economic disparities in diet quality and health: A systematic review and analysis. *Nutrients Review*, *73*(10), 643–660. Epub 2015 Aug 25. PMID: 26307238; PMCID: PMC4586446. https://doi.org/10.1093/nutrit/nuv027

Da Silva, J. G. (2019). Feeding the world sustainably. *United Nations Chronicle*, *49*(1–2). www.un.org/en/chronicle/article/feeding-world-sustainably

Essilfie, G., Sebu, J., & Baako-Amponsah, J. (2024). Does women's empowerment matter for household food security? Evidence from Northern Ghana. *Sage Open*, *14*(2). https://doi.org/10.1177/21582440241245076

FAO. (2009). Global Agriculture Towards 2050. (2009, October 12–13). *High Level Expert Forum*. Rome: FAO. www.fao.org/fileadmin/templates/wsfs/docs/Issues_papers/HLEF2050_Global_Agriculture.pdf

FAO. (2014). Process and scope of the agriculture programme. Chapter 3: Improving infrastructure and trade-related capacities for market access. Rome: FAO. www.fao.org/4/y6831e/y6831e-04.htm

FAO. (2019). The State of Food Security and Nutrition in the World 2019. Safeguarding against economic slowdowns and downturns. Rome: FAO. https://openknowledge.fao.org/server/api/core/bitstreams/16480532-17e9-4b61-b388-1d6d86414470/content

FAO. (2020). Local food systems and COVID-19: A glimpse on India's responses. Rome: FAO. www.fao.org/in-action/food-for-cities-programme/news/detail/en/c/1272232/

Fischer, G., Darkwah, A., Kamoto, J., Kampanje-Phiri, J., Grabowski, P., & Djenontin, I. (2020). Sustainable agricultural intensification and gender-biased land tenure systems: An exploration and conceptualization of interactions. *International Journal of Agricultural Sustainability*, *19*(5–6), 403–422. https://doi.org/10.1080/14735903.2020.1791425

Fischer, T., Byerlee,D., & Edmeades, G. (2014). *Crop Yields and Global Food Security: Will Yield Increase Continue to Feed the World?*. Canberra: Australian Centre for International Agricultural Research.

Gebbers, R., & Adamchuk, V. I. (2010). Precision agriculture and food security. *Science*, *327*(5967), 828–831. PMID: 20150492. https://doi.org/10.1126/science.1183899

Godfray, H. C. J., Beddington, J. R., Crute, I. R., Haddad, L., Lawrence, D., Muir, J. F., ... & Toulmin, C. (2010). Food security: The challenge of feeding 9 billion people. *Science 327*, 812–818. https://doi.org/10.1126/science.1185383

Gulyas, B. Z., & Edmondson, J. L. (2021). Increasing city resilience through urban agriculture: Challenges and solutions in the global north. *Sustainability (Switzerland)*, *13*(3), 1–19. https://doi.org/10.3390/su13031465

Hakkim, V., Joseph, E., Gokul, A., & Mufeedha, K. (2016). Precision farming: The future of indian agriculture. *Journal of Applied Biology and Biotechnology*, *4* (6), 68–72. https://doi.org/10.7324/JABB.2016.40609

Haring, S., Pesci Schmulevich, S., Manser, G. M., & Cooper, M. H. (2023). Rethinking scientists' ongoing participation in "feeding the world." *Frontiers in Sustainable Food Systems*, *7*(July). https://doi.org/10.3389/fsufs.2023.1174704

Hasnat Milton, A., Monroy-Torres, R., Abdullah Al Mamun, M., Keshavarz-Mohammadi, N., Doustmohammadian, A., Mohammadi-Nasrabadi, F., Hajjar, M., Alibeyk, S., & Hajigholam-Saryazdi, M. (2022). Open access edited by community-based participatory interventions to improve food security: A systematic review. *Frontiers in Nutrition: Nutritional Epidemiology*, 9 https://doi.org/10.3389/fnut.2022.1028394

Hawkes, C., Ruel, M. T., Salm, L., Sinclair, B., & Branca, F. (2020). Double-duty actions: Seizing programme and policy opportunities to address malnutrition in all its forms. *Lancet*, *395*, 142–155.

Herrero, M., Henderson, B., Havlík, P., Thornton, P. K., Conant, R. T., Smith, P., Wirsenius, S., Hristov, A. N., Gerber, P., Gill, M., Butterbach-Bahl, K., Valin, H., Garnett, T., & Stehfest, E. (2016). Greenhouse gas mitigation potentials in the livestock sector. *Nature Climate Change*, *6*, 452–461. https://doi.org/10.1038/NCLIMATE2925

HLPE. (2012). Social protection for food security. *A report by the High Level Panel of Experts on Food Security and Nutrition of the Committee on World Food Security*. Rome. Available at www.fao.org/cfs/cfs-hlpe

IFAD. (2021). Annual report 2021. Rome. www.ifad.org/en/annual-report-2021/

IPCC. (2019). Climate Change and Land: an IPCC special report on climate change, desertification, land degradation, sustainable land management, food security, and greenhouse gas fluxes in terrestrial ecosystems. Geneva: IPCC. www.ipcc.ch/site/assets/uploads/2019/11/SRCCL-Full-Report-Compiled-191128.pdf

ISAAA Brief 54. (2018). Global Status of Commercialized Biotech/GM Crops: 2018. Manila: ISAAA. www.isaaa.org/resources/publications/briefs/54/

Jayne, T. S., Snapp, S., Place, F., & Sitko, N. (2019). Sustainable agricultural intensification in an era of rural transformation in Africa. *Global Food Security*, *20*, 105–113. https://doi.org/10.1016/J.GFS.2019.01.008

Kassam, A., Derpsch, R., & Friedrich, T. (2020). Development of conservation agriculture systems globally, (Vol. *21*(1), pp. 31–86). Burleigh Dodds. https://doi.org/10.19103/as.2019.0048.02

Laborde, D., Martin, W., & Vos, R. (2020). *Poverty and Food Insecurity Could Grow Dramatically as COVID-19 Spreads*. IFPRI: International Food Policy Research Institute. Available at: www.ifpri.org/blog/poverty-and-food-insecurity-could-grow-dramatically-COVID-19-spreads

Lajoie-O'Malley, A., Bronson, K., van der Burg, S., & Klerkx, L. (2020). The future(s) of digital agriculture and sustainable food systems: An analysis of high-level policy documents. *Ecosystem Services*, *45*, 101183, ISSN 2212-0416. https://doi.org/10.1016/j.ecoser.2020.101183

Lähde, V., Vadén, T., Toivanen, T., Järvensivu, P., & Eronen, J. T. (2023). The crises inherent in the success of the global food system. *Ecology and Society*, *28*(4). https://doi.org/10.5751/ES-14624-280416

Lipper, L., Thornton, P., Campbell, B., Baedeker, T., Braimoh, A., Bwalya, M., ... & Torquebiau, E. F. (2014). Climate-smart agriculture for food security. *Nature Climate Change*, *4*, 1068–1072. https://doi.org/10.1038/nclimate2437

Lowenberg-DeBoer, J., & Erickson, B. (2019). Setting the record straight on precision agriculture adoption. *Agronomy Journal*, *111*, 1552–1569. https://doi.org/10.2134/agronj2018.12.0779

Maurya, D. K., Maurya, S. K., Mandeep, K., Chaubey, C., Gupta, D., Patel, K. K., Mehta, A. K., & Yadav, R. (n.d.). *View of A Review on Precision Agriculture: An Evolution and Prospect for the Future*. Retrieved May 30, 2024, from https://journalijpss.com/index.php/IJPSS/article/view/4534/8952

Melissa, H., Hoddinott, J., Kumar, N., & Olivier, M. (2018). Social protection, food security, and asset formation. *World Development*, *101*, 88–103. ISSN 0305 750X. https://doi.org/10.1016/j.worlddev.2017.08.014

Naresh, R., Singh, N. K., Sachan, P., Mohanty, L. K., Sahoo, S., Pandey, S. K., & Singh, B. (2024). Enhancing sustainable crop production through innovations in precision agriculture technologies. *Journal of Scientific Research and Reports*, *30*(3), 89–113. https://doi.org/10.9734/jsrr/2024/v30i31861

Nugent, R., Levin, C., Hale, J., & Hutchinson, B. (2020). Economic effects of the double burden of malnutrition. *Lancet*, *395*(10218), 156–164. Epub 2019 Dec 15. PMID: 31852601. https://doi.org/10.1016/S0140-6736(19)32473-0

Oh, S., & Lu, C. (2023). Vertical farming – smart urban agriculture for enhancing resilience and sustainability in food security. *Journal of Horticultural Science and Biotechnology*, *98*(2), 133–140. https://doi.org/10.1080/14620316.2022.2141666

Owino, V., Kumwenda, C., Ekesa, B., Parker, M. E., Ewoldt, L., Roos, N., Lee, W. T., & Tome, D. (2022). The impact of climate change on food systems, diet quality, nutrition, and health outcomes: A narrative review. *Frontiers in Climate*, *4*. https://doi.org/10.3389/fclim.2022.941842

Pingali, P. (2015). Agricultural policy and nutrition outcomes – getting beyond the preoccupation with staple grains. *Food Security*, *7*, 583–591. https://doi.org/10.1007/s12571-015-0461-x

Pingali, P. L. (2012). Green revolution: Impacts, limits, and the path ahead. *Proceedings of the National Academy and Science United States of American*, *109*, 12302–12308.

Pretty, J. (2018). Intensification for redesigned and sustainable agricultural systems. *Science*, *362*, eaav0294.

Qaim, M. (2020). *Role of New Plant Breeding Technologies for Food Security and Sustainable Agricultural Development*. https://doi.org/10.1002/aepp.13044

Raj, S., Roodbar, S., Brinkley, C., & Wolfe, D. W. (2022). Food security and climate change: Differences in impacts and adaptation strategies for rural communities in the global South and North. *Frontiers in Sustainable Food Systems*, *5*(January), 1–18. https://doi.org/10.3389/fsufs.2021.691191

Ray, D. K., Mueller, N. D., West, P. C., & Foley, J. A. (2013). Yield trends are insufficient to double global crop production by 2050. *PLoS ONE*, *8*(6), e66428. https://doi.org/10.1371/journal.pone.0066428

Reardon, T., Echeverria, R., Berdegué, J., Minten, B., Liverpool-Tasie, S., Tschirley, D., & Zilberman, D. (2019). Rapid transformation of food systems in developing regions: Highlighting the role of agricultural research & innovations. *Agricultural Systems,* 172, 47–59. www.sciencedirect.com/science/article/abs/pii/S0308521X17308922

Righettini, M. S., & Bordin, E. (2023). Exploring food security as a multidimensional topic: Twenty years of scientific publications and recent developments. *Quality and Quantity*, *57*(3), 2739–2758. https://doi.org/10.1007/S11135-022-01452-3/FIGURES/3

Ruzzante, S., Labarta, R., & Bilton, A. (2021). Adoption of agricultural technology in the developing world: A meta-analysis of the empirical literature. *World Development*, *146*, 105599. https://doi.org/10.1016/j.worlddev.2021.105599

Shukla, M., Al-Busaidi, K. T., Trivedi, M., & Tiwari, R. K. (2018). Status of research, regulations and challenges for genetically modified crops in India. *GM Crops and Food*, *9*(4), 173–188. https://doi.org/10.1080/21645698.2018.1529518

Tripathi, A., Tripathi, D. K., Chauhan, D. K., Kumar, N., & Singh, G. S. (2016). Paradigms of climate change impacts on some major food sources of the world: A review on current knowledge and future prospects. *Agriculture, Ecosystems & Environment*, *216*, 356–373. https://doi.org/10.1016/J.AGEE.2015.09.034

United Nations. (2018). UN calls for urgent action to feed the world's growing population healthily, equitably and sustainably. UN Department of Economic and Social Affairs News. New York: UNDESA. www.un.org/development/desa/en/news/population/2018-revision-of-world-urbanization-prospects.html

United Nations. (2019). 68% of the world population projected to live in urban areas by 2050, says UN. UN Department of Economic and Social Affairs News. New York: UNDESA. www.un.org/en/desa/un-calls-urgent-action-feed-world%E2%80%99s-growing-population-healthily-equitably-and-sustainably

van Dijk, M., Morley, T., Rau, M. L., & Saghai, Y. (2021). A meta-analysis of projected global food demand and population at risk of hunger for the period 2010–2050. *Nature Food*, *2*(7), 494–501. https://doi.org/10.1038/s43016-021-00322-9

Xie, H., Wen, Y., Choi, Y., & Zhang, X. (2021). Global trends on food security research: A bibliometric analysis. *Land*, *10*(2), 119. https://doi.org/10.3390/LAND10020119

WFP. (2020). The World Food Programme (WFP). New York: UNDESA. https://sdgs.un.org/un-system-sdg-implementation/world-food-programme-wfp-49128

Willett, W., Rockström, J., Loken, B., Springmann, M., Lang, T., Vermeulen, S…& Jonell, M. (2019). Food in the anthropocene: The EAT–lancet commission on healthy diets from sustainable food systems. *Lancet*, *393*, 447–492. https://doi.org/10.1016/S0140-6736(18)31788-4

Wolfert, S., Ge, L., Verdouw, C., & Bogaardt, M. J. (2017). Big data in smart farming – A review. *Agricultural Systems*, *153*, 69–80. ISSN 0308-521X. https://doi.org/10.1016/j.agsy.2017.01.023

Wheeler, T., & von Braun, J. (2013). Climate change impacts on global food security. *Science*, *341*(6145), 508–553. PMID: 23908229. https://doi.org/10.1126/science.1239402

World Bank. (2021). Covid-19 and food protectionism: The impact of the pandemic and export restrictions. Washington, DC: World Bank. https://documents1.worldbank.org/curated/en/417171589912076742/pdf/Covid-19-and-Food-Protectionism-The-Impact-of-the-Pandemic-and-Export-Restrictions-on-World-Food-Markets.pdf

Yuan, G. N., Marquez, G. P. B., Deng, H., Iu, A., Fabella, M., Salonga, R. B., Ashardiono, F., & Cartagena, J. A. (2023). Corrigendum to "A review on urban agriculture: Technology, socio-economy, and policy" [Heliyon 8(11), (2022) Article e11583] (Heliyon (2022) 8(11), (S2405844022028717), (10.1016/j.heliyon.2022.e11583)). *Heliyon*, *9*(2), e13165. https://doi.org/10.1016/j.heliyon.2023.e13165

Zhang, W., Sheng, J., Li, Z., Hu, G., Xuan, J., & Zhao, H. (2021). Integrating rainwater harvesting and drip irrigation for water use efficiency improvements in apple orchards of northwest China. *Scientia Horticulturae*, *275*, 109728. https://doi.org/10.1016/j.scientia.2020.109728

2 Impact of Agriculture Diversity on the Nutritional Status of Children in India

Arpit Singh, Rati Kapoor, and Shambhavi Mishra

2.1 INTRODUCTION

"Nutrition is a desperately neglected aspect of maternal, newborn and child health. More than a third of child deaths and 11% of the total disease burden worldwide are due to maternal and child undernutrition" (Lancet series on Maternal and Child Undernutrition 2008). How we feed the world population, and how governments think of genetically modified food or crops as a technological fix, is an issue. But this is not simple. Malnutrition can be defined as a lack of proper nutrition. The nutritional status of a child, as with any individual, is assessed through dietary, anthropometric, biochemical, and physical observation. Malnutrition affects physical growth, morbidity, mortality, cognitive development, reproduction, and physical work capacity, which in result is an underlying factor for death among under-5 children as well as for many diseases for both children and adults that are highly prevalent in developing countries. Maternal and child undernutrition have both short-term consequences like mortality, morbidity, and disability, and long-term consequences like intellectual ability, economic productivity, and reproductive performance.

India is home to one third of the world's undernourished children, with rates of child undernutrition remaining stubbornly high for decades. Undernutrition is widespread among adults too; one third of all Indian men and women are affected. According to the fifth National Family Health Survey (NFHS-5), 18% of Indian children are born with low birth weight, 36% of children below 3 years of age are stunted, 19% are wasted, and 32% are underweight. Not only are the absolute numbers high, the prevalence of young child undernutrition has changed little over the last two decades. Micronutrient deficiencies are high among children and adults, with 77% of children, 24% of women, and 23% of men being anemic.

While national trends paint a bleak picture, the mosaic of child undernutrition in India reveals five key patterns. First, we find substantial geographic variability with change in the prevalence of various nutrition indicators. Second, trends in stunting by age and gender over the five rounds of the NFHS survey reflect normal global patterns. The greatest declines in height for age occur during the first two years of life, with little change thereafter. Trends in mean weight-for-age scores by child age,

DOI: 10.1201/9781003487227-2

over the five rounds of the NFHS, are like those for height for age. All five rounds of the NFHS data show mean height for age for girls to be similar to or better than that for boys during the first two years. Third, the data on nutrition indicators reveal significant socioeconomic inequalities. The poorest, the scheduled tribes and castes, and those residing in rural areas, bear the highest burden of undernutrition. While undernutrition is higher in children from lower income quintiles, it is substantial in middle income quintiles as well. Approximately half the children in the middle quintile and a quarter in the highest quintile are stunted. Fourth, the level and trends in anemia among both children and adults paint an alarming picture throughout India. The prevalence of anemia among children 12–17 months of age is as high as 80%. Anemia has increased among women who have ever been married from 53.1% in NFHS-4 to 57% in NFHS-5. There is less variability across states and over time, indicating a uniform and static picture of crisis levels in anemia. Fifth, while more than a third of Indian men and more than half of Indian women are too thin, the prevalence of overweight and obesity, currently at 23% (NFHS-5), is rising, increasing the public health importance of associated chronic diseases (Gillespie et al., 2012).

Factors that contribute to malnutrition are many and varied: socioeconomic, demographic, number of members in the family, occupation of parents, education status of parents, family income, maternal nutritional knowledge, resident location, gender, breastfeeding practices, child and maternal care services, dietary intake, etc. Each of these factors affects determinants of malnutrition stated under WHO child growth standards. Child and maternal care services include numerous factors starting from pregnancy and continuing until the child has reached at least the age of 2 years, like antenatal care (ANC), anemia level, deficiency of vitamin A, and iodine at the time of pregnancy, and exclusive breastfeeding, immunization, and dietary intake after the child has been born.

Across the globe, many reforms have taken place to combat malnutrition. The most popular reforms are in maternal and child care services, as within these we have multiple care mechanisms from before the women become mothers until the children reach the age of 5. According to the World Bank and WHO, there are many programs which are ongoing with the help of government agencies and private firms to combat the problem of undernutrition. Within the government plans, promotion of ANC visits and immunization of children are prominent, but dietary intake plays a very important role in determining how well the child or the mother is getting nutrition. In urban areas, it is the dietary pattern that indicates whether mother and child are getting proper micro nutrients, but in rural areas, dietary intake itself depends on the income of the family, crop production, and availability of food. India is a country of vast agricultural diversity, and 70% of the population is associated with agricultural activities. Therefore, improvements in agriculture can lead to improvements in human capital and economic growth, which in turn help to combat the problem of undernutrition.

The track record of the Indian agriculture sector in augmenting the availability of food is noteworthy. The two most prominent examples are the cases of rice and wheat (the Green Revolution) in the 1960s through the 1980s, and of milk from Operation Flood (the White Revolution) during the 1970s through the 1990s. India now needs to manage its economic transformation to ensure that its agriculture sector realizes its potential to reduce poverty and increase access to optimal quality and quantity of foods to nourish its population, on the one hand, and simultaneously to address nutrition and associated chronic diseases, on the other.

2.2 THE ROLE OF AGRICULTURE IN ENHANCING NUTRITION

Mainstreaming nutrition considerations into agricultural operations could increase the availability of and access to nutritious food, which can improve the nutrition status of individuals (Hoddinott, 2012). The world has seen declining rates of hunger over the past three decades. The average per capita calorie consumption in developing countries has risen from 2054 in 1966 to 2803 in 1999, leading to a decline in the number of hungry people from approximately 900 million to approximately 700 million in 2000 (FAO, 2003). Undoubtedly, much of this can be attributed to the successes of the Green Revolution, which contributed to productivity increases and a rise in the quantity of cereal crops available. Yet, despite these accomplishments, the number of those suffering from micronutrient malnutrition remains high, with an estimated 2 billion at risk of iron deficiencies, 1.5 billion at risk of iodine deficiencies, and 0.95 million at risk of vitamin A deficiencies (WHO, 2000). The consequences are seen in human and economic losses for economies, in the form of both current and future productivity losses. Agricultural research can address micronutrient malnutrition by improving both quantity and quality of food intake. Positive effects of agricultural research include decreases in food prices, increased consumption, improved processing and preparation, and better plant breeding.

The prevalence of undernutrition in India has long been thought of as enigmatically high, given the region's income levels and the success of the Green Revolution. However, in recent years the Indian enigma has become even more puzzling. Over the same period, according to the NFHS, the proportion of Indian children that were stunted declined only from 51.0% to 44.9%, and the proportion that were underweight from 42.7% to 40.4% (Bhagowalia et al., 2012). This sluggish nutritional performance in the face of strong economic growth has raised the possibility that undernutrition in India is in some sense disconnected from economic growth in general and perhaps from agricultural growth in particular. These data disconnects mean that existing evidence on the relationship between income, agricultural production, and nutrition is largely unsatisfactory. Perhaps the only existing microeconomic research linking nutrition to household expenditure, agricultural production, and food consumption is work on the Young Lives panel for Andhra Pradesh (Himaz, 2009). That study confirmed the importance of dietary diversity and household wealth, and also used the panel nature of the data to find that the occurrence of drought increased the chances of stunting and underweight by around 6% (Himaz, 2009). However, the sample was representative only for rural areas in Andhra Pradesh. This raises some questions: Is there no relation between economic and agricultural growth and malnutrition? Can better agricultural performance contribute to bringing down malnutrition levels?

A common factor across all such frameworks is the understanding that agriculture can influence nutrition and health through multiple pathways (direct and indirect), and that only one of those relates to the consumption of more food. For example, Headey et al. (2012), Gillespie et al. (2012) and USAID (2013) talk of seven pathways, which include agriculture as the direct and indirect (via income) source of food at household level, macro-level agricultural policy as a driver of prices, and agriculture as an entry-point for enhancing women's control over resources, knowledge, and status.

2.3 ADDRESSING UNDERNUTRITION THROUGH TARGETED AGRICULTURAL INTERVENTIONS

According to the Lancet's series on Maternal and Child Undernutrition 2008 there are many factors which affect the nutritional status of children and women, and in the Lancet's series on Maternal and Child Nutrition 2013 there are many interventions which are combating the problem of undernutrition. However, according to Ruel and Alderman (2013), we need to have more targeted agriculture intervention programs, which gives us the idea that there is still the need for some better interventions to overcome the problem of undernutrition. There are many interventions ongoing, such as biofortification of crops, home gardening, aquaculture, and horticulture, which have a huge impact over the nutritional status of mother and child. Since we do not have any survey which has both data on agricultural diversity and nutritional status, there are difficulties in linking crop production, food intake, economic status, and women's empowerment with the nutritional status of women and children directly.

2.4 IMPACT OF CROP PRODUCTION ON NUTRITIONAL STATUS OF CHILDREN

What is the current scenario of agriculture or, to put it more precisely, how is the production of different crops affecting the nutritional status of children? This chapter explores the distribution of different crop productions across various states of India. It examines the factors determining the nutritional status of children through multilevel modeling. Furthermore, it explores the association between undernutrition (stunting, underweight, and wasting) and the mother's nutritional status as a mediator. It also analyzes the direct and indirect effects on a child's nutritional status and investigates how background characteristics influence the outcome through mediation using structural equation modeling (SEM).

2.5 DATA SOURCES AND METHODOLOGY

There are two data sets used in this study. One is the meso-level dataset for India that contains data about the performance, structure, and dynamics of the agricultural economy at a country level and its disaggregation at state/region, district, and sub-district levels. The dataset maintained by the International Crops Research Institute for Semi-Arid Tropics (ICRISAT), Hyderabad and updated under the Village Dynamics in South Asia (VDSA) project provides a comprehensive one-stop-shop for data related to key agricultural and socioeconomic variables. The all-India database is available from 1950, while the state-level data are from 1966 to 2011. The state data cover 19 major states, namely Andhra Pradesh, Gujarat, Haryana, Karnataka, Madhya Pradesh, Maharashtra, Punjab, Rajasthan, Tamil Nadu, Uttar Pradesh, Bihar, West Bengal, Odisha, Assam, Himachal Pradesh, Kerala, Chhattisgarh, Jharkhand, and Uttarakhand, with district-level data from 1966 onwards for core and additional variables such as area and production (crop-wise), irrigation, land use, wages and prices, input use, census returns (human population and livestock population), infrastructure (roads, markets, banks, and veterinary institutions), and climatic variables. In this study, the district-level data for area and production crop-wise and rainfall are used for the year 2011.

Another set of data which is used in this study for analysis purposes is woman-level data from the fourth round of the District Level Household and Facility Survey (DLHS-4). The DLHS was conducted by the International Institute for Population Sciences, Mumbai with financial support from the Ministry of Health and Family Welfare, Government of India. Bilingual questionnaires in the local language and English pertaining to households and women who had ever been married (age 15–49 years) were canvassed using computer-assisted personal interviewing (CAPI). The sampling design adopted in the DLHS was multistage stratified area probability sampling, which provides reliable estimates at state and district levels and for rural and urban areas. The primary sampling units (PSUs) were census villages for the rural sector and National Sample Survey Office (NSSO) urban frame survey blocks (UFS) for the urban sector. For rural areas of the district, a two-stage sampling design was adopted for normal PSUs. First, PSUs were selected using probability proportional to size (PPS), and then the households were selected using circular systematic sampling (CSS). For large PSUs, three-stage sampling was used, with a first selection by PPS, then selection of one or two segments in the second stage, followed by selection of households using CSS. For urban areas, two-stage stratified sampling design was used for selection of urban frame selection blocks at random in the first stage, and households by CSS in the second stage. The fourth round of person file of DLHS corresponds to the year 2012–13, reflecting multiple levels of hierarchical nesting structure in non-EAG states of India. The woman-level data was then combined with the child-level clinical, anthropometric and biochemical (CAB) component data to get child-level data, which was again combined to village-level data. This process yielded one data set from DLHS round 4 of rural areas, which was child-level data for children aged from 0 to 5 years.

Both the data sets were merged using the district ID. The combined data thus formed cover eight states and their respective districts, with 38,448 children aged 0–5 years across these states and districts, making the data hierarchical in nature. The hierarchical nature of the combined data set can be seen with area and production crop-wise data, along with rainfall data at district level and the data collected for villages in DLHS survey at village or PSU level, and then the individual level. For this study, the nutritional status of children is seen through stunting and underweight, where the height-for-age and weight-for-age indices measures linear growth retardation. Stunting is a small-time anthropometric failure; that is, it is substantially more likely in newborns and decreases with age. Children who are more than two standard deviations below the median of the reference population in terms of height for age are considered short for their age or stunted, and children more than three standard deviations below the median of the reference population median are considered severely stunted. Underweight is defined as low weight for age, a composite measure that takes into account both chronic and acute illness in children. Children more than two standard deviations below the median of the reference median on this index are underweight, and children more than three standard deviations below the median of the reference median are considered severely underweight.

2.6 DATA SET AND APPROACH USED IN THE STUDY

The combined data set contains eight states, 160 districts, and 5033 PSUs, which consist of 27,557 households within which 28,619 women aged 15–49 years have ever been married. The information collected by DLHS 4 (2012–13) and VDSA is used to examine the nutritional status of children. The outcome indicators and explanatory variables are as follows:

Outcome variables:

- Stunting
- Underweight

Level 1: Household or individual-level variables

- Mother's age
- Woman's age at the time of marriage
- Religion
- Caste
- Father's education status
- Mother's education status
- Gravidity
- Delivery place
- Delivery type
- Woman having any problem at time of pregnancy
- Child birth weight
- Child having any problem at time of birth
- Child received vaccination
- Child fed with colostrum

Level 2: Village-level variables

- Distance to nearest district headquarters
- Distance to nearest railway station
- Distance to nearest bus station
- Availability of PHC
- Availability of CHC
- Availability of government hospital

- Availability of ASHA
- Availability of ANM
- Availability of Trained Birth Attendant (TBA)

Level 3: District-level variables

- Area in '000 hectares of cereal production
- Area in '000 hectares of pulse production
- Area in '000 hectares of oil seed production
- Area in '000 hectares of fruit production
- Area in '000 hectares of vegetable production
- Area in '000 hectares of potato production
- Area in '000 hectares of onion production
- Total annual (January to December) rainfall in millimeters

Level 4: State-level variable

- State indicator

Univariate analysis was conducted to filter out the insignificant factors for further analysis. For testing the collinearity of the explanatory variables, we analyzed the magnitude of multicollinearity by considering the size of the variance inflation factor (VIF) (βi). A common rule of thumb is that if VIF (βi)>5 then multicollinearity is high and the relevant variable(s) should be removed. The multilevel modeling approach was also adopted for analyzing the dependent nature of the outcome variable. Our data followed three multilevel models: two-level strict hierarchical structural with district at level one, nested within the state at levels two; three-level strict hierarchical structural with primary sampling unit at level one, nested within district at level two and state at level three; and four-level strict hierarchical structural with household at level one, nested within the primary sampling unit at level two, district at level three, and state at level four. Further, comparison of the three approaches was carried out to evaluate the superiority of one over the others (Goldstein, 2005).

The traditional logistic regression model can be formally expressed as

$$Logit(y_{ij}) = \beta_{0j} + \sum_{n=1}^{p} \beta_{nj}\chi_{nj} + e_{ij}$$

where χ_{nj} are explanatory variables, β_{0j} is the value of E(Y_{ij}) when $\chi_{nj}= 0$, $\forall\ i=1,2,....,p$, e_{ij} = residual variation in y_{ij} that cannot be explained, and $e_{ij} \sim N(0, \sigma^2_e)$. To make this a two-level random intercept model, we let β_{0j} become a random variable, with an assumption that

$$\beta_{0j} = \beta_0 + u_{0j}$$

where u_{0j} is the random part.

The multilevel model is based on a four-level structure of individuals (level 1 denoted by *i* subscript), nested within PSUs (level 2, denoted by *j* subscript), nested within the district (level 3, denoted by *k* subscript), nested within the state (level 4, denoted by *l* subscript). The micro model can be written as

$$Logit(y_{ijkl}) = \beta_{0jkl} + \beta_{1}X_{nijkl} + e_{0ijkl}$$

$$Logit(y_{ijkl}) = \beta_{0jkl} + \sum_{n=1}^{p} \beta_{njkl}\chi_{njkl} + e_{ijkl}$$

with an additional subscript to represent the districts. In addition, there would be a macro model at the PSU level (level 2):

$$\beta_{0jkl} = \beta_{0kl} + u_{0jkl}$$

where u_{0jkl} is the differential for the *j*th PSU in the district nested within the state from average β_{0kl}. There would also be a macro model at the district level (level 3):

$$\beta_{0kl} = \beta_{0l} + u_{0kl}$$

where u_{0kl} is the differential for the *k*th district nested within the state from the average $\beta_{0l.}$ There would also be a macro model at the state level (level 4):

$$\beta_{0l} = \beta_{0} + u_{0l}$$

where u_{0l} is the differential for the *l*th state from the average $\beta_{0.}$

The random effects associated with each level are interpreted as residual differentials for state, district, and PSU and are assumed to be independent and normally distributed with mean 0 and variance σ^2_{l0}, σ^2_{k0}, and σ^2_{j0} respectively. These variances quantify variation between state, between district, and between PSU, respectively, in log odds of being stunted and underweight, conditional on all socio-economic and demographic characteristics along with district-level crop production and rainfall. For binary outcomes, the variance at the lowest level cannot be obtained directly from the model, and all remaining variance is assumed to be simply a function of the binomial distribution. Based on the variance estimates of the random effects, the proportion of variation in log odds of being stunted and underweight is attributable to each level, which is known as the variance partitioning coefficient (VPC) (Browne et al., 2005; Goldstein et al., 2002). For instance, the proportion of the total variation in stunting and underweight (in log odds scale) attributable to districts can be calculated by dividing the between-district variance by the total variance. In calculating the total variance we used the latent variable method approach and treated the between-household variance as having a variance of standard logistic distribution approximated as $\pi^2/3 \cong 3.29$ (Browne et al., 2005; Goldstein et al., 2002). Hence VPC for any level Z is calculated using following formula:

$$VPC_z = \sigma^2_z / (\sigma^2_{l0} + \sigma^2_{k0} + \sigma^2_{j0} + 3.29)$$

The analysis using the four-level model for stunting and underweight was conducted for children aged 0–5 years in rural villages of eight states (Andhra Pradesh, Haryana, Karnataka, Kerala, Maharashtra, Punjab, Tamil Naidu, and West Bengal) for which district-level agriculture data were available, to see the impact of crop production and rainfall on the nutritional status of children. STATA 14.2 was used to obtain results of cross-tabulation and binary logistic regression.

SEM was conducted to examine the association between undernutrition (stunting and underweight), mother's nutritional status as a mediator in the model, and all other predicting variables, for the explanation of the direct and indirect effects on the child's nutritional status. To test the direct and indirect effects of the background variables as well as district variables, path analysis models were constructed. Careful consideration was given to the following criteria of the model fit indices suggested by Hopper et al. (2008) and measuring model fit (Kenny (2015):

a) *p*-values should be less than 0.05.
b) A root mean square error of approximation (RMSEA) less than 0.06 indicates an adequate model fit.
c) A standardized root mean square residual (SRMR, measuring the average distance between the observed and model-implied correlation) less than 0.08 indicates a good fit.

The Akaike information criterion (AIC) value was used for the comparison of the estimated models for goodness of fit of the three cognitive scores to identify the best model. RMSEA, the comparative fit index (CFI), and the Tucker–Lewis Index (TLI) were used to indicate whether the model fits the data. RMSEA measures the degree of model adequacy based on population discrepancy about degrees of freedom; a value less than 0.08 is preferred (acceptable). CFI and TLI are examples of an incremental fit index. These types of indices compare the improvement of the fit of the proposed model over a more restricted model, called an independence or null model, which specifies no relationships among variables. CFI and TLI range from 0 to 1.0, with values closer to 1.0 (or more than 0.80) indicating a better fit (Hu & Bentler, 1999).

2.7 RESULTS

Distribution of crop production across different states

In this study, the distribution of crop-wise production is seen through the production unit per '000 tons, production of fruit and vegetables in an area per '000 hectares, and annual rainfall in millimeters for the year 2011 as per the VDSA using Tableau 10.5 software. Here, we consider the distribution of crop production and annual rainfall over these eight states. The states with the highest level of crop production are marked with darker shades. The VDSA data include various crops like rice, wheat, maize, barley, sorghum, and millet. The data also include the production of different types of pulses and oilseeds production. Figure 2.1 shows production of rice, with West Bengal in the

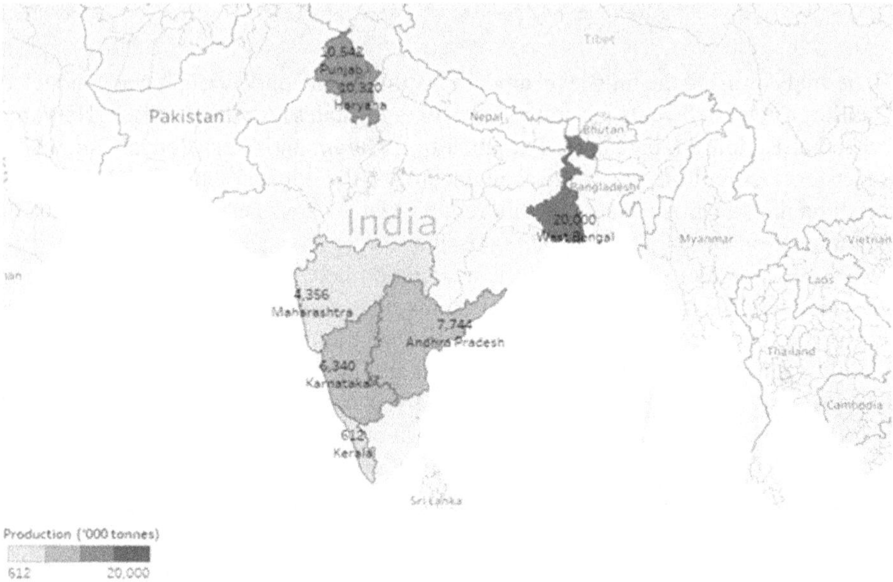

FIGURE 2.1 Rice production across eight states.

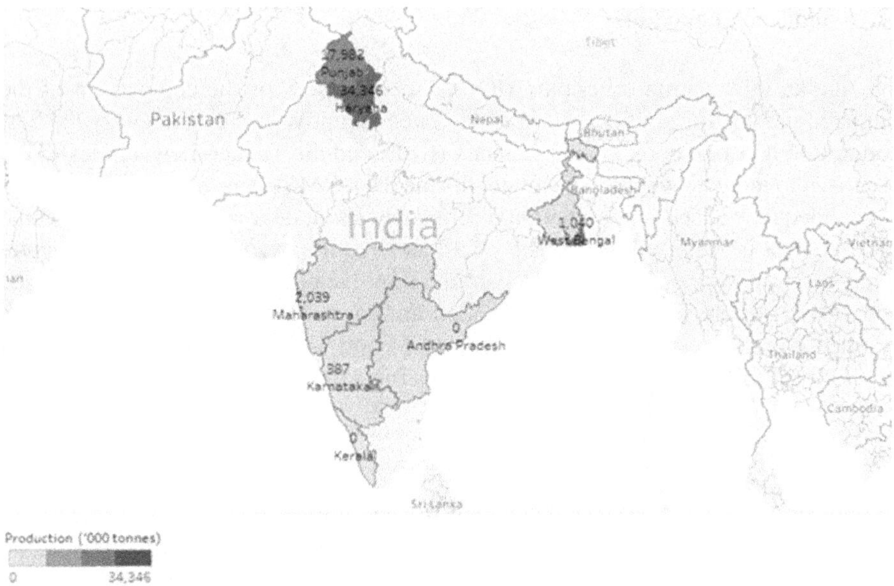

FIGURE 2.2 Wheat production across eight states.

highest position with the largest production in terms of '000 tons, followed by Punjab and Haryana. Figure 2.2 and Figure 2.3 show wheat and maize production, respectively, with Punjab and Haryana highest in wheat production and Karnataka and Maharashtra highest in maize production. Figure 2.4 and Figure 2.5 are about fruit and vegetable production,

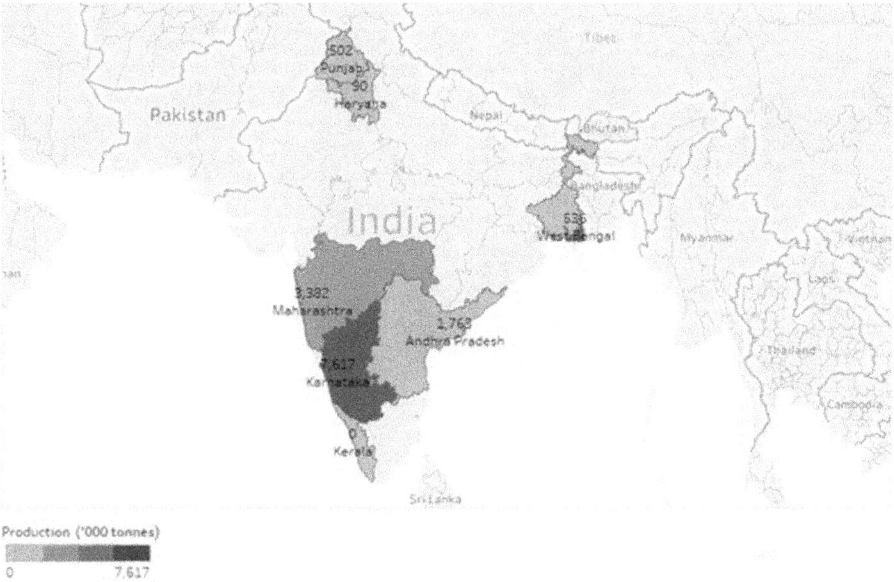

FIGURE 2.3 Maize production across eight states.

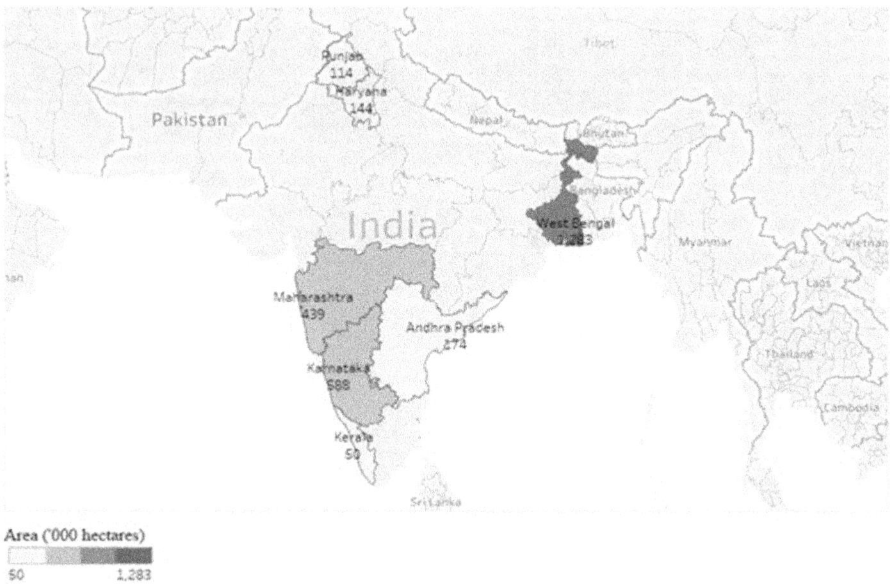

FIGURE 2.4 Vegetable production across eight states.

with West Bengal highest in vegetable production and Maharashtra highest in fruit production. Maharashtra is the leading producer of fruit, oil seed, and pulses (Figure 2.6 and Figure 2.7). Maharashtra also leads in annual rainfall (Figure 2.8), followed by Karnataka, Kerala, and West Bengal.

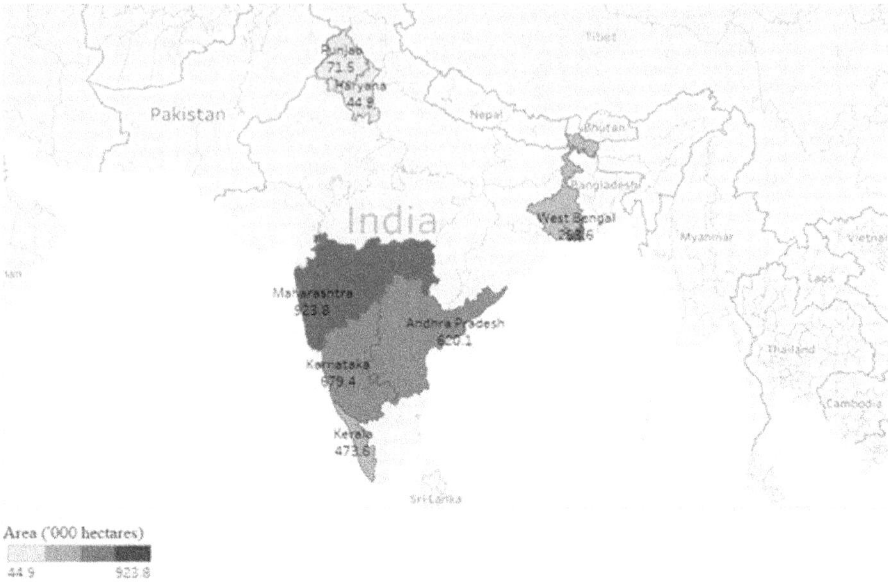

FIGURE 2.5 Fruit production across eight states.

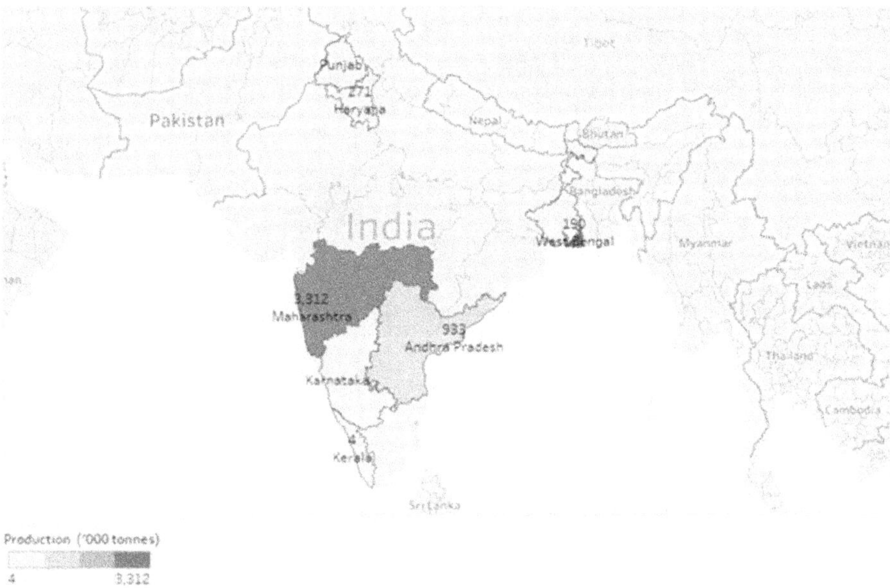

FIGURE 2.6 Pulses production across eight states.

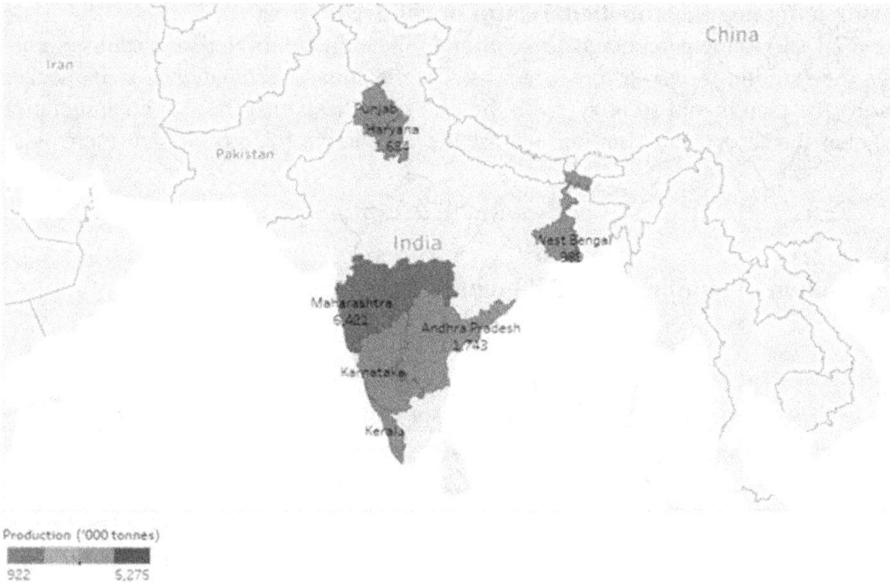

FIGURE 2.7 Oil seed production across eight states.

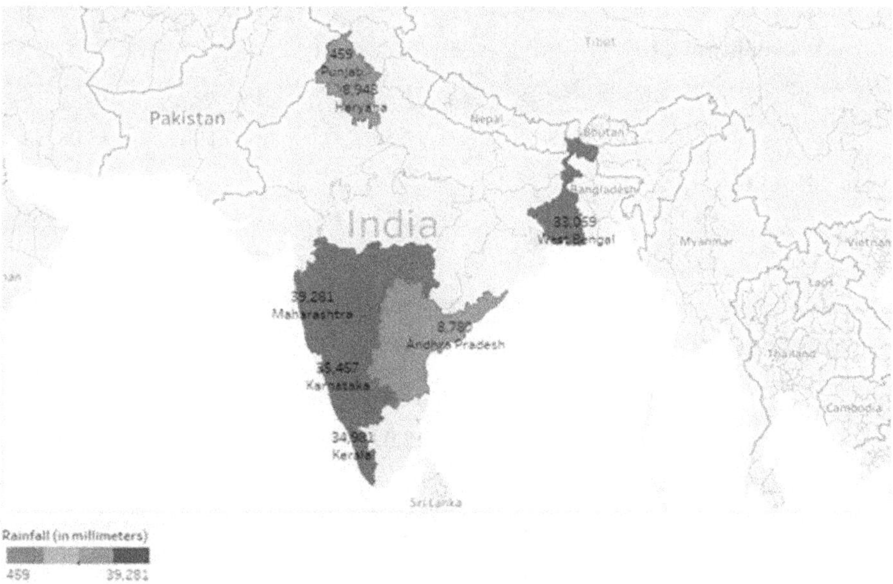

FIGURE 2.8 Annual rainfall in eight states.

Factors affecting the nutritional status of children

Table 2.1 shows the percentage distribution of the indicator of nutrition status of children (i.e., stunting) over different factors. The chi square association is also checked among the factors and stunting, with the null hypothesis that there is no association between the factor and stunting against the alternative hypothesis that there is an

TABLE 2.1
Distribution of Stunting over Different Factors

	Stunting			
Factor	Severely Stunted	Stunted	Normal	Overheight
Availability of Government School				
Yes	13.31	12.48	60.17	14.03
No	11.01	12.50	63.99	12.50
Availability of PHC*				
Yes	12.69	11.75	60.70	14.86
No	13.43	12.69	60.10	13.78
Availability of CHC				
Yes	12.49	11.38	61.76	14.37
No	13.31	12.55	60.16	13.98
Availability of Government Hospital				
Yes	11.13	10.34	62.67	15.87
No	13.35	12.58	60.15	13.92
Availability of ASHA*				
Yes	13.62	12.58	59.98	13.82
No	11.81	12.09	61.34	14.76
Availability of ANM*				
Yes	13.60	12.58	60.02	13.8
No	12.26	12.23	60.92	14.58
Availability of Trained Birth Attendant (TBA)*				
Yes	12.25	11.87	61.05	14.83
No	13.75	12.79	59.85	13.61

TABLE 2.1 (Continued)
Distribution of Stunting over Different Factors

	Stunting			
Factor	Severely Stunted	Stunted	Normal	Overheight
Mother's Age*				
15–20	16.90	12.61	55.32	15.18
21–25	14.68	12.68	57.46	15.17
26–30	12.85	12.35	61.09	13.70
31–35	11.26	12.13	64.15	12.45
36–40	12.50	12.79	61.16	13.55
41–45	12.18	12.88	60.06	14.88
46–50	14.17	12.72	59.55	13.56
Mother's Age at Marriage*				
Below 15	17.93	15.05	56.55	10.48
15–20	13.94	12.96	59.06	14.04
21–25	11.36	11.49	62.55	14.59
26–30	10.75	11.02	63.71	14.52
31–35	10.81	5.95	70.27	12.97
Above 35	10.64	8.51	59.57	21.28
Religion*				
Hindu	13.50	12.76	59.40	14.34
Muslim	13.85	12.75	59.79	13.62
Other	10.95	10.18	67.15	11.72
Caste*				
SC	14.25	13.02	59.86	12.87
ST	14.32	14.47	55.68	15.53
OBC	13.01	12.20	60.86	13.92
General	11.78	11.18	62.05	14.99
Father's Education*				
Illiterate	10.99	12.64	59.89	16.48
Below primary	13.93	13.88	59.62	12.57

(continued)

TABLE 2.1 (Continued)
Distribution of Stunting over Different Factors

	Stunting			
Factor	Severely Stunted	Stunted	Normal	Overheight
Primary to middle	11.89	12.62	61.41	14.07
10th to 12th grade	11.40	11.00	62.31	15.29
Graduate and above	9.57	9.95	64.10	16.38
Mother's Education*				
Illiterate	10.90	14.10	62.18	12.82
Below primary	14.37	13.66	59.74	12.24
Primary to middle	12.87	12.02	60.47	14.64
10th to 12th grade	10.49	10.98	62.88	15.65
Graduate and above	7.89	8.28	67.43	16.40
Mother Having Problem During Pregnancy*				
Yes	13.00	11.81	61.40	13.78
No	13.38	12.75	59.79	14.08
Gravidity				
1	12.51	10.62	59.78	17.10
2	12.61	12.13	61.45	13.81
3	13.83	13.54	59.80	12.83
4	14.98	13.91	59.02	12.09
Delivery Place*				
Government	14.03	12.78	59.41	13.78
Private	11.02	11.08	61.99	15.90
Other	16.12	14.24	57.74	11.90
Delivery Type*				
Normal	13.85	12.86	59.35	13.94
Caesarean	12.11	11.19	61.94	14.76
By instrument	10.54	9.34	67.17	12.95

TABLE 2.1 (Continued)
Distribution of Stunting over Different Factors

	Stunting			
Factor	Severely Stunted	Stunted	Normal	Overheight
Colostrum-Fed				
Yes	13.53	12.44	59.89	14.14
No	13.58	13.54	59.56	13.32
Child Having Birth Problem*				
Yes	15.54	13.38	58.31	12.76
No	13.15	12.43	60.35	14.07
Child Received Vaccination				
Yes	13.34	12.59	60.11	13.96
No	14.87	12.46	57.97	14.70

association. A p-value less than 0.05 indicates an association between stunting and the factor (e.g., mother's age, age at marriage, or availability of ASHA). Similarly Table 2.2 shows the percentage distribution of underweight over different factors.

The associated factors were put into a multilevel model to explore the association of stunting and underweight among the factors within state, district, and PSU-level variables. In Table 2.3, three models are fitted for exploring the association of underweight with different factors. In Model 1 only district-level variables like crop-wise production and annual rainfall are taken, with the variation defined at state and district level. With every unit increase in potato production, the odds of being underweight reduce by 5.3% (OR: 0.947). Similarly, the odds of being underweight increase by 0.7% in castor production (OR: 1.007), 0.9% in safflower production (OR: 1.009), and 0.2% in maize production (OR:1.002), with VPC 2.3% at state level and 0.6% at district level. In Model 2 both the district-level and PSU-level variables are taken into account, which results in addition of odds of being underweight by 0.2% per unit increase in distance to nearest railway station (OR: 1.002), with VPC 1.4% at state level, 0.4% at district level, and 7.4% at PSU level. In Model 3 the individual variables are also taken into account with district and PSU-level variables, which results in odds of being underweight by 36% if mother's education is below primary (OR: 1.36) and 25% if it is primary to middle (OR: 1.249) compared to mother's education to 10th–12th grade. There is also an increase in the odds of being underweight by 81% if delivery is done by any instrument (OR: 1.817) compared to normal delivery. With a per unit increase in child birth weight, the odds of being underweight

TABLE 2.2
Distribution of Underweight over Different Factors

	Underweight			
Factor	**Severely Underweight**	**Underweight**	**Normal**	**Overweight**
Availability of Government School				
Yes	9.78	16.92	70.42	2.87
No	8.08	16.92	73.02	1.98
Availability of PHC*				
Yes	9.15	16.18	71.42	3.25
No	9.92	17.12	70.21	2.75
Availability of CHC				
Yes	8.37	15.92	72.62	3.10
No	9.84	16.97	70.35	2.84
Availability of Government Hospital				
Yes	7.93	16.25	72.48	3.34
No	9.83	16.95	70.39	2.83
Availability of ASHA*				
Yes	9.85	17.12	70.29	2.74
No	9.36	16.08	71.23	3.32
Availability of ANM*				
Yes	9.92	17.09	70.23	2.76
No	9.28	16.43	71.16	3.13
Availability of Trained Birth Attendant (TBA)				
Yes	9.98	17.15	69.75	3.12
No	9.64	16.81	70.82	2.73
Mother's Age*				
15–20	11.05	18.25	67.35	3.34
21–25	10.29	17.13	69.64	2.94

TABLE 2.2 (Continued)
Distribution of Underweight over Different Factors

	Underweight			
Factor	Severely Underweight	Underweight	Normal	Overweight
26–30	9.22	16.65	71.40	2.73
31–35	9.48	16.54	71.09	2.89
36–40	10.86	17.70	68.39	3.05
41–45	9.38	17.45	69.95	3.23
46–50	9.54	16.73	71.33	2.40
Mother's Age at Marriage*				
Below 15	12.28	21.11	64.66	1.95
15–20	10.30	18.18	68.72	2.80
21–25	8.18	14.30	74.43	3.10
26–30	8.76	13.49	74.21	3.55
31–35	10.75	16.67	70.97	1.61
Above 35	6.25	16.67	77.08	0.00
Religion*				
Hindu	9.95	17.36	69.77	2.92
Muslim	9.59	18.00	70.05	2.37
Other	8.41	12.60	76.25	2.75
Caste*				
SC	10.68	17.72	68.84	2.76
ST	13.09	20.66	63.71	2.54
OBC	8.91	16.91	71.13	3.05
General	8.19	13.85	75.16	2.80
Father's Education*				
Illiterate	11.35	16.76	69.73	2.16
Below primary	10.38	18.52	68.71	2.39
Primary to middle	9.03	16.37	71.62	2.98
10th to 12th grade	8.15	14.50	74.22	3.13

(continued)

TABLE 2.2 (Continued)
Distribution of Underweight over Different Factors

	Underweight			
Factor	Severely Underweight	Underweight	Normal	Overweight
Graduate and above	5.71	11.06	78.72	4.51
Mother's Education*				
Illiterate	10.53	20.39	67.11	1.97
Below primary	9.97	18.90	68.66	2.47
Primary to middle	9.17	16.68	71.27	2.88
10th to 12th grade	7.22	13.65	75.85	3.28
Graduate and above	5.02	8.53	81.43	5.02
Woman Having Problem During Pregnancy*				
Yes	9.16	15.84	72.17	2.84
No	9.99	17.34	69.81	2.86
Gravidity*				
1	8.80	13.66	73.69	3.85
2	8.97	16.45	71.88	2.70
3	10.46	18.30	68.65	2.58
4	11.59	19.70	66.35	2.36
Delivery Place*				
Government	10.28	17.80	69.36	2.56
Private	7.50	13.23	75.59	3.68
Other	13.25	20.88	64.04	1.82
Delivery Type				
Normal	10.72	17.79	68.97	2.51
Caesarean	6.64	13.43	75.92	4.01
By instrument	5.14	13.60	79.46	1.81
Colostrum-Fed*				
Yes	9.88	16.92	70.41	2.79
No	11.11	17.98	68.51	2.40

TABLE 2.2 (Continued)
Distribution of Underweight over Different Factors

	Underweight			
Factor	Severely Underweight	Underweight	Normal	Overweight
Child Having Birth Problem*				
Yes	11.89	16.98	68.28	2.86
No	9.64	16.92	70.59	2.86
Child Received Vaccination*				
Yes	9.66	17.01	70.58	2.75
No	12.37	17.32	67.63	2.68

TABLE 2.3
Multilevel Model for Factors Associated with Underweight

Underweight	Model 1	Model 2	Model 3
District-Level Variable			
Vegetable production	1.001 (0.009)	1.003 (0.010)	0.998 (0.009)
Potato production	0.947 (0.030)*	0.945 (0.030)*	0.980 (0.028)
Onion production	0.997 (0.009)	0.994 (0.011)	1.000 (0.009)
Castor production	1.007 (0.002)*	1.007 (0.002)*	1.006 (0.002)*
Linseed production	0.998 (0.013)	0.989 (0.012)	0.990 (0.012)
Sunflower production	0.997 (0.003)	0.998 (0.003)	1.000 (0.003)
Sesamum production	1.006 (0.011)	1.005 (0.011)	1.005 (0.012)
Safflower production	1.009 (0.003)*	1.011 (0.003)*	1.009 (0.003)*
Maize production	1.002 (0.001)*	1.002 (0.001)*	1.001 (0.001)
Pulse production	1.000 (0.001)	0.999 (0.000)	1.000 (0.000)
Annual rainfall	1.000 (0.000)	1.000 (0.000)	1.000 (0.000)
PSU-Level Variable			
Distance to nearest district headquarters		1.001 (0.001)	1.001 (0.001)
Distance to nearest railway station		1.002 (0.001)*	1.000 (0.001)
Distance to nearest bus station		1.001 (0.002)	0.999 (0.003)
Availability of PHC		1.061 (0.06)	1.103 (0.074)
Availability of CHC		0.963 (0.107)	0.980 (0.134)
Availability of ASHA		0.953 (0.066)	0.961 (0.083)
Availability of ANM		1.031 (0.065)	1.062 (0.084)
Availability of TBA		0.953 (0.054)	0.926 (0.066)

(continued)

TABLE 2.3 (Continued)
Multilevel Model for Factors Associated with Underweight

Underweight	Model 1	Model 2	Model 3
Individual-Level Variable			
Mother's education (Ref: 10th–12th grade)			
Illiterate			0.766 (0.439)
Below primary			1.362 (0.083)*
Primary to middle			1.249 (0.071)*
Graduate and above			0.767 (0.148)
Delivery type (Ref: normal)			
Caesarean			0.874 (0.086)
By instrument			1.817 (0.32)*
Delivery place (Ref: government hospital)			
Private hospital			0.740 (0.068)*
Other			1.039 (0.116)
Child birth weight			0.643 (0.056)*
Mother's age (Ref: 25–30 years)			
15–20			1.207 (0.175)
21–25			1.053 (0.067)
31–35			1.202 (0.095)*
36–40			0.969 (0.169)
41–45			0.810 (0.509)
46–50			3.062 (0.730)
Cons	0.372 (0.215)	0.329 (0.214)	1.122 (0.246)
Random part			
Variance (state)	0.078 (0.068)	0.052 (0.047)	0.000 (0.000)
VPC (%)	2.300	1.432	0.000
Variance (district)	0.022 (0.010)	0.016 (0.009)	0.009 (0.010)
VPC (%)	0.648	0.440	0.272
Variance (PSU)		0.271 (0.074)	0.009 (0.093)
VPC (%)		7.467	0.272

are reduced by 35%. In this model, VPC turns out to be 0.2% at district and PSU level, and we observe no variance at state level.

In Table 2.4, three models are fitted to see the association of the factors with stunting, similar to Table 2.3. Model 1 defines a district variable where with a per unit increase in vegetable production the odds of being stunted increase by 3% (OR:1.034) with no variation at state or district level. In Model 2 the odds of being stunted increase by 0.3% with a per unit change in distance to nearest district headquarters and decrease by 0.3% with a per unit change in distance to nearest railway station. No variation is observed at state or district level; the only variation observed

TABLE 2.4
Multilevel Model for Factors Associated with Stunting

Stunting	Model 1	Model 2	Model 3
District-Level Variable			
Cereal production	1.000 (0.000)	1.000 (0.000)	1.000 (0.000)
Fruit production	1.001 (0.001)	1.001 (0.001)	1.002 (0.001)*
Vegetable production	1.034 (0.005)*	1.029 (0.005)*	1.021 (0.006)*
Potato production	0.894 (0.013)*	0.907 (0.014)*	0.934 (0.018)*
Onion production	0.965 (0.005)*	0.969 (0.005)*	0.977 (0.007)*
Annual rainfall	1.000 (0.000)	1.000 (0.000)	1.000 (0.000)
PSU-Level Variable			
Distance to nearest district headquarters		1.003 (0.001)*	1.002 (0.001)*
Distance to nearest railway station		0.997 (0.001)*	0.996 (0.001)*
Individual-Level Variable			
Mother's education (Ref: 10th–12th grade)			
Illiterate			0.926 (0.342)
Below primary			1.307 (0.067)*
Primary to middle			1.178 (0.062)*
Graduate and above			0.877 (0.113)
Delivery place (Ref: government hospital)			
Private			0.879 (0.057)*
Other			1.058 (0.080)
Child having birth problem (Ref: no)			
Yes			1.28 (0.094)*
Mother's age (Ref: 25–30 years)			
15–20 years			0.875 (0.174)
21–25 years			1.116 (0.056)*
33–35 years			0.888 (0.083)
36–40 years			1.018 (0.141)
41–45 years			0.875 (0.423)
46–50 years			7.272 (0.698)*
Religion (Ref: Hindu)			
Muslim			0.955 (0.102)
Other			1.021 (0.094)
Cons	0.259 (0.079)	0.241 (0.084)	0.246 (0.108)
Random part			
Variance (state)	0.000 (0.000)	0.000 (0.000)	0.000 (0.000)
VPC (%)	0.000	0.000	0.000
Variance (district)	0.000 (0.000)	0.000 (0.000)	0.000 (0.000)
VPC (%)	0.000	0.000	0.000
Variance (PSU)		0.026 (0.064)	0.005 (0.083)
VPC (%)		0.784	0.150

is at PSU level, with VPC 0.78%. In Model 3 (Table 2.4) individual-level variables are taken into consideration, which results in an increase of 30% in the odds of being stunted if the mother's education is below primary level (OR: 1.30) and an 18% increase if it is primary to middle level (OR:1.18), with reference to mother's education level at 10th–12th grade. There is a 12% reduction in the odds of being stunted if the delivery place is private (OR: 0.879), compared to a government-run place of delivery. If the child has problems at the time of birth, the odds of being stunted increase by 28% compared to a child having no problem at the time of birth (OR: 1.28). There is no state or district-level variation; only PSU-level variation is present, with VPC 0.15%.

Representation of factors associated with nutritional status of children using SEM

SEM was performed using the SEM Builder in Stata 14.2. The path diagrams for stunting and underweight show that each model provides a good fit with the data and provides a better model when compared with a multilevel model of the same outcome. Though the initial model did not fit the data well, stunting and underweight were seen to be directly associated with crop production, annual rainfall, PSU-level variables (distance to nearest district, bus station, railway station, etc.) and individual-level variables, while path diagrams Figure 2.9 and Figure 2.10 have the intermediate

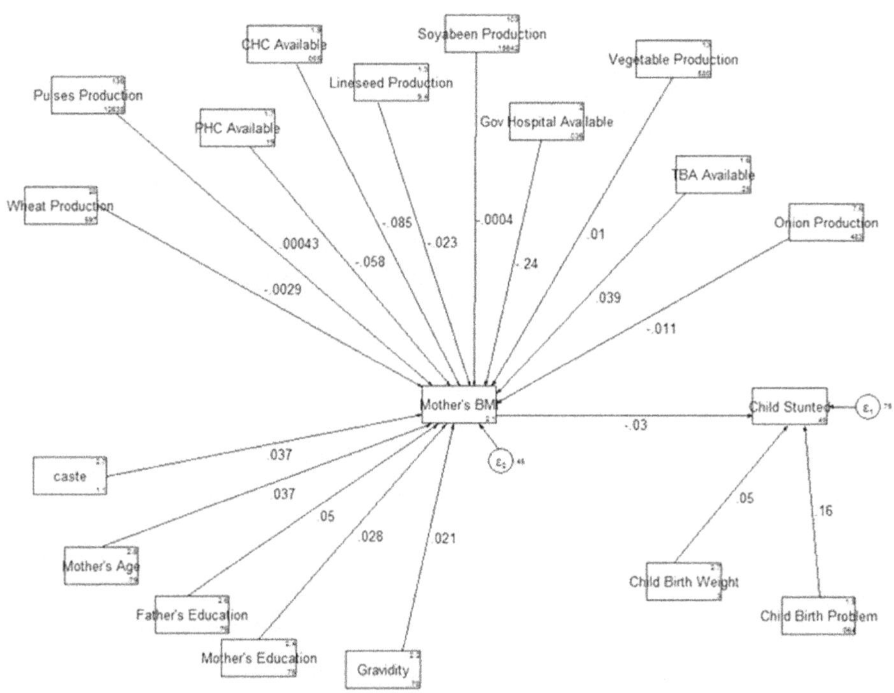

FIGURE 2.9 Path model for stunting.

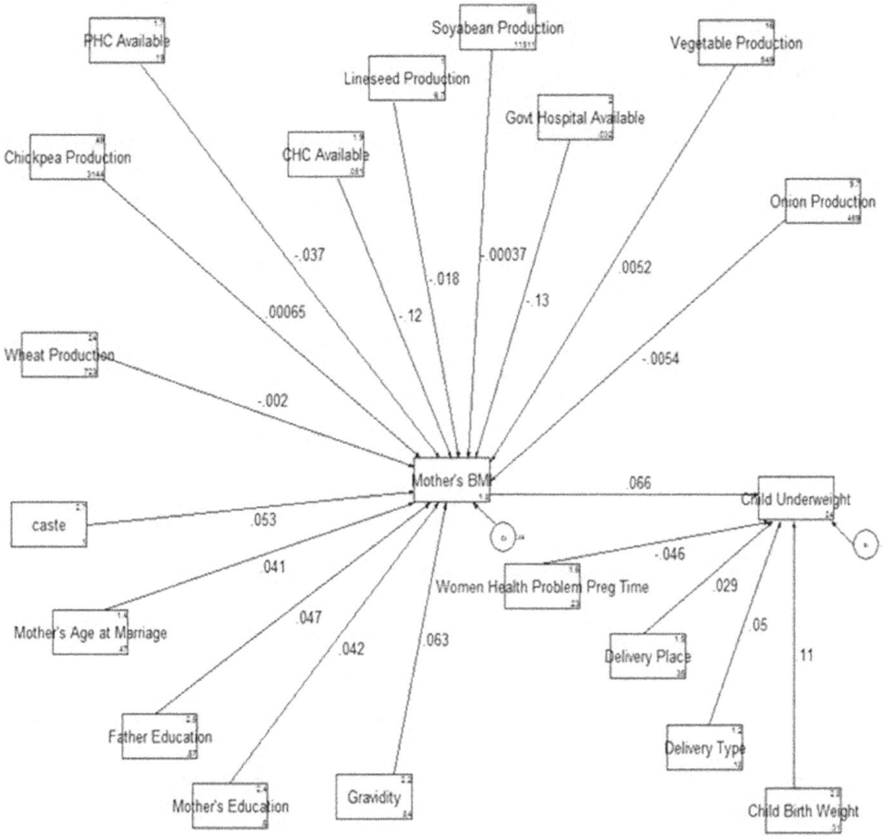

FIGURE 2.10 Path model for underweight.

variable of nutritional status, which is determined by the woman's BMI. The association of district-level, PSU-level, and individual-level variables with mother's BMI was found to be significant and positively associated with stunting and underweight. The major point to keep in mind is that although the *p*-values for the path coefficients were significant (i.e., less than 0.05), we could not find the indirect links or the covariance which are significantly associated among the factors.

For the model shown in Figure 2.9, the RMSEA value is 0.029, which is less than 0.08 and indicates the model is a good fit; the CFI value is 0.835, which is greater than 0.8 and indicates good model fit (Table 2.5). For the model shown in Figure 2.10, the RMSEA value is 0.042, which is less than 0.08 and indicates good model fit; the CFI value is 0.672, which is less than 0.8 but lies between 0 to 1, which indicates that the model is a moderately good fit (Table 2.6).

TABLE 2.5
Goodness of Fit of Path Model for Stunting

Fit Statistic	Value	Description
Likelihood Ratio		
chi^2_ms(17)	94.042	Model vs. saturated
p-value	0	
chi^2_bs(35)	503.172	Baseline vs. saturated
p-value	0	
Population Error		
RMSEA	0.029	Root mean squared error of approximation
90% CI, lower bound	0.024	
upper bound	0.035	
p-value	1	Probability RMSEA $\leq$ 0.05
Information Criteria		
AIC	386527.9	Akaike's information criterion
BIC	386672.6	Bayesian information criterion
Baseline Comparison		
CFI	0.835	Comparative fit index
TLI	0.661	Tucker–Lewis index
Size of Residuals		
SRMR	0.01	Standardized root mean squared residual
CD	0.074	Coefficient of determination

TABLE 2.6
Goodness of Fit of Path Model for Underweight

Fit Statistic	Value	Description
Likelihood Ratio		
chi^2_ms(18)	301.612	Model vs. saturated
p-value	0	
chi^2_bs(37)	900.413	Baseline vs. saturated
p-value	0	
Population Error		
RMSEA	0.042	Root mean squared error of approximation
90% CI, lower bound	0.038	
upper bound	0.046	
p-value	0.999	Probability RMSEA $\leq$ 0.05
Information Criteria		
AIC	654927.2	Akaike's information criterion
BIC	655090.3	Bayesian information criterion
Baseline Comparison		
CFI	0.672	Comparative fit index
TLI	0.325	Tucker–Lewis index
Size of Residuals		
SRMR	0.014	Standardized root mean squared residual
CD	0.058	Coefficient of determination

2.8 CONCLUSION

Determining the nutritional status of children is a complex task, as it depends on many factors such as the child's health after birth, the mother's health status during pregnancy, the mother's education, the availability of health facilities in the village, the mother's age at time of marriage, and so the list goes on. This study considers factors like mother's age, parents' education status, availability of health facilities, availability of other necessary facilities in villages, crop production, and annual rainfall in the area. Multilevel modeling is fitted in order to reveal the factors which were associated with the nutritional status of children, adjusted for different levels in the model. The models for stunting and underweight showed some common factors that affect the nutritional status of children, including vegetable production, potato production, and onion production at district level; of these, the potato production results turn out to be significant in both models. At the PSU level, distance to the nearest district headquarters and distance to the nearest railway station are the associated factors, with distance to the nearest railway station having a significant impact on stunting and underweight. In the stunting model, a child having birth problems had significant impact on stunting but was not present in models for underweight. In the underweight model, delivery type was shown to have a significant impact on underweight. In the SEM, the impact on the nutritional status of children is seen with the mediating effect of the mother's nutritional status, which is captured through the mother's BMI. The factors from district, PSU, and individual levels were seen to have direct associations with the mother's BMI, which is also seen to have an impact on the child's nutritional status. Seen through the previous objective of the multilevel modeling approach, there is an increase in the number of factors which are now associated with the mother's BMI and result in an impact on the child's nutritional status.

Thus, the SEM approach seems to show a clearer picture of how the nutritional status of children is being affected, and it also helps in understanding the areas we can work upon. Child nutritional status might not be directly affected by crop production, as with an increase in crop production there is an increase in crop consumption and also an increase in the economic value of the family. This study aims to clarify how the present level of crop production, its economic value, and consumption have an impact on the nutritional status of children. Agriculture has never had a direct effect on the nutritional status of children.

The limitations of this study are that the data are limited to eight states, with information on production of different crops and annual rainfall only. The data do not contain information regarding food consumption or dietary intake in a household, as many of the families have a variety of production that is totally cash-based. There is a dire need for detailed data regarding crop production and consumption in the form of a national survey so that we can see what the current scenario of agriculture and nutrition in India is.

REFERENCES

Ajayi, R.O., Matthews, B.G., Taylor, M., Kvalsvig, D.J., Davidson, L., Kauchali, S., Mellins, C., 2017. Structural equation modeling of the effects of family, preschool, and stunting on the cognitive development of school children. Front. Nutr*i*. 4, Article 17.

Bhagowalia, P., Headey, D., Kadiyala, S., 2012. Agriculture, income, and nutrition linkages in India, insights from a nationally representative survey. *IFPRI Discussion Paper 01195, July 2012*. Washington, DC: IFPRI.

Browne, W.J., Subramanian, S.V., Jones, K., Goldstein, H., 2005. Variance partitioning in multilevel logistic models that exhibit overdispersion. *J. R. Stat. Soc.: Ser. A* 168 (3), 599–613.

Bryce, J., Coitinho, D., Darnton-Hill, I., Pelletier, D., Pinstrup-Andersen, P., for the Maternal and Child Undernutrition Study Group, 2008. Maternal and child undernutrition: Effective action at national level. *Lancet*. 371 (9611), 510–526.

Food and Agriculture Organization (FAO), 2003. *World agriculture: Towards 2015/30. An FAO perspective*. Rome: FAO.

Gillespie, S., Harris, J., Kadiyala, S., 2012. The agriculture–Nutrition disconnect in India, What do we know? *IFPRI Discussion Paper 01187, June 2012*.

Goldstein, H., 2005. *Multilevel models*. Oxford: Wiley Online Library.

Goldstein, H., Browne, W., Rasbash, J., 2002. Partitioning variation in multilevel models. *Understanding Stat.: Stat. Issues Psychol. Educ. Soc. Sci.* 1 (4), 223–231.

Headey, D., 2012. *Turning economic growth into nutrition-sensitive growth*. Paper delivered at 2020 Conference: Leveraging Agriculture for Improving Nutrition and Health, February 10–12, New Delhi. Washington, DC: IFPRI.

Hooper, D., Coughlan, J., Mullen, M.R., 2008. Structural equation modelling: guidelines for determining model fit. *Electronic Journal of Business Research Methods* 6 (1), 53–60. Available online at www.ejbrm.com

Hu L., Bentler P.M., 1999. Cutoff criteria for fit indexes in covariance structure analysis: Conventional criteria versus new alternatives. *Struct. Eq. Modeling: Multidiscip. J.*, 6, 1–55.

Kenny, A.D., 2015. Measuring model fit. Retrieved from http://davidakenny.net/cm/fit.htm.

Himaz, R., 2009. Persistent stunting in middle childhood: The case of Andhra Pradesh using longitudinal data. *IDS Bull.* 40 (4), 30–38.

Hoddinott, J., 2012. *Agriculture, health and nutrition. Reshaping agriculture for nutrition and health*. Washington, DC: IFPRI.

World Health Organization (WHO), 2000. *Nutrition for health and development. A global agenda for combating malnutrition*. Geneva: WHO.

3 Uncovering the Hurdles of Food Security

A Journey Towards Sustainable Food Production

Harika Vasa, Chhavi Taliwal, and Maheshwar Mekam

3.1 INTRODUCTION

Access to fundamental requirements like food, shelter, and clothing is crucial for human survival, with food being a fundamental metabolic need (Dutta & Saikia, 2018). The world's population has surpassed 8.1 billion, according to the United Nations, and it is projected to increase by almost 2 billion in the next 30 years. China and India currently have a population of 1.4 billion, consolidating their positions as the most populated nations in the world. (Global Issues | United Nations, n.d.).As the population continues to increase, meeting basic needs thereafter may become more challenging.

Humans rely on natural resources for survival. The effective utilization of these resources is crucial for ensuring food security (Rabbi et al., 2021). Despite significant advancements made over the years, the world is still facing the triple challenge of undernourishment, overweight/obesity, and nutritional deficiencies linked to insufficient consumption of essential nutrients (Shoba Suri, 2024). Hunger remains a significant issue worldwide. In the year 2022, an approximate range of 691 to 783 million individuals worldwide have encountered hunger, and it is projected that by 2030, nearly 600 million people will suffer from chronic undernourishment. An alarming number of nearly 2.4 billion people, primarily women and the rural population, face inadequate access to sufficient, safe, and nutritious food (The State of Food Security and Nutrition in the World 2023). This situation is exacerbated by factors such as low food availability, rising prices, limited access to fresh and potable water, sanitation, nutrition resources, and the impact of climate change. These interconnected factors contribute to an increasing state of food insecurity (Wheeler & Von Braun, 2013).

Eradicating hunger and ensuring food security will require sustained and focused endeavors, especially in regions in Asia and sub-Saharan Africa, where the world's largest populations are experiencing chronic hunger. The reduction of undernutrition holds immense potential for improving health outcomes and alleviating poverty (Shoba Suri, 2024). Therefore, managing limited resources wisely is important to meet present needs and future generations. Optimal use of these resources, adopting

DOI: 10.1201/9781003487227-3

sustainable practices for food production and consumption, is the key to bolstering food security globally (Rabbi et al., 2021).

3.2 FOOD SECURITY

Food security is a versatile concept, which has led to numerous attempts to define it in different ways to cater for the needs of researchers and policymakers. Since the 1990s, approximately 200 definitions have been proposed to address this area (Dutta & Saikia, 2018). The most comprehensive definition among these is the one that was accepted by the World Food Summit in 1996 and put forth by the Food and Agriculture Organization (FAO): "Food security exists when all people, at all times, have physical, social and economic access to sufficient, safe and nutritious food that meets their dietary needs and food preferences for an active and healthy life" (Food Security | IFPRI: International Food Policy Research Institute, 2021). From this definition, four dimensions were identified: availability, access, utilization, and stability (Manikas et al., 2023).

Domains of food security

The four domains of food security are availability, access, utilization and stability, as represented in Figure 3.1.

1) *Availability:* The food availability domain is an essential component that significantly impacts food security. It primarily focuses on the supply side of food, encompassing various factors that influence accessibility and stability within the food system. This dimension of food security is intricately tied to the production estimates, trade dynamics, and stock levels of crucial food commodities.
2) *Access:* Having a sufficient amount of food accessible at the national or international level is one of the major components to increase food security; this provision alone will not guarantee food security at the household level.

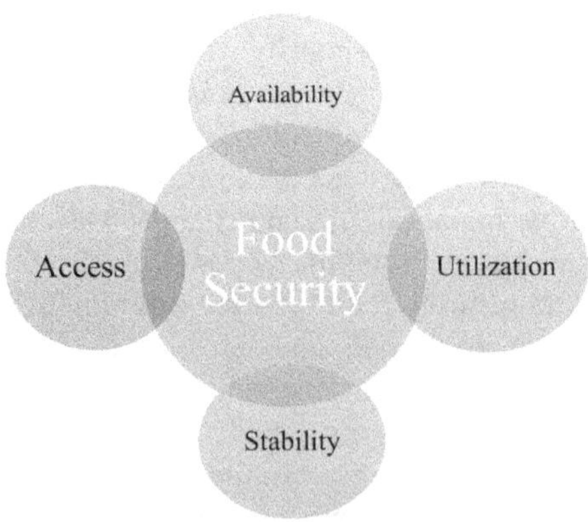

FIGURE 3.1 Four domains of food security.

Therefore, the focus has shifted towards acknowledging that limited access to food is a major challenge that necessitates the implementation of strategic policies. These policies are designed to tackle various aspects, such as income disparities, expenditure patterns, market dynamics, and price fluctuations, all of which play a vital role in attaining the ultimate goal of food security. In essence, while the availability of food resources is vital, attention must also be directed towards enhancing access to these resources at the individual and family levels.

3) *Utilization:* Utilization is a crucial factor that pertains to the body's efficient use of various nutrients for sustaining health and well-being. The nutritional status of individuals is influenced by both the quality of food consumed and its utilization. Factors such as malnutrition, prevalence of various diseases, levels of morbidity, and rates of mortality within a population all contribute significantly to determining the level of utilization and, thus, overall food security.
4) *Stability:* A nation, community, or person can still be considered food-insecure if there is insufficient access to food and a decline in nutritional well-being. Beyond these factors, external circumstances such as economic downturns, the occurrence of natural disasters, and high rates of unemployment can significantly contribute to the worsening state of food security (FSC Indicators Handbook, 2020; Indicators of Food Security – Humanitarian Global, 2021).

Food insecurity

Food insecurity, as described by the FAO, occurs if an individual does not have consistent access to an adequate quantity of nutritious and safe food, which is needed for proper growth, development, and overall well-being. This lack of access may be due to food unavailability or insufficient resources to acquire food (Ritchie & Roser, 2024).

Indicators of food security

Researchers and various international organizations have developed numerous indicators to measure food security.

There are two essential challenges when it comes to measuring food security: identifying what exactly has to be measured, and determining the method of measurement. The first challenge involves selecting suitable indicators for various dimensions (such as availability, access, utilization, and stability) and components (safety, quality, quantity, and cultural acceptability/preference). The second challenge pertains to the methodology used to calculate these indicators, which encompasses data, methods, and models (Manikas et al., 2023). Here are a few important indicators that the international agencies developed:

I. *Food Consumption Score (FCS):* This indicator was given by the World Food Programme (WFP) in the year 1996 and serves as a pivotal tool to gather data on consumption of food at the household level. It tracks food consumption over the seven days preceding the survey, with a detailed analysis of the food consumption frequency, dietary diversity, and nutritional importance of food (Data4Diets | INDDEX Project, 2023). The steps to calculate the score are as follows:

a. Categorize food items into designated food categories, excluding condiments.
b. Determine the total frequency of consumption for food items within the identical group.
c. Multiply the consumption frequency of every food category by its weight, as shown in Table 3.1.
d. Add up the weighted scores of the food groups to calculate the food consumption scores.
e. Evaluate the food consumption status of the household by considering the designated thresholds. If the FCS is 0–21, then they are categorized as poor consumption status; if the score is 21.5–35, they are categorized as borderline; and if the score is >35, then they fall under acceptable consumption status (World Food Programme, 2015; Data4Diets | INDDEX Project, 2023).

This index serves as a reliable measure to gauge the adequacy and quality of food intake, making it an indispensable instrument in monitoring and addressing nutritional challenges at the household level.

II. *Household Food Insecurity Access Scale (HFIAS):* In 2006, the Food and Nutrition Technical Assistance Project, funded by the United States Agency for International Development (USAID) in collaboration with the Academy for Educational Development, released a tool designed to evaluate the access aspect of household food insecurity (Gebreyesus et al., 2015). This tool is a simple and easy-to-use method for evaluating the effects of development food aid initiatives on the accessibility aspect of food insecurity at the household

TABLE 3.1
Standard Food Categories and Their Weights Used for the Determination of the Food Consumption Score

Food Category	Weight
Main staples/cereals	2
Pulses	3
Vegetables	1
Fruits	1
Animal foods (meat and fish)	4
Dairy (milk)	4
Sugars	0.5
Oils	0.5
Condiments	0

Source: Data4Diets | INDDEX Project (n.d.).

level. The guide consists of a well-designed questionnaire and instructions for data collection and analysis. The HFIAS comprises nine questions that have been utilized in various countries and have been shown to differentiate between food-insecure and food-secure households in diversified cultural settings. The data obtained through this scale can be utilized in determining the prevalence of household food insecurity (access component) and to identify changes in a population's food insecurity status over time (Indicator Guide | Food and Nutrition Technical Assistance III Project (FANTA), n.d.).

III. *Prevalence of Undernourishment (PoU):* Prevalence of Undernourishment (PoU) serves as a vital metric that measures the proportion of individuals within a population who do not have sufficient food intake on a regular basis to sustain a healthy and active lifestyle. It is quantified as a percentage. This metric plays a pivotal role in monitoring advancements towards the achievement of Target 2.1 of the Sustainable Development Goals (SDGs) (Food and Agriculture Organization, n.d.), which seeks to eradicate hunger, ensure food security, and improve nutrition (Goal 2 | Department of Economic and Social Affairs, n.d.). The PoU is recognized globally and is utilized by various international organizations, NGOs, and government bodies. It is calculated in terms of percentage of the total number of undernourished individuals (SDG Meta data, 2023). This indicator is derived by the FAO and produces information every year (Data4Diets | INDDEX Project, 2023). Data collection involves individual dietary intake surveys and anthropometric measurements on a group of people which represents the total population. While these surveys can be costly, a well-designed household survey focusing on food acquisitions could provide a reliable estimate of PoU at a reasonable cost and frequency to support UN SDG monitoring efforts (SDG Meta data, 2023).

IV. *Food Insecurity Experience Scale (FIES):* Food insecurity can manifest in varying degrees of severity, which are measured by the Food Insecurity Experience Scale (FIES). The FIES is a tool which is developed by FAO that measures and assesses the household food insecurity levels (moderate or severe) (The DHS Program, 2020). By utilizing the FIES, we can estimate the proportion of the population facing challenges in obtaining sufficient, safe, and nutritious food for their well-being and development. This provides information on the prevalence rate of food insecurity at moderate and severe levels (Figure 3.2). The Food Security Questionnaire is employed to collect data (Ritchie & Roser, 2024). This questionnaire consists of eight questions to which respondents are asked to self-report their access to food in regard to both quantity and quality over the past 12 months. The questions primarily focus on the lack of financial means and resources to acquire food (The DHS Program, 2020). The scale enables the assessment of food insecurity at both individual and household levels, considering varying degrees of severity. This allows for comparisons between countries and specific subpopulations rather than solely focusing on national trends (Ritchie & Roser, 2024).

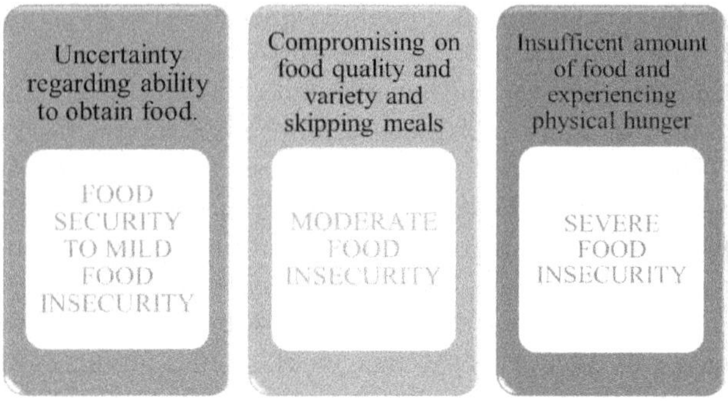

FIGURE 3.2 Food Insecurity Experience Scale. (Adapted from Hunger I FAO I Food and Agriculture Organization of the United Nations, n.d.)

V. *Global Food Security Index (GFSI):* The Global Food Security Index (GFSI) is a comprehensive indicator developed by the Economist Intelligence Unit (EIU) to track national food security progress. Since 2012, this index has been published annually and covers over 113 countries. The EIU prioritized countries with higher populations to ensure a broader coverage of the worldwide population. This index identifies the country's most and least susceptible to food insecurity (Izraelov & Silber, 2019). To assess different aspects of food security, EIU uses 28 unique indicators. The GFSI stands out due to its comprehensive evaluation of food security across the three internationally recognized dimensions of affordability, availability, and quality and safety. This approach goes beyond addressing hunger to consider the underlying factors that results in food insecurity (The Global Food Security Index I UNCCD, n.d.). The affordability category consists of six parameters that examine a country's ability to afford food and the financial challenges faced during normal circumstances and food-related crises. In addition to the annual baseline score, quarterly adjustments are made to reflect changes in incomes, exchange rates, and food prices globally. The availability category, with 11 indicators, evaluates components influencing supply and accessibility of food. It analyzes how structural elements impact the ability of country to produce and distribute food, and identifies potential risks to availability. The quality and safety category, with 11 indicators, focuses on the nutritional aspects of diets and food safety standards of every country (Izraelov & Silber, 2019). The EIU uses various databases from the World Bank, the FAO, and the WFP. The GFSI demonstrates strong statistical characteristics and maintains statistical consistency (Thomas et al., 2017).

A comprehensive indicator for food security should cover all four dimensions of food security at the individual level, according to the food security definition which was established during the 1996 World Food Summit (Manikas et al., 2023).

3.3 CHALLENGES IN ACHIEVING FOOD SECURITY

Food security will remain a global concern for the next 50 years and beyond. Achieving food security at both local and international levels is a complex task, as various challenges need to be overcome. These obstacles include ensuring access to affordable and nutritious food for every individual, implementing sustainable agricultural practices to protect the environment, addressing issues related to food waste and loss throughout the supply chain, and promoting equitable distribution of resources to minimize hunger and malnutrition. Additionally, factors such as climate change, natural disasters, and socioeconomic disparities further complicate efforts to establish food security. Various issues related to food security are explained below. (see also Figure 3.3).

Population growth

Population growth is a complex global issue that connects with food security. Ensuring food security becomes ever more challenging as the population expands. The world population is estimated to increase to 9.7 billion by 2050. This significant expansion of population can be attributed mainly to the rising number of individuals reaching reproductive age, the gradual extension of human life expectancy, the increase in urbanization, and the rapid pace of migration. In countries like India, which are already the most populated, a slight increase in population can also make a difference; it is estimated that there can be a rise of 15% of the current population by the year 2050 (Table 3.2). A rapid increase in population is estimated in some parts of Africa, which are already food-insecure, making it more challenging to ensure food availability (Global Issues | United Nations, n.d.). The migration of rural inhabitants to urban areas due to urbanization has resulted in the desertion of large

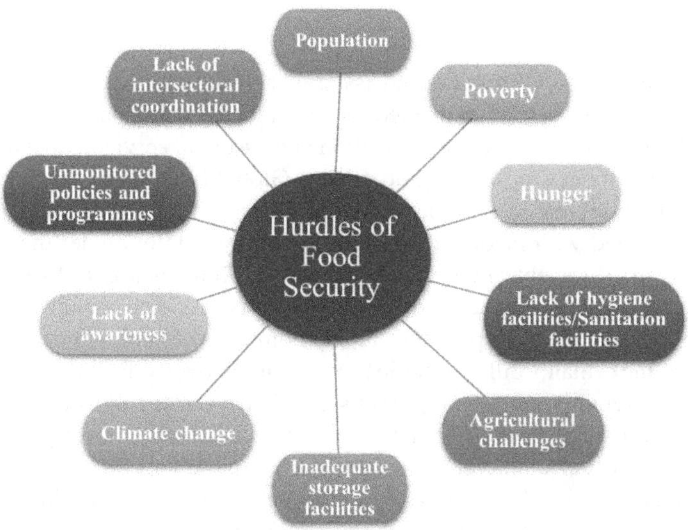
Population
Poverty
Hunger
Lack of hygiene facilities/Sanitation facilities
Agricultural challenges
Inadequate storage facilities
Climate change
Lack of awareness
Unmonitored policies and programmes
Lack of intersectoral coordination
Hurdles of Food Security

FIGURE 3.3 Hurdles to achieving food security.

TABLE 3.2
Top 10 Countries by Population

No.	Name	Population in 2024	Estimated Population by 2050	Percentage Change (%)
1	India	1,441,719,852	1,670,490,596	15.86
2	China	1,425,178,782	1,312,636,325	–7.90
3	United States of America	341,814,420	375,391,963	9.82
4	Indonesia	279,789,049	317,225,213	13.38
5	Pakistan	245,209,815	367,808,468	49.99
6	Nigeria	229,152,217	377,459,883	64.72
7	Brazil	217,637,297	230,885,725	6.087
8	Bangladesh	174,701,211	203,904,900	16.72
9	Russia	143,957,079	133,133,035	–7.52
10	Mexico	129,388,467	143,772,364	11.12

Source: World Population Clock: 8.1 billion People (LIVE, 2024) – Worldometer (n.d.).

areas of cultivated land, consequently causing a decline in the capacity of regional food production, which can again result in food insecurity (Kang et al., 2023). The correlation between population growth and food security underscores the necessity of proactive measures to improve agricultural productivity, mitigate food waste, and enhance distribution systems. By recognizing the intricate relationship between these two factors, policymakers, scientists, and communities can work together to develop strategies that promote equitable access to nutritious food while striving to maintain environmental sustainability in the face of a growing population.

Poverty

Poverty is a complex and multifaceted issue worldwide that encompasses not only the lack of income and resources needed for sustainable livelihoods but issues such as hunger, malnutrition, low access to education and essential services, social marginalization, and lack of decision-making processes (Global Issues I United Nations, n.d.). Moreover, due to increased food demand and decreased crop productivity, elevated food prices coupled with income disparities could potentially hinder the access and availability of food for poor households (Pawlak & Kołodziejczak, 2020). A person living by spending less than 2.15 dollars per day is presently defined as living in extreme poverty (Goal 2 I Department of Economic and Social Affairs, n.d.). From 1990 to 2014, more than 1 billion people moved out of poverty, leading to a significant reduction in extreme poverty on a global scale. However, the COVID-19 pandemic has resulted in a surge in the population residing in extreme poverty, marking the first occurrence of such an increase in a generation. In the year 2020, a major setback was noticed as the crisis led to an additional 71 million people residing in extreme poverty in comparison to the previous year. This setback has caused a reversal of progress in crucial areas like childhood vaccination and income equality among nations, something that has not been witnessed in the past 30 years. If the current trajectory persists, it is estimated that by 2030, a staggering 575 million people will still be trapped in extreme poverty, and 84 million children will not be able to attend school (Global Issues | United Nations, n.d.).

Poverty and food security are interconnected issues that have significant implications for individuals, communities, and societies. Addressing this requires a comprehensive approach encompassing economic development, social safety nets, and sustainable agriculture practices. It is essential to secure substantial mobilization of resources from diverse channels, such as improved development cooperation, to ensure that developing countries, especially the least developed ones, have sufficient and reliable funding to carry out initiatives and strategies aimed at eradicating poverty in all its forms (Sustainable Development Goals | United Nations Development Programme, 2024).

Hunger

Food security and hunger are closely connected and are considered major global issues. Hunger is a distressing physical sensation arising from inadequate dietary energy consumption (Hunger | FAO, n.d.). Based on the 2023 Global Hunger Index (GHI) scores and preliminary classifications, 43 countries are facing severe or alarming levels of hunger. Among them, nine countries (Burundi, Central African Republic, Democratic Republic of the Congo, Lesotho, Madagascar, Niger, Somalia, South Sudan, and Yemen) are experiencing alarming levels of hunger, while 34 countries have a severe level of hunger. Additionally, 18 countries are dealing with moderate hunger levels. According to GHI projections, 58 countries are projected to fall short of achieving low hunger by 2030 if the current trend persists (Von Grebmer et al., 2023a).

GHI scores are presented on a 100-point scale, where 0 represents the best score (indicating no hunger) and 100 represents the worst score, as shown in Figure 3.4. A value of 100 on the scale would indicate extremely alarming levels of undernourishment, child wasting, child stunting, and child mortality (Von Grebmer et al., 2023b).

In the past few years, hunger has worsened in numerous nations. Hunger levels have risen in nearly 18 countries since 2015, as indicated by moderate, severe, or alarming 2023 GHI rankings. The severity of hunger has been exacerbated by a combination of crises, such as the consequences of the COVID-19 pandemic, the conflict between Russia and Ukraine, as well as various violent conflicts and climate-related

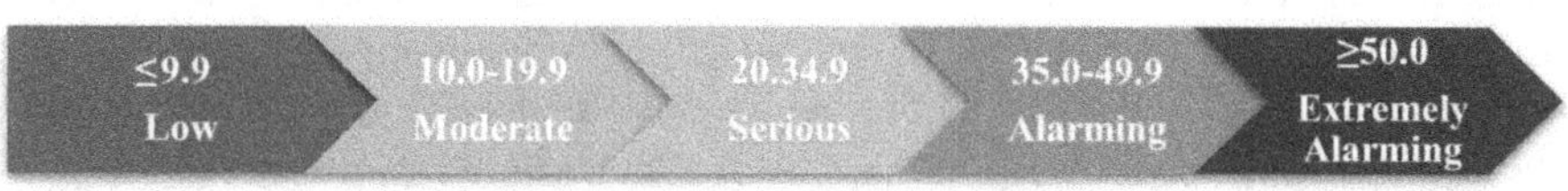
≤9.9
Low
10.0-19.9
Moderate
20.34.9
Serious
35.0-49.9
Alarming
≥50.0
Extremely Alarming

FIGURE 3.4 Global Hunger Index showing severity of hunger on a 100-point scale. (Adapted from Methodology – Global Hunger Index (GHI) – Peer-Reviewed Annual Publication Designed to Comprehensively Measure and Track Hunger at the Global, Regional, and Country Levels, n.d.)

disasters globally. This has led to certain nations facing food shortages, while others have shown greater resilience (Von Grebmer et al., 2023a).

The 2023 edition of the State of Food Security and Nutrition in the World (SOFI) report reveals that an additional 122 million people are now experiencing hunger compared to 2019, before the pandemic (The State of Food and Agriculture, 2023). Countries with low and middle income levels, which are usually more susceptible to crises, have been disproportionately affected in comparison to high-income countries. Various underlying factors, including state fragility, inadequate governance, inequality, and persistent poverty, heavily influence the ability of nations to bounce back from these shocks (Von Grebmer et al., 2023b).

If current trends persist, the objective of achieving the SDG of eradicating hunger by 2030 will not be attained (World Health Organization, 2023). This highlights the critical need to implement holistic approaches that tackle the underlying factors contributing to food insecurity, including poverty, conflict, and climate change. It underscores the significance of collaborative efforts between governments, international organizations, and local communities in formulating effective policies and programs.

Lack of hygiene/sanitation facilities

Access to safe and fresh drinking water, proper and adequate sanitation, and hygiene facilities are necessary for reducing food security risks. Implementing good sanitation practices, such as safe water supply and hygienic waste disposal, is important in preventing food contamination and related health issues (Vuong et al., 2022).

Approximately 2.2 billion people across the globe still lack access to clean drinking water, while almost half of the world's population lacks access to safe sanitation. Moreover, 2 billion people do not have access to handwashing facilities with soap, and 419 million people are still practicing open defecation. These practices can result in the spread of various neglected tropical diseases (NTDs) like soil-transmitted helminths, trachoma, and schistosomiasis (Water, Sanitation and Hygiene (WASH), n.d.). Practicing food safety through safe water, sanitation, and hygiene (WASH) practices can decrease fecal food contamination by approximately 96% (Global Food Security: The Critical Role of Water, Sanitation, and Hygiene (WASH) | Food Security and Nutrition Network, n.d.). Water is required not only for health but also for food security, poverty reduction, peace and human rights, ecosystems, and education. In order to accomplish SDG 6, which aims to provide access to water and sanitation to all by 2030, there needs to be a significant increase in the current global rates of progress. Specifically, a six-times increase is required for drinking water, a five-times increase for sanitation, and a three-times increase for hygiene (Water | UNICEF, n.d.).

It is imperative for governments to guarantee the resilience and continuity of water and sanitation services, as well as promote proper hygiene practices and facilities, in the face of climate-related disasters. This is crucial in safeguarding public health amidst an unpredictable future (Water | UNICEF, n.d.). Moreover, the integration of WASH initiatives with food security programs can significantly bolster resilience against climate change and other environmental adversities. Ultimately, the WASH and food security initiatives together can foster sustainable development.

Agricultural challenges

Agriculture, being a vital sector, holds fundamental importance for developing countries because a properly functioning agricultural sector is crucial in ensuring food security and agricultural products serve as a significant contributor to national income. This sector plays a strategic role in enhancing food availability and achieving overall food security (Smutka et al., 2016; Wegren & Elvestad, 2018).

Agricultural obstacles such as decreased crop and livestock productivity, escalating expenses of fertilizer and seeds, soil deterioration, alterations in land use caused by desertification, pest invasions, limited availability of resources like water, salinity, and climate change impact food accessibility and lead to higher food costs, potentially plunging millions of people further into poverty (Agriculture and Food Security The IAEA Contribution, n.d.). Moreover, crises like COVID-19 (Carducci et al., 2021; Fan et al., 2021) and the war between Ukraine and Russia (Behnassi & El Haiba, 2022; Osendarp et al., 2022) have introduced additional shocks to the resilience of the agricultural and food system. These shocks have had detrimental effects on prices, food security, and social stability.

Despite the anticipated rise increased global food demand in the coming years, uncertainties persist about whether global agriculture can meet this demand by increasing food production (Pawlak & Kołodziejczak, 2020). Enhancing food provision through improved agricultural productivity and expanding the usage of agricultural land appears to be a viable approach to combat hunger (Smyth et al., 2015). Nevertheless, low-income developing nations may face challenges in producing sufficient food due to limited technology and knowledge. This underscores the importance of boosting investments in agricultural research and extension systems to enhance agricultural productivity. Research on sub-Saharan Africa highlights the necessity of directing investments towards elevating agricultural productivity in this region without causing significant environmental harm (Pawlak & Kołodziejczak, 2020).

The increasing need for food has already reduced natural resources, causing soil erosion, loss of diverse landscapes, and environmental pollution worldwide. This has introduced new challenges in ensuring food safety and sustainable food production (Garcia et al., 2020). Furthermore, transboundary diseases and disasters also pose a significant risk to food security and safety. Natural disasters such as floods and fires create pathways for pathogens, heavy metals, chemicals, and other pollutants to contaminate the air, water, and the environment where food is grown (Wu et al., 2017; Andrade et al., 2018).

In addressing these challenges, investment in research and education, promoting small-scale farming initiatives, and implementing policies that support food production and distribution are essential steps towards achieving sustainable food security solutions.

Inadequate storage facilities and food wastage

Insufficient storage facilities pose a serious threat to food security, as they can lead to spoilage and waste of essential food sources. A lack of proper infrastructure may lead to an increase in the vulnerability of communities to hunger and malnutrition. As the population is growing, sustaining the current food production levels to meet the requirements of the growing global population becomes infeasible. This challenge is further exacerbated by the seasonal nature of crop growth, which contrasts with the year-round demand for food. These circumstances highlight the importance of our endeavors to achieve global food security. Nonetheless, food security cannot be achieved solely through increased production. It is equally crucial to address food wastage by implementing effective food preservation and storage methods, ensuring that food remains available for consumption beyond the production area (Food Security: Improve with Better Storage Solutions, n.d.).

The wastage of food occurs throughout the entire process of food cultivation, from its origin to consumption. The amount of food lost varies and depends on its form (Ayomide et al., 2022). One of the significant factors that contributes to global food insecurity is post-harvest losses. These losses result in both physical and quality deterioration of food, reducing its economic value and rendering it unsuitable for human consumption. While efforts are primarily focused on improving food storage facilities at the farmer and national levels, it is equally important to promote household-level food storage. This would enhance the food availability to the consumers and contribute to food security (Afriyie et al., 2023). Utilizing appropriate food storage solutions plays a crucial role in achieving this. Additionally, a barrier to achieving food security is the disproportionate allocation of resources. Over the past 30 years, 95% of investments in food science research have been directed towards increasing food productivity, while only 5% have been allocated to reducing food losses (Food Security: Improve with Better Storage Solutions, n.d.).

Although proper storage facilities may ensure that the food stocks are available, this is not enough to guarantee that those food stocks are accessible to the most vulnerable in society. Therefore, it is crucial to implement mechanisms that not only maintain optimal storage levels but also ensure proper distribution. A sufficient food supply is important, but it is not the only factor in achieving food security. Income inequality plays a significant role in perpetuating food insecurity, as low-income groups often struggle to access the necessary nutrition (Lynn Kennedy et al., 2019). Addressing the issue of inadequate storage facilities is imperative in safeguarding food security and ensuring access to nutritious meals for all members of society.

Climate change

Climate change poses a major risk to global food security due to its impact on agricultural productivity, food distribution systems, and water availability. The increasing temperatures and changing weather patterns resulting from climate change are disrupting traditional farming practices and leading to decreased crop yields in many regions.

From the mid-20th century onwards, there has been a notable increase in the world's population and individual consumption levels, leading to a significant surge in the manufacturing of products and services (Arrieta & Aguiar, 2023). Currently, the actions of the growing population have surpassed the Earth's ability to sustain the resources we utilize and manage the waste we produce. This has resulted in a range of biophysical transformations occurring at an unprecedented pace in the history of our planet (Lewis & Maslin, 2015). Such biophysical transformations are taking place in six dimensions:

a) modification of the global climate system;
b) extensive contamination of air, water, and soil;
c) accelerated decline of biodiversity;
d) restructuring of the biogeochemical cycles of carbon, nitrogen, and phosphorus;
e) alterations in land use and land cover; and
f) exhaustion of resources, such as freshwater and arable land (Steffen et al., 2015).

The interaction between these dimensions is intricate and ever-changing, leading to disruptions in fundamental factors affecting human health. This includes the deterioration of air quality, water quality, nutritional value of food, increased risk of infectious diseases, as well as exposure to extreme weather events like heat waves, droughts, fires, and tropical storms (Myers, 2017). As a result, the well-being of humanity and the environment are closely interlinked and cannot be separated for much longer (Myers & Frumkin, 2020; Portner et.al, 2023).

Climate change poses a threat to distinctive ecosystems, results in increasingly severe weather phenomena, diminishes biodiversity, and threatens our present lifestyle in numerous ways (O'Neill et al., 2017). The consumption of food within households is responsible for over 60% of worldwide greenhouse gas emissions and accounts for about 50% to 80% of overall resource utilization (Ivanova et al., 2016). Therefore, the need to promote environmentally sustainable eating habits among individuals is increasingly crucial (Magrini et al., 2018; Hedin et al., 2019). Understanding the relationship between climate change and food security is essential to develop effective adaptation and mitigation strategies to ensure sustainable food production.

Lack of awareness

Awareness is one of the key factors in ensuring food security. Insufficient awareness regarding food security issues can significantly increase the risks and challenges associated with maintaining a stable and dependable food supply for individuals and communities. This lack of awareness can result in inadequate access to vital resources, limited understanding of sustainable agricultural practices, and inadequate preparedness for potential food crises. Farmers from different regions of the world may not be familiar with sustainable agriculture technologies and the SDGs, which directly or indirectly contribute to food insecurity (Mabe et al., 2021). Facilitating the transfer of technology from developed to developing countries is crucial to assist these processes to bridge technology gaps, and overcome knowledge barriers (Pawlak & Kołodziejczak, 2020). By increasing education and understanding about food security issues, communities can work towards developing more resilient and sustainable food systems that provide everyone with an adequate and nutritious food supply.

Unmonitored policies and programs

To alleviate food insecurity, it is essential to have well-crafted food and nutrition security programs and policies in place. Policies that focus on fundamental rights to food issues have widespread political and social support, and are effectively executed are more effective in combating hunger and malnutrition. National policies and programs should align with international, legally binding agreements pertaining to the human right to sufficient food that has been endorsed by the country of which the country is a party. Implementation strategies of policies and specific actions should cater to each vulnerable group and tackle the various root causes of food insecurity and malnutrition (Food and Agricultural Organization, n.d.).

Food and nutrition security policies are set with certain objectives, and time-bound goals and benchmarks have been designed. As well as designing policies and programs, monitoring is equally important. Monitoring is conducted simultaneously with the implementation of policies, programs, and projects. It involves collecting, processing, and analyzing information to assess whether they are progressing as intended in terms of time, cost, efficiency, and, more importantly, if they are contributing to the desired outcomes and objectives. It is a dynamic and adaptable process that enables necessary adaptations and adjustments to enhance the effectiveness of actions towards achieving the desired results and objectives (Food and Agricultural Organization, n.d.).

Insufficient monitoring within a nutrition program can greatly contribute to the exacerbation of issues related to food insecurity. In the absence of proper oversight and guidance, nutrition programs can unintentionally worsen the prevalence of food insecurity within communities, thereby placing vulnerable populations at an even higher risk of malnutrition and hunger. For instance, in India, the Public Distribution System (PDS) plays a vital role in partially fulfilling the essential food and fuel requirements of various households. However, while the PDS effectively safeguards households by providing basic entitlements at affordable prices and convenient locations, it falls short of meeting the complete food needs of any household and serves as a supplementary measure. Numerous studies have examined the efficacy of the PDS (Gupta & Mishra, 2018; Pradhan & Rao, 2018). Each of these studies has indicated that the PDS is not functioning effectively, as a significant amount of food fails to reach the intended recipients, resulting in substantial wastage and high costs for limited benefits (George & McKay, 2019). The barriers have to be identified, and stringent actions have to be implemented.

Hence, it is crucial to establish robust monitoring frameworks that ensure transparency, accountability, and equitable distribution of food resources to safeguard against the detrimental impacts of unmonitored policies on food security.

Lack of intersectoral coordination

The absence of effective intersectoral coordination, where various sectors and stakeholders work together seamlessly, often leads to challenges in ensuring food security for vulnerable populations. Food and nutrition security encompasses multiple sectors, including health, environment and agriculture, and entails an intricate, cross-sectoral, and interdisciplinary relationship between them (Durojaye & Chilemba, n.d.).

While it is crucial for various programs addressing health determinants to have regional cooperation and support for multisector collaboration, the majority of actions are carried out at the national level. The World Health Organization has consistently stressed the significance of multisectoral collaboration in enhancing health outcomes. Nevertheless, effective allocation of resources and setting priorities across sectors necessitates the establishment of mechanisms and initiatives that facilitate the articulation of interdependencies, harmonization of strategies, and development of pathways for change.

By connecting various sectors and promoting a unified strategy, communities can more effectively tackle the underlying issues of food insecurity and establish long-lasting measures that enhance the availability of healthy food for everyone. Ultimately, encouraging collaboration across sectors is crucial in creating comprehensive solutions that prioritize food security as a basic human right and guarantee that every individual can obtain a sufficient and nutritious diet.

In order to address these obstacles effectively, it is crucial for governments, organizations, and individuals to collaborate and implement sustainable solutions. Furthermore, raising awareness about food insecurity and advocating for policies that support food sovereignty are essential steps in creating a more food-secure world for future generations. Ultimately, by recognizing and actively working to overcome the challenges in achieving food security, we can strive towards a more equitable and sustainable global food system.

3.4 STRATEGIES TO IMPROVE FOOD SECURITY

Solutions to the challenges of food security are crucial in addressing the complex issues surrounding the availability of sufficient, safe, and nutritious food for all individuals. Implementing sustainable agricultural practices, promoting equitable distribution systems, enhancing food storage and preservation technologies, and supporting small-scale farmers can significantly contribute to improving food security on a global scale. Additionally, investing in research and development to enhance crop yields, advocating for policies that prioritize food security, and raising awareness about the importance of nutrition and balanced diets are essential components of a comprehensive approach to addressing food security challenges.

Sustainable agriculture practices

Agriculture plays a major role in reducing food insecurity and promoting a healthy lifestyle. With the increasing global population, there is a growing need to produce more food to meet the demand. Hence, it becomes imperative to adopt a different approach to farming in order to achieve both food security and a healthy lifestyle. Sustainable agricultural practices play an important role in this scenario by advocating for environmentally friendly methods that guarantee the long-term availability of nutritious food (Colson, 2022). When evaluating sustainable food production, it

TABLE 3.3
Benefits of Sustainable Agricultural Practices

Environmental Benefits	• Protects and improves soil health • Improves soil porosity • Protects water quality • Reduces nutrient leaching • Enhanced soil microbial activity • Landscape diversification • Minimal chemical use • Reduces climate change • Prevents pollution • Biodiversity conversion • Mitigation of greenhouse gas emissions
Economic Benefits	• Low economic losses • Can be implemented at lower expense than conventional farming • More profits
Social Benefits	• Increases food security • Consistent access to affordable food • Fosters stronger connections between farmers and consumers • Supports small-scale farmers • Creates a more equitable food system

is important to take a holistic approach that addresses three key dimensions concurrently: economic, social, and environmental (Qu et al., 2024). The benefits of sustainable agricultural practices are listed in Table 3.3. Sustainable agriculture plays a crucial role in conserving natural resources, fostering social equity, and guaranteeing economic viability (Rehman et al., 2022; The Role of Sustainable Agriculture Practices in Driving Food Security, 2023).

Sustainable agriculture increases crop production and improves the quality of produce for consumers by minimizing the environmental effects of conventional farming practices. Its goal is to safeguard essential resources such as soil fertility, which is integral to the long-term viability of farming operations.

It is possible to implement sustainable agriculture practices at any level. Techniques like utilizing renewable energy sources, crop rotation, organic farming, soil enrichment, integrated pest management, agroforestry, mixed cropping, permaculture, hydroponics, urban agriculture, and growing cover crops can be adopted. Education and awareness are vital in promoting sustainable agriculture methods and encouraging individuals to opt for sustainable food choices. By offering information and resources, people can make well-informed decisions about their food consumption and actively support sustainable farming practices (The Role of Sustainable Agriculture Practices in Driving Food Security, 2023).

Investing in sustainable agriculture plays a vital role in enhancing people's food security by utilizing local resources. This is accomplished through several means.

a) Firstly, the implementation of sustainable agriculture practices in local production not only enhances food availability but also creates job opportunities within the economy, thereby promoting economic growth.
b) Secondly, sustainable agriculture enables the production of a greater quantity of food per acre by adopting efficient practices. This not only increases crop yield but also ensures the cultivation of more nutritious produce, ultimately leading to a larger supply of food.
c) Lastly, organic farming techniques, such as crop rotation and crop selection, contribute to the production of healthier and more flavorful crops. By maintaining high quality standards, farmers can sustain their yield while providing nutritious food to the population (Colson, 2022).

Through sustainable practices, food production becomes more efficient and less dependent on harmful practices, leading to healthier ecosystems and a more secure food supply for current and future generations. In essence, the adoption of sustainable agriculture practices is essential for combating food insecurity and creating a more sustainable and equitable food system globally.

Crop diversification

Crop diversification involves transitioning from growing low-income traditional crops to more profitable ones. It is considered a practical and effective method to address uncertainties in agriculture, especially in light of climate change. By diversifying crops, second-generation issues like soil degradation, salinity, pests, diseases, pollution, profit decline, nutrient imbalances, and climate change can be minimized. Additionally, crop diversification enhances the resilience of farms, allowing agroecosystems to recover their productivity levels following disturbances through increased biodiversity across different locations and seasons (Barman et al., 2022).

Crop diversification refers to the practice of enhancing crop diversity through methods such as multiple cropping, intercropping, or crop rotation, which focuses on specialized farming practices. The primary objective of crop diversification is to enhance productivity, sustainability, and the availability of ecological systems (Wezel et al., 2014; Garbach et al., 2017). This may signify a step in the direction of fostering sustainable production systems, value chains for minor crops, and gaining socioeconomic advantages (Meynard et al., 2018; Feliciano, 2019). Enhanced agricultural variety, improved crop rotation diversity, mixed cropping (Bedoussac et al., 2015), incorporation of leguminous crops in predominantly cereal-based systems (Watson et al., 2017), perennial leys or grassland (Haughey et al., 2018), and locally adapted varieties or variety combinations are all examples of agricultural diversification strategies. Within developing nations, crop diversification is characterized as the replacement of one or more agricultural products with another.

Crop diversification is a goal-oriented strategy that responds to demand, is tailored to specific needs, and is pursued at a national level. It involves dynamic and iterative processes that integrate spatial, temporal, value addition, and resource-complementary techniques while also transitioning away from traditional and less profitable crops. As highlighted by Barman et al. (2022), crop diversification holds great potential in achieving objectives such as ensuring nutritional security, increasing income, enhancing food security, generating employment opportunities, and promoting sustainable agricultural development.

Improving purchasing power

Enhancing the ability of individuals and communities to make purchases can significantly contribute to enhancing food security. By increasing purchasing power, individuals are better equipped to access a wider variety of nutritious food options, ultimately bolstering food security within households and communities. This boost in purchasing power enables individuals to make more informed and healthier food choices, thereby improving overall well-being and nutritional outcomes.

A case study carried out by Ayaviri-Nina et al. (2022) in Chambo, Ecuador, regarding the purchasing power of rural families has demonstrated a correlation between the total income of the family and food security at the household level. The findings of this study provide statistical proof that the purchasing power of a household, as indicated by the monthly family income, has a positive impact on food security. Families with higher incomes are shown to have a higher likelihood of being food-secure, whereas those with lower incomes are more susceptible to food insecurity.

In underdeveloped areas, governments can implement various policies to boost the purchasing power of the population. These policies may include initiatives to increase employment opportunities, such as job training programs and support for small businesses. Additionally, improving access to financial services and promoting financial literacy can empower individuals to make informed spending decisions and manage their resources more effectively. Overall, a comprehensive approach that addresses various aspects of economic development is key to increasing purchasing power in underdeveloped and developing countries to promote sustainable growth.

Monitoring and timely evaluation of nutritional programs

The significance of nutritional programs in enhancing food security cannot be overstated, as these initiatives play a crucial role in guaranteeing that every individual and communities get sufficient amounts of food. Many international organizations and institutions have initiated projects aimed at improving food security at the global level. The FAO of the United Nations is investing in rural infrastructure to enhance agricultural practices. Similarly, the WFP is striving to improve food security by distributing food in areas facing shortages and also supporting refugees by providing them with nutritious food. The WFP operates the Food for Assets program, where participants acquire new skills or contribute to infrastructure renovation in exchange for food, thereby enhancing food security (Food Security: Sufficient Safe and Healthy Food for Everyone – WUR, n.d.).

The issue of food and nutrition security in rural communities of India has been identified as a major problem by the WHO. In response, the government has planned to implement various schemes and programs to tackle this issue. The government of India introduced several initiatives in 2016 with the goal of doubling farmers' income by 2022. These initiatives include the National Food Security Mission and the Integrated Schemes on Oilseeds, Pulses, Palm Oil, and Maize (ISOPOM) Rashtriya

Krishi Vikas Yojana (RKVY). These programs aim to overcome obstacles and enhance agricultural productivity, particularly in rainfed areas. In the last 20 years, the Indian authorities have made substantial strides and executed diverse initiatives to address the issue of food and nutritional security in rural areas. Notable endeavors encompass the initiation of mid-day meals in educational institutions, the establishment of Anganwadi systems to distribute rations to expectant and nursing mothers, and the provision of subsidized grain to individuals living below the poverty threshold via a public distribution system. The National Food Security Act (NFSA) of 2013 is a significant initiative designed to guarantee food and nutrition security for vulnerable populations by implementing various schemes and programs (Naik & Yarazari, 2019).

Continuous monitoring and timely evaluation of such nutritional programs play a pivotal role in enhancing food security by effectively assessing the impact and outcomes of the initiatives implemented. By evaluating the efficiency of these programs, valuable insights can be gained to ensure that the identified targets are being met and that the overall nutritional needs of the population are adequately addressed. Additionally, through regular assessment and adjustment based on the evaluation results, necessary improvements can be made to optimize the effectiveness of the food security initiatives. Such strategic monitoring and evaluation processes not only provide a means to track progress but also enable stakeholders to make informed decisions and undertake corrective actions promptly, thereby reinforcing the overall success and impact of nutritional programs aimed at the enhancement of food security for individuals and communities.

Community participation

Community participation plays a crucial role in the enhancement of food security within a region. When community members actively engage in initiatives that are framed to improve food security, they contribute to the development of sustainable solutions that benefit everyone. Through collaboration and involvement in projects such as community gardens, food banks, and educational programs, individuals come together to address food insecurity issues at the grassroots level. The involvement of beneficiaries and local stakeholders is a key element for the success of community-based nutrition interventions (Robert & Feijoo, 2022).

Involving the community members as collaborators in interventions to decrease health disparities, as suggested by community-based participatory intervention theory, is powerful on multiple levels (Tremblay et al., 2017). Various types of community-based participatory interventions, categorized under agricultural and nutritional groups, have been implemented successfully. Agricultural workshops, soil and seed improvement, and agroecological practices are popular strategies that show promise in reducing food insecurity in developing countries (Doustmohammadian et al., 2022). Therefore, fostering community participation in policy implementation is not just beneficial but essential for creating lasting and impactful changes in food security at the grassroots level.

Along with the aforementioned strategies, food security can be facilitated by implementing measures to minimize food waste, promoting advancements in food production techniques, enhancing agricultural research and development efforts, uplifting rural communities, addressing the issues arising from climate change, raising awareness about population growth, reducing poverty and hunger levels, and fostering economic connections between rural and urban areas.

3.5 SUSTAINABLE DEVELOPMENT GOALS AND FOOD SECURITY

The United Nations adopted the Sustainable Development Goals (SDGs), also referred to as the Global Goals, in 2015. These goals serve as a universal call to action, which aims to eradicate poverty, safeguard the environment, and promote peace and prosperity for all people by 2030. The 17 SDGs are interconnected, acknowledging that progress in one domain will have an impact on other areas. Furthermore, they emphasize the importance of achieving a harmonious balance between social, economic, and environmental sustainability in the pursuit of development (THE 17 GOALS | Sustainable Development, n.d.).

Food security is a vital component of the SDGs and plays a pivotal role in enhancing human well-being and eliminating poverty (Ana Tomicic, 2023). The SDGs encompass a wide range of interconnected targets pertaining to agriculture and food, emphasizing their importance in achieving sustainable development (Brooks, 2016).

SDG 1: No Poverty. Food security is intricately linked to the elimination of poverty. Providing adequate and healthy food to everyone can help in disrupting the cycle of poverty.

SDG 2: Zero Hunger. SDG 2 specifically targets ending hunger, achieving food security, improving nutrition, and promoting sustainable agriculture. The achievement of this objective heavily relies on the effective management of food systems, encompassing all stages from production to consumption.

SDG 3: Good Health and Well-being. Access to healthy food is important for promoting optimal health and overall well-being. Sufficient nutrition plays a significant role in preventing diseases, supporting growth, and enhancing cognitive development. On the other hand, when individuals face food insecurity, it can result in malnutrition, stunting, and a range of health problems. By prioritizing food security, we have the ability to have a positive effect on people's health and well-being.

SDG 5: Gender Equality. Gender equality is closely interlinked with food security. In many developing nations, women always have a vital role in the production, processing, and distribution of food. By empowering women in agriculture, decreasing gender-based inequalities, and challenging social norms, food security can be strengthened.

SDG 8: Decent Work and Economic Growth. The food systems sector offers substantial employment opportunities for a major portion of the global population. Encouraging sustainable agriculture practices and creating decent work within the food industry can contribute to economic growth and alleviate poverty.

SDG 10: Reduced Inequalities. Addressing inequalities is essential for attaining food security. Risk groups, including small-sector farmers and marginalized communities, mostly encounter obstacles when it comes to accessing resources and markets.

SDG 13: Climate Action. Climate change presents significant challenges to food security. Unpredictable weather patterns, shifting environmental conditions, and extreme events all have an impact on crop yields, damage the food production systems, and threaten livelihoods.

SDG 14: Life Below Water. Food systems can have negative effects on marine ecosystems and fisheries sustainability. Issues such as overfishing, pollution, and habitat destruction can lead to a decrease in fish availability, and marine biodiversity, and, in turn, lead to food insecurity.

SDG 15: Life on Land. Biodiversity loss and land degradation have a direct impact on food security, making sustainable land use practices, conservation efforts, and biodiversity preservation crucial for maintaining a resilient food system.

Food security is a key aspect of sustainable development and is closely connected to various SDGs. By recognizing these linkages and implementing specific strategies, we can progress towards zero hunger and establish a food-secure global community. As countries aim to reach the targets outlined in the SDGs, they are also making strides towards ensuring food security for everyone (Ana Tomicic, 2023).

3.6 CONCLUSION

Uncovering the hurdles of food security is an intricate process that involves analyzing various factors contributing to the global challenge of ensuring everyone has access to safe and nutritious food. Achieving sustainable food production is required to ensure food security for present and future generations. This journey towards sustainable food production encompasses not only the identification of obstacles but also the development of innovative solutions and strategies and also creating awareness among general population which will finally promotes the long-term food security worldwide.

Addressing issues such as poverty, hunger, and climate changes that impact agricultural productivity, as well as enhancing food distribution systems and advancing agricultural technologies like crop diversification, crop rotation, mulching, soil management, compost application, and agroforestry, can increase product variety, stability, and improved yield. These practices are helpful in transitioning agricultural and food systems to achieve global food and nutrition security and in building a sustainable food system. This journey is multidimensional and requires collaboration among stakeholders at local, national, and international levels. Continuous implementation and monitoring of policies and programs to ensure food security are imperative to the success of these efforts.

By navigating through these complexities and forging partnerships across sectors, we can pave the way towards a resilient and food-secure future. It is imperative to prioritize investments in sustainable agriculture, foster innovation, and promote inclusive policies to build a more equitable and sustainable food system. By approaching these issues holistically and inclusively, we can effectively overcome the challenges related to food security and strive towards a shared goal of providing everyone with access to the necessary food resources to lead healthy, fulfilling lives and making a solid foundation for a brighter and more nourished future for generations to come.

REFERENCES

Afriyie, E., Zurek, M., Asem, F. E., Okpattah, B., Ahiakpa, J. K., & Zhu, Y. G. (2023). Consumer food storage practices and methods at the household-level: A community study in Ghana. *Frontiers in Sustainable Food Systems*, 7. https://doi.org/10.3389/fsufs.2023.1194321

Agriculture and Food Security The IAEA Contribution. (n.d.). www.unep.org/Documents.Multilingual/Default.asp?DocumentID=589&Articl

Ana Tomicic. (2023, July 28). Connecting the Dots: How Food Systems Impact Multiple SDGs | FEAST. https://feast2030.eu/connecting-the-dots-how-food-systems-impact-multiple-sdg

Andrade, L., O'Dwyer, J., O'Neill, E., & Hynds, P. (2018). Surface water flooding, groundwater contamination, and enteric disease in developed countries: A scoping review of connections and consequences. *Environmental Pollution*, 236, 540–549. https://doi.org/10.1016/j.envpol.2018.01.104

Arrieta, E. M., & Aguiar, S. (2023). Healthy diets for sustainable food systems: A narrative review. *Environmental Science: Advances*, 2(5), 684–694. Royal Society of Chemistry. https://doi.org/10.1039/d2va00214k

Ayaviri-Nina, V. D., Quispe-Fernández, G. M., Vanegas, J. L., Ortega-Mejía, V., & Cordero-Ahiman, O. V. (2022). Importance of purchasing power and education in the food security of families in rural areas—Case study: Chambo, Ecuador. *Sustainability*, 14(10), 6068. https://doi.org/10.3390/su14106068

Ayomide, A., Ajimati, V., Oladayo, T., David Miteu, G., Anyanwu Nkiruka, J., Ilupeju, D., Falope, J., Agboola, O., Christiana Ojeokun, O., Olayinka, T., & Oghale Benneth, E. (2022). The impact of high technology storage facilities on food security in Nigeria-Nigeria case study: Mini review. *African Journal of Food Science and Technology*, 13(6), 1–4. https://doi.org/10.14303//ajfst

Barman, A., Saha, P., Patel, S., & Bera, A. (2022). Crop diversification an effective strategy for sustainable agriculture development. In *Sustainable Crop Production – Recent Advances*. IntechOpen. https://doi.org/10.5772/intechopen.102635

Bedoussac, L., Journet, E.-P., Hauggaard-Nielsen, H., Naudin, C., Corre-Hellou, G., Jensen, E. S., Prieur, L., & Justes, E. (2015). Ecological principles underlying the increase of productivity achieved by cereal-grain legume intercrops in organic farming. A review. *Agronomy for Sustainable Development*, 35(3), 911–935. https://doi.org/10.1007/s13593-014-0277-7

Behnassi, M., & El Haiba, M. (2022). Implications of the Russia–Ukraine war for global food security. *Nature Human Behaviour*, 6(6), 754–755. https://doi.org/10.1038/s41562-022-01391-x

Brooks, J. (2016). Food security and the sustainable development goals. In P. Love (Ed.), *Debate the Issues: New Approaches to Economic Challenges* (pp. 143–146). OECD Publishing.

Carducci, B., Keats, E. C., Ruel, M., Haddad, L., Osendarp, S. J. M., & Bhutta, Z. A. (2021). Food systems, diets and nutrition in the wake of COVID-19. *Nature Food*, 2(2), 68–70. https://doi.org/10.1038/s43016-021-00233-9

Colson, D. (2022, March 20). How Does Sustainable Agriculture Promote Food Security? https://walterschindler.com/agricultural-sustainability-articles/promoting-food-security/

Data4Diets | INDDEX Project. (n.d.). 2023. Retrieved May 6, 2024, from https://inddex.nutrition.tufts.edu/data4diets

Doustmohammadian, A., Mohammadi-Nasrabadi, F., Keshavarz-Mohammadi, N., Hajjar, M., Alibeyk, S., & Hajigholam-Saryazdi, M. (2022). Community-based participatory interventions to improve food security: A systematic review. *Frontiers in Nutrition*, 9. https://doi.org/10.3389/fnut.2022.1028394

Durojaye, E., & Chilemba, E. M. (n.d.). Food Security SA Working Paper Series: #003 Accountability and the Right to Food: A Comparative Study of India and South Africa. www.foodsecurity.ac.za

Dutta, H., & Saikia, A. A. (2018). Food security: A review on its definition, levels and evolution. *Asian Journal of Multidimensional Research (AJMR)*, *7*(7), 111–122.

Fan, S., Teng, P., Chew, P., Smith, G., & Copeland, L. (2021). Food system resilience and COVID-19 – Lessons from the Asian experience. *Global Food Security*, 28, 100501. https://doi.org/10.1016/j.gfs.2021.100501

Feliciano, D. (2019). A review on the contribution of crop diversification to sustainable development goal 1 "No poverty" in different world regions. *Sustainable Development*, 27(4), 795–808. https://doi.org/10.1002/sd.1923

Food and Agricultural Organization. (n.d.). *Policy and Programme | The Right to Food*. Food and Agriculture Organization of the United Nations. Retrieved May 6, 2024, from www.fao.org/right-to-food/areas-of-work/policy-programme/en/

Food and Agriculture Organization. (n.d.). 2.1.1 Prevalence of Undernourishment. Retrieved May 6, 2024, from www.fao.org/sustainable-development-goals-data-portal/data/indicators/2.1.1-prevalence-of-undernourishment/en

Food Security | IFPRI: International Food Policy Research Institute. (n.d.). Retrieved May 5, 2024, from www.ifpri.org/topic/food-security

Food Security: Improve with Better Storage Solutions. (n.d.). Retrieved May 6, 2024, from https://sourcetrace.com/blog/food-security-storage-solutions/

Food Security: Sufficient Safe and Healthy Food for Everyone – WUR. (n.d.). Retrieved May 6, 2024, from www.wur.nl/en/show/food-security-11.htm

FSC Indicators Handbook. (2020). https://fscluster.org/handbook/content.html

Garbach, K., Milder, J. C., DeClerck, F. A. J., Montenegro de Wit, M., Driscoll, L., & Gemmill-Herren, B. (2017). Examining multi-functionality for crop yield and ecosystem services in five systems of agroecological intensification. *International Journal of Agricultural Sustainability*, 15(1), 11–28. https://doi.org/10.1080/14735903.2016.1174810

Garcia, S. N., Osburn, B. I., & Jay-Russell, M. T. (2020). One health for food safety, food security, and sustainable food production. In *Frontiers in Sustainable Food Systems* (Vol. 4). Frontiers Media S.A. https://doi.org/10.3389/fsufs.2020.00001

Gebreyesus, S. H., Lunde, T., Mariam, D. H., Woldehanna, T., & Lindtjørn, B. (2015). Is the adapted Household Food Insecurity Access Scale (HFIAS) developed internationally to measure food insecurity valid in urban and rural households of Ethiopia? *BMC Nutrition*, 1(1). https://doi.org/10.1186/2055-0928-1-2

George, N. A., & McKay, F. H. (2019). The public distribution system and food security in India. *International Journal of Environmental Research and Public Health*, 16(17), 3221. https://doi.org/10.3390/ijerph16173221

Global Food Security: The Critical Role of Water, Sanitation, and Hygiene (WASH) | Food Security and Nutrition Network. (n.d.). Retrieved May 6, 2024, from www.fsnnetwork.org/resource/global-food-security-critical-role-water-sanitation-and-hygiene-wash

Global Issues | United Nations. (n.d.). Retrieved May 5, 2024, from www.un.org/en/global-issues/

Goal 2 | Department of Economic and Social Affairs. (n.d.). Retrieved May 6, 2024, from https://sdgs.un.org/goals/goal2

Gupta, A., & Mishra, D. K. (2018). Public distribution system in Uttar Pradesh: Access, utilization and impact. *Indian Journal of Human Development*, 12(1), 20–36. https://doi.org/10.1177/0973703018774668

Haughey, E., Suter, M., Hofer, D., Hoekstra, N. J., McElwain, J. C., Lüscher, A., & Finn, J. A. (2018). Higher species richness enhances yield stability in intensively managed grasslands with experimental disturbance. *Scientific Reports*, 8(1), 15047. https://doi.org/10.1038/s41598-018-33262-9

Hedin, B., Katzeff, C., Eriksson, E., & Pargman, D. (2019). A systematic review of digital behaviour change interventions for more sustainable food consumption. *Sustainability*, 11(9), 2638. https://doi.org/10.3390/su11092638

Household Food Insecurity Access Scale (HFIAS) for Measurement of Food Access: Indicator Guide | Food and Nutrition Technical Assistance III Project (FANTA). (n.d.). Retrieved May 6, 2024, from www.fantaproject.org/monitoring-and-evaluation/household-food-insecurity-access-scale-hfias

Hunger | FAO | Food and Agriculture Organization of the United Nations. (n.d.). Retrieved May 5, 2024, from www.fao.org/hunger/en/

Indicators of Food Security – Humanitarian Global. (2021, November 26). Humanitarian global. https://humanitarianglobal.com/indicators-of-food-security/

Ivanova, D., Stadler, K., Steen-Olsen, K., Wood, R., Vita, G., Tukker, A., & Hertwich, E. G. (2016). Environmental impact assessment of household consumption. *Journal of Industrial Ecology*, 20(3), 526–536. https://doi.org/10.1111/jiec.12371

Izraelov, M., & Silber, J. (2019). An assessment of the global food security index. *Food Security*, 11(5), 1135–1152. https://doi.org/10.1007/s12571-019-00941-y

Kang, J., Duan, X., & Yun, R. (2023). The impact of urbanization on food security: A case study of Jiangsu Province. *Land*, 12(9). https://doi.org/10.3390/land12091681

Lewis, S. L., & Maslin, M. A. (2015). Defining the anthropocene. *Nature*, 519(7542), 171–180. https://doi.org/10.1038/nature14258

Lynn Kennedy, P., Schmitz, A., & van Kooten, G. C. (2019). Food security and food storage. In P. Ferranti, E.M. Berry, & J.R. Anderson (eds.), *Encyclopedia of Food Security and Sustainability* (pp. 433–443). Elsevier. https://doi.org/10.1016/B978-0-08-100596-5.22251-8

Mabe, F. N., Mumuni, E., & Sulemana, N. (2021). Does smallholder farmers' awareness of Sustainable Development Goal 2 improve household food security in the Northern Region of Ghana? *Agriculture & Food Security*, 10(1), 9. https://doi.org/10.1186/s40066-020-00281-7

Magrini, M.-B., Anton, M., Chardigny, J.-M., Duc, G., Duru, M., Jeuffroy, M.-H., Meynard, J.-M., Micard, V., & Walrand, S. (2018). Pulses for sustainability: Breaking agriculture and food sectors out of lock-in. *Frontiers in Sustainable Food Systems*, 2. https://doi.org/10.3389/fsufs.2018.00064

Manikas, I., Ali, B. M., & Sundarakani, B. (2023). A systematic literature review of indicators measuring food security. In *Agriculture and Food Security* (Vol. 12, no. 1). BioMed Central Ltd. https://doi.org/10.1186/s40066-023-00415-7

Methodology – Global Hunger Index (GHI) – Peer-Reviewed Annual Publication Designed to Comprehensively Measure and Track Hunger at the Global, Regional, and Country Levels. (n.d.). Retrieved May 7, 2024, from www.globalhungerindex.org/methodology.html

Meynard, J.-M., Charrier, F., Fares, M., Le Bail, M., Magrini, M.-B., Charlier, A., & Messéan, A. (2018). Socio-technical lock-in hinders crop diversification in France. *Agronomy for Sustainable Development*, 38(5), 54. https://doi.org/10.1007/s13593-018-0535-1

Myers, S., & Frumkin, H. (2020). *Planetary Health*. Island Press. https://doi.org/10.5822/978-1-61091-966-1

Myers, S. S. (2017). Planetary health: Protecting human health on a rapidly changing planet. *The Lancet*, 390(10114), 2860–2868. https://doi.org/10.1016/S0140-6736(17)32846-5

Naik, M., & Yarazari, S. (2019, November). Government initiatives for food and nutritional security for rural communities in India. Paper delivered at *ISEE National Seminar -2019 on Socio-Digital Approaches for Transforming Indian Agriculture, Hisar.*

O'Neill, B. C., Oppenheimer, M., Warren, R., Hallegatte, S., Kopp, R. E., Pörtner, H. O., Scholes, R., … & Yohe, G. (2017). IPCC reasons for concern regarding climate change risks. *Nature Climate Change*, 7(1), 28–37. https://doi.org/10.1038/nclimate3179

Osendarp, S., Verburg, G., Bhutta, Z., Black, R. E., de Pee, S., Fabrizio, C., Headey, D., … & Ruel, M. T. (2022). Act now before Ukraine war plunges millions into malnutrition. *Nature*, 604(7907), 620–624. https://doi.org/10.1038/d41586-022-01076-5

Pawlak, K., & Kołodziejczak, M. (2020). The role of agriculture in ensuring food security in developing countries: Considerations in the context of the problem of sustainable food production. *Sustainability (Switzerland)*, 12(13). https://doi.org/10.3390/su12135488

Portner et al. (2023). *Climate Change 2022 – Impacts, Adaptation and Vulnerability*. Cambridge University Press. https://doi.org/10.1017/9781009325844

Pradhan, M., & Rao, N. (2018). Gender justice and food security: The case of public distribution system in India. *Progress in Development Studies*, 18(4), 252–266. https://doi.org/10.1177/1464993418786795

Qu, B., Xiao, Z., Upadhyay, A., & Luo, Y. (2024). Perspectives on sustainable food production system: Characteristics and green technologies. *Journal of Agriculture and Food Research*, 15. https://doi.org/10.1016/j.jafr.2024.100988

Rabbi, M. F., Hasan, M., & Kovács, S. (2021). Food security and transition towards sustainability. *Sustainability (Switzerland)*, 13(22). https://doi.org/10.3390/su132212433

Rehman, A., Farooq, M., Lee, D.-J., & Siddique, K. H. M. (2022). Sustainable agricultural practices for food security and ecosystem services. *Environmental Science and Pollution Research*, 29(56), 84076–84095. https://doi.org/10.1007/s11356-022-23635-z

Ritchie, H., & Roser, M. (2024). How is Food Insecurity Measured? Our World in Data. https://ourworldindata.org/food-insecurity

Robert, R. C., & Feijoo, B. L. (2022). Beneficiary and local stakeholder participation in community-based nutrition interventions. *Current Developments in Nutrition*, 6(9), nzac131. https://doi.org/10.1093/cdn/nzac131

SDG Meta Data. (2023). Prevalence of Undernourishment: Percent (%) Number of undernourished People: Millions (of People) 2.c. Classifications (CLASS_SYSTEM). https://esa.un.org/unpd/wpp/Download/Standard/Population/

Shoba Suri. (2024). Halfway to 2030: Unravelling Global food security challenges. www.orfonline.org/expert-speak/halfway-to-2030-unravelling-global-food-security-challenges#ftn1

Smutka, L., Steininger, M., Maitah, M., & Škubna, O. (2016). The Czech Agrarian Foreign Trade Development in 21st Century. https://cabidigitallibrary.org

Smyth, S. J., Phillips, P. W. B., & Kerr, W. A. (2015). Food security and the evaluation of risk. *Global Food Security*, 4, 16–23. https://doi.org/10.1016/j.gfs.2014.08.001

Steffen, W., Richardson, K., Rockström, J., Cornell, S. E., Fetzer, I., Bennett, E. M., Biggs, R., … & Sörlin, S. (2015). Planetary boundaries: Guiding human development on a changing planet. *Science*, 347(6223). https://doi.org/10.1126/science.1259855

Sustainable Development Goals | United Nations Development Programme. (n.d.). Retrieved May 6, 2024, from www.undp.org/sustainable-development-goals

THE 17 GOALS | Sustainable Development. (n.d.). Retrieved May 6, 2024, from https://sdgs.un.org/goals#history

The DHS Program – Search Results. (2020). https://dhsprogram.com/searchresults.cfm?q=Food+Insecurity+Experience+Scale+%28FIES%29%3A+#gsc.tab=0&gsc.q=Food%20Insecurity%20Experience%20Scale%20(FIES)%3A%20&gsc.page=1https://dhsprogram.com/pubs/pdf/DHSQM/DHS8-Module-FAO-FIES-Instructions-EN-16Oct2020-DHSQM.pdf

The Global Food Security Index | UNCCD. (n.d.). Retrieved May 6, 2024, from www.unccd.int/resources/knowledge-sharing-system/global-food-security-index

The Role of Sustainable Agriculture Practices in Driving Food Security. (2023, July 27). https://thesunmediafoundation.org/2023/06/27/the-role-of-sustainable-agriculture-practices-in-driving-food-security/

The State of Food and Agriculture 2023. (2023). *In the State of Food and Agriculture 2023*. FAO. https://doi.org/10.4060/cc7724en

The State of Food Security and Nutrition in the World 2023. (2023). *In the State of Food Security and Nutrition in the World 2023*. FAO; IFAD; UNICEF; WFP; WHO. https://doi.org/10.4060/cc3017en

Thomas, A. C., D'Hombres, B., Casubolo, C., Kayitakire, F., & Saisana, M. (2017). *The Use of the Global Food Security Index to Inform the Situation in Food Insecure Countries*. JRC Science Hub, European Union. https://doi.org/10.2760/83356

Tremblay, M., Martin, D. H., Macaulay, A. C., & Pluye, P. (2017). Can we build on social movement theories to develop and improve community-based participatory research? A framework synthesis review. *American Journal of Community Psychology*, 59(3–4), 333–362. https://doi.org/10.1002/ajcp.12142

Von Grebmer, K., Bernstein, J., Wiemers, M., Reiner, L., Bachmeier, M., Hanano, A., Chéilleachair, R. N., … & Ndlovu, M. (2023a). *Global Hunger Index the Power of Youth in Shaping Food Systems a Peer-Reviewed Publication*. Bonn: Welthungerhilfe, Concern International. www.globalhungerindex.org

Von Grebmer, K., Bernstein, J., Wiemers, M., Reiner, L., Bachmeier, M., Hanano, A., Chéilleachair, R. N., … & Ndlovu, M. (2023b). *Global Hunger Index the Power of Youth in Shaping Food Systems a Peer-Reviewed Publication*. Bonn: Welthungerhilfe, Concern International. www.globalhungerindex.org

Vuong, T. N., Van Dang, C., Toze, S., Jagals, P., Gallegos, D., & Gatton, M. L. (2022). Household water and food insecurity negatively impacts self-reported physical and mental health in the Vietnamese Mekong Delta. *PLoS ONE*, 17(5 May). https://doi.org/10.1371/journal.pone.0267344

Water | UNICEF. (n.d.). Retrieved May 6, 2024, from www.unicef.org/wash/water

Water, sanitation and hygiene (WASH). (n.d.). Retrieved May 6, 2024, from www.who.int/health-topics/water-sanitation-and-hygiene-wash#tab=tab_1

Watson, C. A., Reckling, M., Preissel, S., Bachinger, J., Bergkvist, G., Kuhlman, T., Lindström, K., … & Stoddard, F. L. (2017). *Grain legume production and use in European agricultural systems. Advances in Agronomy*, 144, 235–303. https://doi.org/10.1016/bs.agron.2017.03.003

Wegren, S. K., & Elvestad, C. (2018). Russia's food self-sufficiency and food security: An assessment. *Post-Communist Economies*, 1–23. https://doi.org/10.1080/14631377.2018.1470854

Wezel, A., Casagrande, M., Celette, F., Vian, J.-F., Ferrer, A., & Peigné, J. (2014). Agroecological practices for sustainable agriculture. A review. *Agronomy for Sustainable Development*, 34(1), 1–20. https://doi.org/10.1007/s13593-013-0180-7

Wheeler, T., & Von Braun, J. (2013). Climate change impacts on global food security. In *Science* (Vol. 341, no. 6145, pp. 508–513). American Association for the Advancement of Science. https://doi.org/10.1126/science.1239402

World Food Programme. (2015, February 3). *Meta Data for the Food Consumption Score (FCS) Indicator*. World Food Programme. www.wfp.org/publications/meta-data-food-consumption-score-fcs-indicator

World Health Organization. (2023, July 12). 122 Million More People Pushed into Hunger Since 2019 Due to Multiple Crises, Reveals UN Report. www.who.int/news/item/12-07-2023-122-million-more-people-pushed-into-hunger-since-2019-due-to-multiple-crises--reveals-un-report

World Population Clock: 8.1 Billion People (LIVE, 2024) – Worldometer. (n.d.). Retrieved May 7, 2024, from www.worldometers.info/world-population/

Wu, L., Taylor, M. P., & Handley, H. K. (2017). Remobilisation of industrial lead depositions in ash during Australian wildfires. *Science of The Total Environment*, 599–600, 1233–1240. https://doi.org/10.1016/j.scitotenv.2017.05.044

4 Empowering Women for Improved Nutritional Well-being

Strategies to Address Anemia and Enhance Food Security in India

Neha Goyal, Jagriti Jaiswal, and Lochan Sharma

4.1 INTRODUCTION

Proper nutrition is highly valued, similar to maintaining good health. Nutrition encompasses more than just the absence of malnutrition or nutritional deficiency illness. Similarly, health goes beyond simply the absence of sickness and includes a positive physiological state of well-being. In order to have improved health of women, children, and adolescents in the future, it is crucial to prioritize investments in nutrition. Investment in nutrition yields significant human, social, and economic advantages. There are clear global commitments to take action, with specific goals to monitor progress. To transform these promises into tangible results, it is imperative that all stakeholders, ranging from the government to the general public, collaborate harmoniously. Improving the quality of the diet is crucial, along with protecting, promoting, and supporting breastfeeding. It is important to ensure that everyone has access to key nutrition interventions, sufficient water and sanitation, and adequate education and information (Branca et al., 2015).

The health of the population is influenced by multiple factors, including economic efficiency, educational status, and access to basic health services, political stability, and social and cultural development. It is essential to prioritize adequate food intake as a fundamental aspect of human well-being. Enhancing nutritional intake has a positive impact on productivity, leading to higher levels of economic growth. Similar to previous findings, a rise in economic growth has the potential to greatly enhance the nutritional status of a nation (Dube & Phiri, 2015; Ghosh, 2018).

Proper nutrition is essential for maintaining optimal human well-being. It is widely acknowledged that having access to an adequate food supply is a fundamental human right that holds great significance in today's world. Recognizing the importance of reasonable nutrition, investing in human capital becomes crucial for the overall well-being of individuals and society. It plays a vital role in laying the groundwork for

DOI: 10.1201/9781003487227-4

economic development and making significant contributions to the well-being of households and society (Grosso et al., 2020).

There exist significant urban and rural inequalities in nutritional well-being and also nutrition status disparity among states. The gap between affluent and poor has grown because of the negative health effects of poverty and hunger. The impact of poverty and malnutrition on health has led to a significant disparity between different socioeconomic groups. According to the UNCTD's 2000 evaluation, inequality in the global economy is on the rise. Based on this, it was claimed that differences in development levels exist even within Indian states, and that although hunger and malnourishment are widespread in India, the occurrence and trends vary by state (Antony & Laxmaiah, 2008).

Investment in human capital and working towards economic growth while ignoring half of the population will be an injustice. Studies show women influence the health of the whole family, especially the children. But there is a significant disparity between men and women in nutrition intake, and many cultural, social, and political factors influence this disparity in food consumption and different nutritional attainment of women and men. There is plentiful evidence of gender bias in health and other forms of care.

In societies that are more egalitarian, it is found that the gap in nutrition status is less in relative terms and also in absolute terms: women are more healthy and nourished. Working towards the improvement of women health's and nutritional well-being is understood as a welfare approach to development which India adopted in its first few five-year plans. Women are considered recipients, and policies are made concerning their basic needs like food, shelter, and safety rather than considering them as active agents of change and also overlooking the dual link between gender and development (Moser, 2012). Everyday responsibilities, like meal preparation, water collection, field work, and managing family businesses, can place substantial demands on a woman's time and energy. Ensuring that nutritional, health, and agricultural investments are structured to empower women and promote gender equality enables women to allocate time for the care of their children and other family members. In the grand scheme of things, enhancing women's understanding of nutrition and promoting healthier eating habits and hygiene practices can play a significant role in combating undernutrition.

Furthermore, early marriage and childbirth have a significant impact on women's health and contribute to the existing disparities in socioeconomic status (Santhya et al., 2010). The inefficient use of health facilities and the prevalence of anemia among women of reproductive age have contributed to a significant increase in maternal mortality rates. There is a correlation between the health and nutrition of women and the likelihood of giving birth to low-weight infants. Women may struggle to provide food and adequate care for their children. Ultimately, the economic well-being of a household is influenced by the health of women. When women experience poor health, their productivity in the labor force may be negatively impacted.

Empowering women and reducing inequalities improves nutrition well-being and also make women better economic agents, as nutrition is directly linked to human capabilities. It will not just help in easily doing economic activities but also activities linked with reproduction, like pregnancy, child rearing, and breast feeding. It is clear that women's nutritional well-being has a significant bearing on children's health. Hence, investing in women's nutrition can have multiple effects on society as whole. Lack of agency, resources, autonomy, and achievements, considered as dimensions of empowerment (Kabeer, 2021) among women, influence their calorie intake and overall health (DeRosa et al., 2000). Women in agricultural and allied activities require special attention in the context of nutrition, as the tasks require more physical activities, and as female deprivation in terms of calorie intake and nutritional well-being is worse in rural than urban areas.

The impact of low nutritional value among women on human development are numerous and build up over time. For example, maternal malnutrition has been found to be associated with a higher risk of maternal mortality. Maternal short stature and iron deficiency contribute significantly to the risk of maternal mortality during delivery, accounting for at least 20% of such cases (Black et al., 2008). In addition, the impact of maternal malnutrition extends to crucial factors such as intrauterine growth retardation, child malnutrition, and the increasing prevalence of chronic diseases. These issues are closely interconnected and have been extensively studied by researchers (Victora et al., 2008).

Interestingly, more than half of the women aged 15–49 experience iron deficiency. In contrast to the pronounced disparity between rural and urban areas in chronic energy deficiency (CED), the regional gap in anemia is smaller. Therefore, over 50% of women, regardless of where they live, experience varying degrees of anemia, ranging from mild to severe. Over 15% of women in both rural and urban India are affected by the two most serious forms of anemia. The prevalence of anemia among pregnant women is significantly higher, with nearly 59% affected. More than half of these cases are classified as moderate or severe. It is evident that a significant number of malnourished women, specifically over 77% with CED and 70% with any anemia, reside in rural India. This highlights the higher occurrence of malnutrition among rural women. There is a strong possibility that a considerable number of women who experience CED may also have anemia.

Measuring empowerment is difficult, as it is a multidimensional concept and indicators change with time and space. However, for the sake of comparison, policy-making, and implementation, a few international organizations like UNDP, WHO, and WEF release yearly data of women's empowerment indicators and gender indices. These data will be discussed later on in this chapter, and a link between women's nutrition and women's empowerment will be assessed.

There is no universal solution that can be applied to every situation. Instead, there are numerous interventions that are tailored to specific contexts. It is crucial to include young women in the development programs for all these initiatives and make sure their perspectives are incorporated into policy formation. Recognizing the substantial contribution of women in the agricultural and food systems of developing countries, it is crucial to implement food policy, nutritional schemes, health services, and agricultural projects that take gender into account. This approach can empower women by allowing them to maintain control over resources and participate in decision-making regarding crop selection. The government of India has implemented schemes like

ICDS, POSHAN Abhiyaan, National Food Security Mission, Pradhan Mantri Matru Vandana Yojana, and National Rural Livelihood Mission in the past few years.

Against this backdrop, this chapter also assesses the interventions and strategies adopted by the government of India to enhance the nutritional well-being of women. It focuses on the research question of how empowering women can improve nutritional well-being and also gender indices in India. This question raises other considerations, such as the strategies or government intervention needed to enhance women's nutrition, particularly in addressing anemia, and to improve their inclusion in sustainable development goals.

So, the research question stipulated above suggests the objectives of the sections that follow: to assess the status of the nutritional diet pattern among adult women; to analyze the status of women through gender indices; and to evaluate government strategies to improve the nutritional intake and reduce the prevalence of anemia among women. The chapter's objectives are achieved using secondary data that is based on a timeline. Information is obtained from various reliable sources such as governmental sites and survey reports like NFHS, the World Bank, WHO, and FAO.

The framework of this chapter is centered on theoretical and critical research, examining various factors such as female nutritional diet, workforce participation, food consumption, and government strategies (policies) aimed at reducing undernutritional conditions among women. This chapter focuses on a secondary database and provides an explanatory approach. Therefore, descriptive statistical tools are utilized, with a focus on graphical presentation to effectively convey the key factors of the variables and facilitate critical analysis. In addition, basic inferential statistics are utilized to uncover the relationship between causes and effects.

4.2 GENDER IN THE CONTEXT OF HEALTH AND FOOD INSECURITY

SDG 2 is a broad target to eradicate hunger, achieve food security, and improve nutrition, while promoting sustainable agriculture, as has become a global challenge. With a recent spurt of events globally, such as consistently occurring infectious diseases, economic depression, and war and conflict, the loss of quality of human life has further increased the need to emphasize this pressing issue. Moreover, it is important to understand the contextual realities and challenges, as issues are as pressing in terms of the degree of harm to individuals as poor health and nutrition and food insecurity. The classic literature brings out the dynamics of caste, class, and socioeconomic profile to compare and analyze the effects of gender-wise comparison and analysis, but the need to do this more rigorously has increased (WHO, 2023). Addressing nutrition issues for everyone, particularly women and children, is essential in successfully achieving larger SDG goals. In India, anemia and food insecurity are serious matters that greatly affect the health of Indian women and therefore the overall well-being of the family and community at large.

A recently published critical review, which aims to measure the depth of food insecurity in India, shows that with the transitioning economy, the overall production and quantity of food has increased. Over the past 30 years, India has transformed from a food-deficit nation to a self-sufficient food-producing country (Nutrition and Food Security, n.d.), but this has not yet translated into gains for the general population. This review studied cross-sectional information from across communities and contexts; in seven of the studies identified, the respondents were women, entailing their experiences and journeys taken to live through the challenges of food insecurity (McKay et al., 2023). Similarly, in other studies (Masa et al., 2017; Tadesse et al., 2017; Joshi et al., 2019) across different contexts, when researched on the lines of food insecurity, the narration has primarily come through women, indicating their key role in channelizing food-related situations. Agarwal (2018) conducted a study to examine the abilities and limitations of SDG 5 (pertaining to gender equality) and its role in achieving household food security in the Indian context. It brings out the significant potential that lies in meticulous examination of women's ability to access land and natural resources. This consideration has the potential to significantly enhance women's ability to generate and acquire food. But limitations to this approach surface when discussing the social constraints faced by women in the community, namely its lack of clarity regarding the need for accessible resources for women. While women are at the forefront of channelizing food insecurity, they have also shielded their families from the repercussions of it. Women's experiences of the negative impacts of food insecurity and obesity are experientially very different from those of men, but the causes are still under-researched (Sims et al., 2021). Feeding India remarks that with the unspoken rules in a patriarchal context, traditional households tend to save the larger share of the bread earned for men, whereas children and women get what is left after everyone else has finished (Feeding India, 2022). The situations of insecurity and hunger lead to elevated risks of developing deficiencies and undernourishment, the most prevalent being iron deficiency. The degrading health and nutritional profile heightens the risk for intergenerational transfer of poor health and nutritional deficiencies (Sims et al., 2021).

Furthermore, there is evidence in the literature that suggests a clear link between malnutrition and anemia in women. Research evidence has explored the condition of women with anemia in association with their empowered roles, especially in terms of their engagement into economic activities and decision-making roles within the household. A study by Mishra et al. (2021) focuses on anemia and its correlation with dietary patterns among the Garhwals of the Himalayan region, highlighting the critical importance of addressing the nutritional needs of anemic individuals in that region.

Despite several international bodies identifying the significance of gender equality in food systems, efforts to improve local food systems continue to lack a strong gender perspective. Almost 46% of reports offering potential solutions to hunger in the COVID-19 pandemic did not abide by that perspective (Visser & Wangu, 2021). The role that women play in the context of food security has been recognized by several international bodies, acknowledging them as primary producers of food, primary caretakers of the household, and contributors in activities related to agricultural development. On the other hand, men's role is more focused towards cash crops, which have a direct influence on household-level food security.

Therefore, concerning their counterparts, women are more likely to be affected by any contextual change in the direct familial environment or larger community-level shifts, for example in terms of increased family responsibilities and reduced productivity, affecting the possibility of using opportunities to be more reliant and empowered.

4.3 WOMEN'S NUTRITION AND WOMEN'S EMPOWERMENT: A SYNCHRONIZED PHENOMENON

Globally, 60% of all working women are engaged in agricultural activities, with little or no access to credit, loans, or technology, which ultimately pins down to increasing the risks of hunger, illness, infections, and lack of productivity (UN Women, n.d.). While we understand now that women, being the core of family and larger social networks, can channel the contextual consequences to the wider social environment, it is also important to understand that the implications for women themselves are multiple and have a high risk of being intergenerational, genetically or behaviorally.

Understanding the crucial role that women play in household nutrition and food security, their empowerment status is one of the important variables in tackling these challenges effectively. As mentioned earlier, talks across international bodies and agencies discussing the security of food nutrition and health for a larger population have been gender-blind in their frameworks (Njuki et al., 2022). Thus, creating space to emphasize the drawing of more comprehensive and analytical frameworks of research is crucial.

Baye (2017), through careful observation, has highlighted the significance and need for adopting a different mindset and executing policies and programs effectively. One crucial thing to note here is that the correlation between contextual realities, and thereby the nutritional profile of women and women's empowered role in society, is tough to describe directionally, as in what causes what. Wilunda et al. (2023) explored the relationship between empowerment of women and the nutritional and health profile of their children, particularly in terms of anemia and hemoglobin concentration in the sub-Saharan African context. Not only did they find a positive correlation between women's empowerment and reduced rates of anemia, along with increased hemoglobin concentration in children, but they also stood against social evils, for example by changing attitudes towards violence, being participatory in decision-making events, and being socially independent. This link between women's empowerment and children's nutritional status has also been identified by Yaya et al. (2019) as having significant effects on the development of human labor supply and their productivity, economic growth, and development. Lufuke et al. (2022) also investigated the impact of women's empowerment on household dietary patterns, nutrition improvement, and diet-related health outcomes in the African context.

The findings in the literature support the argument of a positive connection between women's empowerment and food security and dietary improvement, but there is a lack of extensive research in this domain exploring the impact of women's empowerment on increased demand for certain food categories. It is crucial to develop and implement strategies that promote women's empowerment and examine its influence on nutrition intake to address the issue of anemia. With an empowered role of women, food systems could be significantly strengthened to fight hunger and malnutrition (Yila & Sylla, 2020). Henceforth, the analytical comprehensive framework must bring to light innovations and interventions that emphasize significantly the component of women's empowerment.

There could be different facilitators to empower women such as education and entrepreneurship, but researchers have suggested that, in some cases, businesses which are small and home-based would generate little profit but would come as an additional burden on women, especially when the spousal support is limited (Malapit et al., 2019; Njuki et al., 2022). Women would often also be restricted on grounds of social norms, social identity, socioeconomic status in the family, and lack of decision-making and leadership roles to execute their skills in an entrepreneurial capacity. Some investment models could be investments in maternal education, particularly counseling and education focusing on nutrition-related knowledge; in interventions that enhance their decision-making skills and leadership roles in the family; in larger food systems; and in promoting equal and equitable gender norms (Njuki et al., 2022).

4.4 ANTHROPOMETRIC TRANSITIONS AND THE GENDERED DIVIDEND: EVIDENCE FROM NFHS, DHS, AND NNMB

The data from NFHS across the years 1998–99 (NFHS 2), 2005–06 (NFHS 3), 2015–16 (NFHS 4), and 2020–21 (NFHS 5) reveal significant trends in food consumption, women's health, and nutrition in India (Table 4.1). There has been a steady increase in milk consumption, from 55% in 1998–99 to 72.2% in 2020–21, and a consistently high consumption of pulses, increasing slightly from 87.8% to 92.9% over the same period. Fruit consumption has also risen significantly, from 33% to 49.7%. Vegetable consumption has remained relatively stable, slightly decreasing from 92.9% in 2005–06 to 90.8% in 2020–21. Chicken or meat consumption shows an overall increase from 31.9% in 1998–99 to 35.9% in 2020–21, despite a dip to 22.7% in 2005–06. Figure 4.1 and Figure 4.2 represent the percentage consumption of the food products consumed and the percentage of women facing anemia and undernutrition.

In terms of women's health, the percentage of women below 145 cm in height has decreased from 13.2% in 1998–99 to 11.5% in 2020–21, indicating improvements in stature. The mean BMI has gradually increased from 20.3 to 22.4, suggesting better nutritional status. Poor nutritional value, according to WHO, is linked with poor

TABLE 4.1
Percentages of Women Eating Specific Foods in India

Year	Milk	Pulses	Fruit	Vegetables	Chicken or Beat
1998–99	55	87.8	33	85.2	31.9
2005–06	55.4	89.5	45.7	92.9	22.7
2015–16	68	89.9	45.7	85.5	32.5
2020–21	72.2	92.9	49.7	90.8	35.9

Source: National Health Family Surveys, Ministry of Health and Family Welfare.

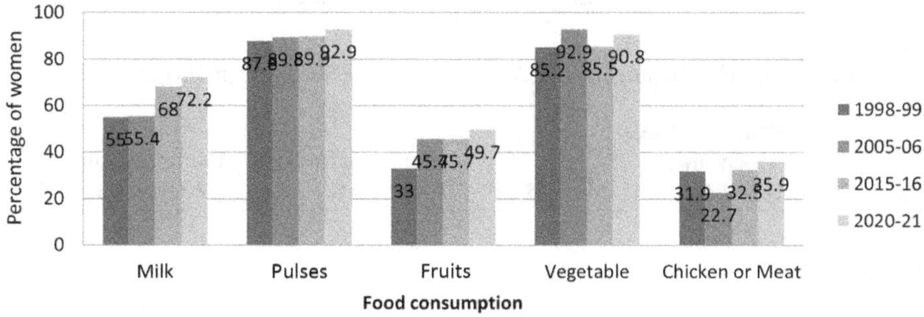

FIGURE 4.1 Percentage of consumption of food products by women. (Data from National Health Family Surveys, Ministry of Health and Family Welfare.)

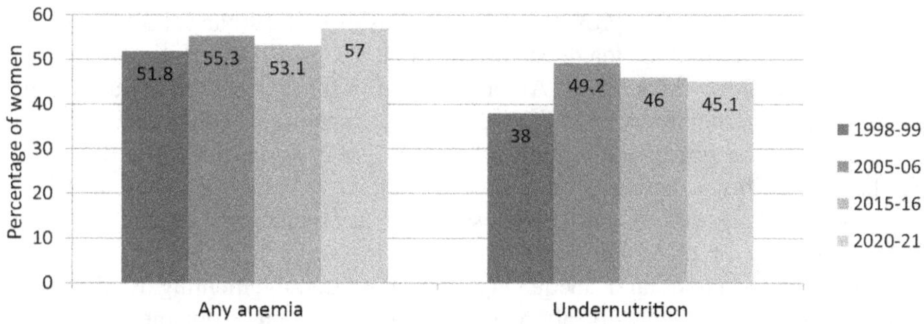

FIGURE 4.2 Percentage of women facing anemia and undernutrition. (Data from National Health Family Surveys, Ministry of Health and Family Welfare.)

standard of living. It is also a deprivation of the dimension of health in measuring multidimensional poverty (Ramya, 2021). However, the prevalence of anemia among women has worsened, rising from 51.8% in 1998–99 to 57% in 2020–21 (Table 4.2).

The rate of undernutrition (being either thin or obese) among women increased from 38% in 1998–99 to 49.2% in 2005–06 and then slightly improved to 45.1% in 2020–21 (Table 4.2). Obesity is a big problem nowadays due to undernourishment and also due to a sedentary lifestyle (Park et al., 2020). According to the National Nutrition Monitoring Bureau (2017) urban nutrition report, around 44% of adult women are overweight and obese, much higher than adult men (34%) (pooled data from 16 states). While there have been positive trends in the consumption of nutritious foods and some aspects of women's health, challenges such as anemia and undernutrition remain significant issues.

India has witnessed "limited progress" in meeting diet-related non-communicable disease (NCD) targets. Currently, 6.2% of adult women and 3.5% of adult men are living with obesity. Additionally, 9% of adult women and 10.2% of adult men are affected by diabetes (Global Nutrition Report, 2022).

TABLE 4.2
Prevalence of Undernutrition and Anemia Among Women in India

Year	Women Below 145 cm in Height (%)	Mean BMI	Women with Any Anemia (%)	Women with Undernutrition (%)
1998–99	13.2	20.3	51.8	38
2005–06	11.4	20.5	55.3	49.2
2015–16	11.2	21.9	53.1	46
2020–21	11.5	22.4	57	45.1

Source: National Health Family Surveys, Ministry of Health and Family Welfare.

Agarwal and Sethi (2013) provide a detailed analysis of the urban subset of the third round of the Demographic Health Survey of India, focusing on nutrition disparities among women within urban areas. Among women in the poorest urban quartile, the prevalence of maternal thinness and moderate/severe anemia was significantly higher as compared to the rest of the urban population. The importance of utilizing urban data that is specific to the needs of the poor for effective planning was emphasized. Several suggestions were made to address this issue, including conducting regular field assessments of maternal nutritional status in outreach programs, enhancing access to food subsidies and adequately iodized salt, implementing food supplementation programs, exploring alternative methods of iron supplementation, and establishing counseling days as a regular practice.

4.5 INDICES HINT: INEQUALITY AND POOR DEVELOPMENT OF WOMEN

The data on GDI, GII, and GGGI over various years show trends in gender equality. The GDI has shown a steady improvement, starting at 0.545 in 2000 and increasing to 0.586 in 2005, 0.594 in 2010, and significantly jumping to 0.795 in 2015. By 2020, the GDI further rose to 0.82, indicating substantial progress in gender development. The GII, available from 2010 onwards, initially recorded a high value of 0.748, suggesting significant gender inequality. However, by 2015, the GII had improved to 0.563, reflecting a reduction in gender inequality. The GGGI, first recorded in 2005 at 0.601, showed gradual progress, rising to 0.615 in 2010, 0.664 in 2015, and reaching 0.668 by 2020. These data collectively indicate positive strides towards gender equality over the two decades, with improvements in gender development and reductions in gender inequality. Table 4.3 shows the gender-related indices of India.

GDI does not take into account any nutrition indicators for its measurement. GDI and GII both have life expectancy as one of their indicators, which is undoubtedly related to the nutritional aspect; malnutrition, obesity, and undernutrition are connected with low life expectancy (Zheng et al., 2014; Shetty, 2013). In this context, life expectancy is closely tied to factors such as nutritional intake and access to healthcare services. According to a report by WHO (1998), it is suggested that health expectancy

TABLE 4.3
Gender-Related Indices, India (2000–20)

Year	GDI	GII	GGGI
2000	0.545	—	—
2005	0.586	—	0.601
2010	0.594	0.748	0.615
2015	0.795	0.563	0.664
2020	0.820	0.488	0.668

Source: World Economic Forum (2020).

Note: GDI = Gender Development Index, GII = Gender Inequality Index, GGGI = Global Gender Gap Index.

holds greater significance than life expectancy. The maternal mortality ratio (MMR) and the adolescent fertility rate (AFR) are the two indicators of the reproductive health dimension of GII. Nutrition had a crucial role in declining MMR globally; long-term as well short-term daily calorie intake and balanced diet can remarkably influence MMR (Manfredini, 2020). The risk of death is generally linked with severe anemia among mothers (Daru et al., 2018). Nevertheless, the GDI, which evaluates Healthy Diet Index (HDI) components separately for males and females, has faced significant criticism for not accounting for women's nutritional intake. While SDG 5 places a strong emphasis on achieving gender equality and empowering women and girls, it also recognizes the importance of addressing disparities and promoting inclusivity in different areas, such as nutrition. Similarly, the MPI, unlike the HDI, considers maternal health and nutrition under the subheading of health indicators.

4.6 LINK BETWEEN WOMEN'S EMPOWERMENT AND NUTRITION: AN ANALYSIS OF WENI, WEAI, AND RELATED INDICES

The Women's Empowerment and Nutrition Index (WENI) is a multidimensional index that integrates literature on the drivers of nutrition and empowerment, alongside multisite formative research from rural South Asia. It consists of 40 indicators across the domains of food, health, and institutions, expanding to 50 indicators to include the fertility domain for younger women. These indicators are categorized into three dimensions of empowerment: knowledge, resources, and agency. The indicators were selected from an initial set of 128 candidates through normative and statistical evaluations and are aggregated using the Alkire–Foster (A–F) method for constructing multidimensional indices (Alkire & Foster, 2011). This approach underpins many well-known indices, such as the MPI and the WEAI. The A–F indices are advantageous because they are additive and decomposable, enabling analysis of the contributions of each domain and dimension to the overall index and allowing examination of results for various subpopulations of interest.

Narayanan et al. (2019) introduced an index that focuses on assessing women's empowerment in relation to nutrition. They described nutritional empowerment as the method through which individuals gain the ability to achieve proper nourishment and good health, in a situation where this ability was previously withheld from them. The index is developed based on extensive research conducted in South Asia, taking into account various factors that impact nutritional outcomes. The index was constructed using data from two sites in India and validated by estimating two nutritional outcomes, BMI and anemia, based on the index. The study revealed a strong correlation between our index and these outcomes, suggesting that the WENI can be a valuable tool for researchers seeking to comprehend the nutritional well-being of women and their families in rural South Asia (Lentz et al., 2021; Saha & Narayanan, 2022).

The original WEAI module, developed by IFPRI, USAID, and OPHI, was adapted to the local context. The WEAI is calculated as a weighted sum of two subindicators: the 5 Domains of Empowerment (5DE) index and the Gender Parity Index (GPI). The 5DE subindex evaluates women's empowerment across five domains: production, resources, income, leadership, and time. The GPI measures the gap in empowerment levels between the index woman and man within the household (Alkire et al., 2013; Malapit et al., 2014).

There is a strong relationship between women's empowerment in the agricultural sector and their nutritional well-being, and this is captured by WEAI. Gupta et al. (2019) studied the relationship between women's empowerment in agriculture and their iron deficiency. Relationships between WEAI and per capita calorie availability, dietary diversity, and adult BMI were examined and it was found that increases in women's empowerment are positively associated with calorie availability and dietary diversity at the household level (Sraboni et al., 2014; Tsibo et al., 2018).

Some other indices related to this debate are the Empowerment in WASH Index (EWI) and Women Empowerment in Livestock Index (WELI), developed recently and much used in gender analysis. EWI is a new survey-based tool to measure women's empowerment and gender outcomes in the WASH (Water, Sanitation and Hygiene) sector. Dickin (2019) showed that empowered women used improved sanitation facilities and, hence, greater progress can be made towards universal access to WASH services and reducing related gender disparities (Heckert et al., 2023; Dery et al., 2020). In WELI, an index proposed by Galiè et al. (2019), decision related to nutrition is an indicator showing the inextricable link in question (Dery et al. 2020; Kaluwa et al., 2022).

4.7 STRATEGIES TO ENHANCE NUTRITION AND FOOD SECURITY

Strategies by the government of India to deal with low nutritional well-being can be considered alongside policies like removal of taxes on unprocessed food and taxing unhealthy and unhygienic foods (as in the UK, Mexico, France, and Norway). Education and awareness regarding nutrition in particular and health in general also help in coping with this issue (Shahid & Bishop, 2019).

Government strategies for dealing with women's undernutrition affecting their empowerment and decision-making power to access infrastructure and policy benefits have been injected through policies like schemes like ICDS, POSHAN Abhiyaan, National Food Security Mission, Pradhan Mantri Matru Vandana Yojana, and National Rural Livelihood Mission in the past few years. One major potential strategy is women's education, and Rao (2010) discusses how the literacy level of women can impact various aspects of their lives, including reproductive behavior, contraceptive use, child health and upbringing, hygiene practices, employment opportunities, and overall societal status. According to World Bank data for 2022, only 69% of Indian women were literate.

According to an NHM report accessed on May 18, 2024, the Anemia Mukt Bharat strategy aims to address the issue of anemia among six specific beneficiary groups. These groups include children aged 6–59 months, children aged 5–9 years, adolescents aged 10–19 years, pregnant and lactating women, and women of reproductive age (15–49 years). The strategy focuses on implementing six interventions in a life cycle approach to effectively reduce anemia.

Through a comprehensive analysis of various factors, strategic intervention can effectively contribute to the achievement of the objectives set by SDGs, MPI, HDI, and other economic indicators. This approach allows for substantial advancements towards these objectives. Khandelwal et al. (2014) conducted a thorough examination of the government programs for women and children in India. On analyzing the results, it was discovered that of the 33 MCHN interventions, six were identified as direct nutrition interventions that could potentially make a difference during the 1000-day period. Upon conducting a thorough examination of these interventions, it has become evident that there are areas that could benefit from improvement and valuable lessons to be learned. The Indian government has implemented various interventions that have had a substantial impact on the 1000-day period. However, there is room for improvement in the nutrition component, with interventions that prioritize healthcare needs, immunization, cash transfers, and other related areas. The importance of nutrition was only recognized in terms of ensuring the availability of sufficient food, without taking into account the specific details of macro and micro nutrient content. This aspect could benefit from some improvements in the interventions. Additionally, Ghosh et al. (2020) highlight the importance of nutritional intervention as an indicator of the utilization of prenatal and postnatal healthcare services for both the mother and child. Receiving antenatal care (ANC) and delivering at a health facility with skilled assistance play a crucial role in addressing malnutrition and reducing infant and child mortality rates. Several studies have highlighted the impact of ANC and skilled delivery on these important health outcomes. The low proportion of institutional deliveries (that is, deliveries at a healthcare facility), along with inadequate health assistance, contribute significantly to the rates of maternal and child mortality. The rate of institutional deliveries has risen significantly, from 39% to 79%, between 2004–06 and 2015–16. Enhancing antenatal care coverage yields a notable effect on boosting institutional deliveries. It is concerning to see such a significant difference in institutional deliveries among states, even though the reproductive child health program initiative has been in place since the 1990s (Figure 4.3). Proper antenatal

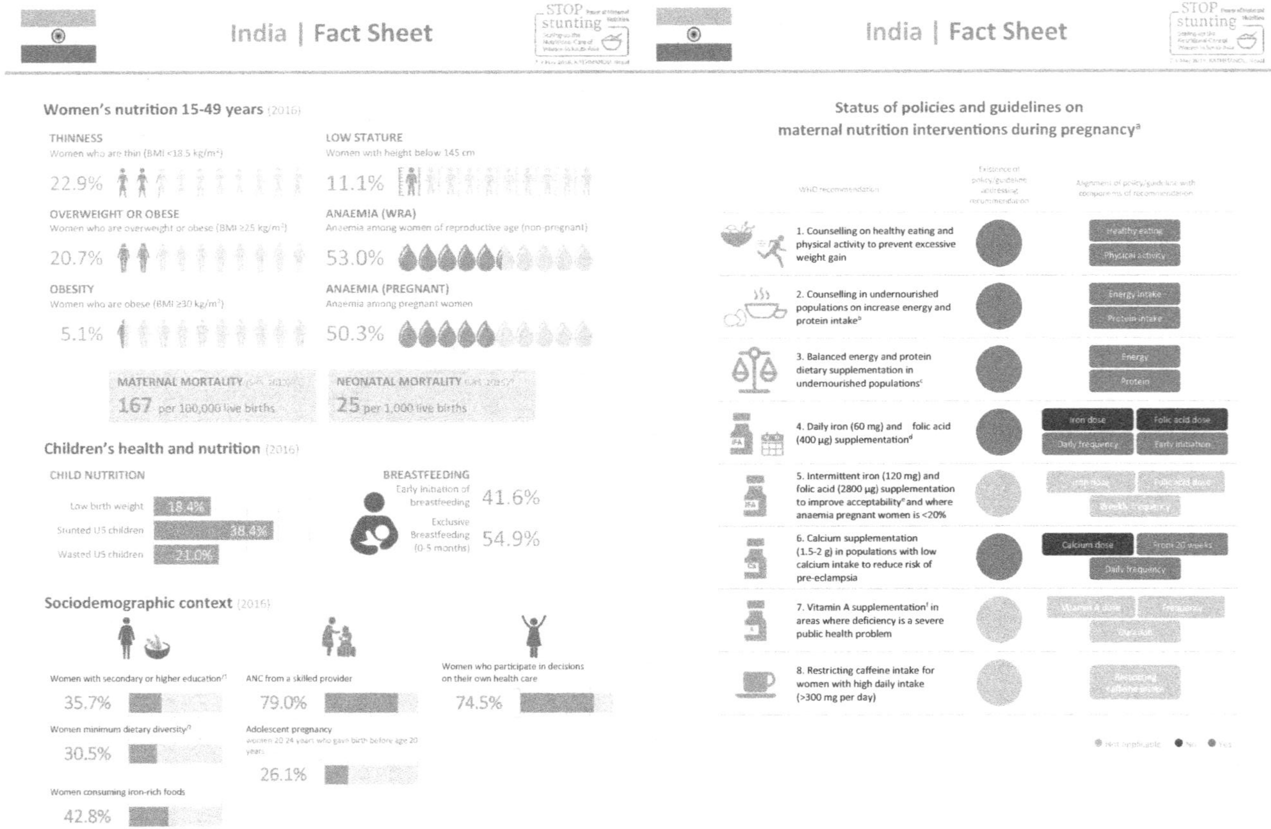

FIGURE 4.3 Nutritional care of pregnant women in South Asia: policy environment and program action. (UNICEF, 2019.)

check-ups have been shown to reduce the risk of infant mortality for mothers of all age groups, according to UNICEF (2019).

India's ICDS (integrated child development services) scheme is the world's largest community-based program (Sachdev & Dasgupta, 2001) and was introduced on October 2, 1975. The major focus of the scheme is to target children who are 6 years old or less, pregnant and lactating mothers, and women aged between 16 and 44. This policy aims to improve education and awareness regarding health, nutrition, and education, popularly known as knowledge, attitude, and practices (KAP) of the target community. This policy was introduced into the local community through a focal point, or "Anganwadi", located within the range of convenient reach. The Anganwadi system is managed by the female Anganwadi worker (AWW) appointed by a committee constituted by the state government/ UT administration on an honorary basis, performing as a key-level functionary. The Anganwadi center serves as a central point for immunization, distribution of vitamin A, iron and folic acid tablets, and treatment of small ailments and first aid. It is also the functionary center for activities performed by auxiliary nurses and midwives (ANM). It incorporates health check-up and referral services, which include regular check-ups, body weight recording, immunization, and management of malnutrition, diarrhea, deworming, and other general ailments. To attain the policy objectives, AWW uses a certain day for an immunization session or a "take home" collection day for growth-monitoring activities. Chart is prepared for growth recording to identify undergrowth or malnutrition, if any. However, this scheme was not able to perform at the benchmark due to poor understanding of methodology and technicality (including in relation to weight recording), and paucity of time. To overcome these challenges it requires good training, supervision, and support. Moreover, it is observed in many areas that ICDC progress is not good and other plateau effects are significant after the initial elevation. This situation can be explained by diversified geographical and socioeconomic conditions across the country, which include local customs, whims and fancies, poor community mobilization and participation, insufficient logistical support, irregular supply, inadequate staff, inappropriate time budgeting, and erroneous understanding of the major targets of ICDS service components (Gupta et al., 2013).

Another government strategy to target nutritional uplift among women is POSHAN Abhiyaan, which was launched on March 8, 2018 in the Jhunjhunu district of Rajasthan. Its objective is to reduce malnutrition by using a life cycle concept adopting a synergized and result-oriented approach. This policy intervention works based on five pillars. The first pillar, known as ICDS, uses the common application software CAS to trigger action for service providers facilitating better outreach to beneficiaries for the first 3 years (1000 days). The second pillar is convergence action planning, which includes development and operationalization of a convergence nutritional action plan at state, district, and block level by integrating coordinated and cross-sectional efforts to improve the nutritional outcomes. The third pillar is capacity building of ICDS officials/functionaries through an incremental learning approach focused on progressive learning and understanding the actions and their contribution to maternal, infant, and young child nutrition. The fourth pillar is centered around Jan Andolan, which involves behavior change communication and community mobilization. This pillar focuses on creating awareness among beneficiaries about important technical areas such as antenatal care, institutional delivery, breastfeeding, complementary feeding, growth monitoring and promotion, immunization and vitamin A, prevention of anemia, management of diarrhea, and hygiene and sanitation practices. This is achieved through the development and implementation of mid-media, mass media, and community-based multisectoral campaigns. The last pillar provides performance incentives to encourage governments to increase nutritional incentives for frontline officials to achieve objectives. Additionally, monthly monetary incentives are given to the AWWs for implementing the ICDS-CAS. However, in order to accomplish the goals set out by all five pillars, there is one hurdle that must be overcome: the requirement to accurately monitor India's progress in addressing undernutrition at the district, state, and national levels using relevant and high-quality data (Pooja, 2022).

Even after so many efforts by government and non-government sectors, the situation has not changed much, and has even degraded in many states, as nutrition is not a priority for the government. The Mid-Day Meal Scheme has positively impacted the enrolment ratio in primary school and benefited socially disadvantaged groups, especially girls (Paul & Mondal, 2012; Kaur, 2021). However, there have been many incidents reported in the media of children and adults becoming sick after eating the mid-day meal, which is distributed for the purpose of providing nutrition. No proper measures of hygiene and health are being followed while preparing and distributing the food (Deodhar et al., 2007). Even the nutritional value of food items served as part of the mid-day meal are not at par with the recommended nutritional daily allowances (RDA) stipulated by ICMR (Deodhar et al., 2010).

The National Food Security Mission is a policy-level strategy implemented in 2007–08 to ensure food security for all. Its main objective is to increase the production of rice, wheat, and pulses by 10, 8, and 2 million tonnes respectively by the end of the XI Plan. This will be achieved through expanding agricultural areas, improving productivity, restoring soil fertility, creating employment opportunities, and boosting the farm-level economy. The Mission will be maintained throughout the 12th Five Year Plan with the goal of producing an extra 25 million tonnes of food grains. This will include 10 million tonnes of rice, 8 million tonnes of wheat, 4 million tonnes of pulses, and 3 million tonnes of coarse cereals by the conclusion of the XII Plan. Under the XI Plan, the National Food Security Mission for Rice (NFSM-Rice) was carried out in 144 districts across 16 states. Similarly, the NFSM for Wheat (NFSM-Wheat) was implemented in 142 districts across 9 states, while the NFSM for Pulses (NFSM-Pulses) was executed in 468 districts across 16 states. Starting from the year 2012–13, the states of Arunachal Pradesh, Manipur, Meghalaya, Mizoram, Nagaland, and Sikkim have been included in the NFSM-Rice program. Two hill states have also been included (Naik & Nethrayini, 2019; Jose et al., 2020).

Another popular and crucial government policy is the National Rural Livelihoods Mission. Launched in June 2011, this initiative aims to provide institutional platforms for the rural poor. Its objective is to empower people to enhance their family incomes by providing assistance for their livelihoods and facilitating access to financial services. The brief assesses the accomplishments of the project throughout its first decade. The analysis reveals that the mission has achieved some accomplishments in enhancing the well-being of rural women, who play a crucial role in the initiative, and subsequently their families. The accomplishments primarily focus on the development of social connections, the activation of community involvement, and a certain level of availability of financial resources. The NRLM acknowledges that the means of earning a living for the three different categories of impoverished individuals, namely the "least poor", "middle poor", and "poorest/vulnerable poor", are not the same. To target them effectively, it is necessary to thoroughly analyze their livelihoods, vulnerabilities, and social circumstances, and thereafter develop methods to address these particular weaknesses (Mishra et al., 2020; Vir, 2023). Various policies and initiatives have been implemented to address and narrow this gap, but still there is scope for improvement, and making it a national priority is necessary (Shankar et al., 2017).

4.8 CONCLUSION

With a detailed and in-depth understanding captured across evidence from the literature, we explored the association between nutritional security, impacts on the overall health and nutritional status of women, and opportunities to empower them from all walks of life. We looked across conceptual literature, a secondary database for health and nutrition variables and indices, and evaluated the state-led interventions and other implementation models to develop and strengthen this association. The theoretical and conceptual framework used for this study examined indicators such as nutritional diet, workforce participation, food consumption, and state-led interventions in particular. Literary evidence clearly and repeatedly emphasizes the positive relation between the food and nutritional security of the household and the empowered profile of women, which has been implicated due to gender equality across food systems globally. Databases and trends over time have suggested an improvement in the food consumption and anthropometric profile of women, but even then malnutrition and anemia remain at significantly high levels. Although women are facilitating a multi-actor role in the food systems, their empowered role in society, uplifting them above the social norms, identities, and customary suppression, would lead to improved growth and development indices in national and global contexts. International frameworks intervening in solutions towards food security need to encourage a gender-neutral and equity-oriented lens. The need is also for strategic intervention, cutting across intersections of vulnerabilities, livelihood, and social circumstances that cripple the resources required for food and nutrition security of the community, and food systems at large.

REFERENCES

Agarwal, B. (2018). Gender equality, food security and the sustainable development goals. *Current Opinion in Environmental Sustainability*, 34, 26–32.

Agarwal, S., & Sethi, V. (2013). Nutritional disparities among women in urban India. *Journal of Health, Population, and Nutrition*, 31(4), 531

Alkire, S., & Foster, J. (2011). Counting and multidimensional poverty measurement. *Journal of Public Economics*, 95(7–8), 476–487.

Alkire, S., Meinzen-Dick, R., Peterman, A., Quisumbing, A., Seymour, G., & Vaz, A. (2013). The women's empowerment in agriculture index. *World Development*, 52, 71–91.

Antony, G. M., & Laxmaiah, A. (2008). Human development, poverty, health & nutrition situation in India. *Indian Journal of Medical Research*, 128(2), 198–205.

Baye, K. (2017). The Sustainable Development Goals cannot be achieved without improving maternal and child nutrition. *Journal of Public Health Policy*, 38, 137–145.

Black, R. E., Allen, L. H., Bhutta, Z. A., Caulfield, L. E., De Onis, M., Ezzati, M., ... & Rivera, J. (2008). Maternal and child undernutrition: Global and regional exposures and health consequences. *The Lancet*, 371(9608), 243–260.

Branca, F., Piwoz, E., Schultink, W., & Sullivan, L. M. (2015). Nutrition and health in women, children, and adolescent girls. *BMJ*, 351. doi: https://doi.org/10.1136/bmj.h4173

Daru, J., Zamora, J., Fernández-Félix, B. M., Vogel, J., Oladapo, O. T., Morisaki, N., ... & Khan, K. S. (2018). Risk of maternal mortality in women with severe anaemia during pregnancy and post partum: A multilevel analysis. *The Lancet Global Health*, 6(5), e548–e554.

Deodhar, S. Y., Mahandiratta, S., Ramani, K. V., Mavalankar, D. V., Ghosh, S., & Braganza, V. S. (2007). Mid day meal scheme: Understanding critical issues with reference to Ahmedabad city. *Working paper 2007-03-03*. Indian Institute of Management Ahmedabad.

Deodhar, S. Y., Mahandiratta, S., Ramani, K. V., Mavalankar, D., Ghosh, S., & Braganza, V. (2010). An evaluation of mid day meal scheme. *Journal of Indian School of Political Economy*, 22(1–4), 33–49.

DeRosa, L., Das, M., & Millman, S. (2000). Does female disadvantage mean lower access to food? *Population and Development Review*, 26(3), 517–547.

Dery, F., Bisung, E., Dickin, S., & Dyer, M. (2020). Understanding empowerment in water, sanitation, and hygiene (WASH): A scoping review. *Journal of Water, Sanitation and Hygiene for Development*, 10(1), 5–15.

Dickin, S., & Bisung, E. (2019). *Empowerment in WASH Index*. Stockholm Environment Institute. www.jstor.org/stable/resrep22981

Dube, W., & Phiri, A. (2015). Nutrition and economic growth in South Africa: A threshold co-integration approach. *Journal of Economic Studies*, *42*(1), 138–156.

FeedingIndia. (2022). Women Are Hungrier: How Gender Plays A Part In Food Insecurity Retrieved from www.feedingindia.org/blog/how-gender-plays-a-part-in-food-insecurity/

Galiè, A., Teufel, N., Korir, L., Baltenweck, I., Webb Girard, A., Dominguez-Salas, P., & Yount, K. M. (2019). The women's empowerment in livestock index. *Social Indicators Research*, 142(2), 799–825.

Ghosh, S. (2018). India: Nutrition intake and economic growth, a causality analysis. *Development Studies Research*, *5*(1), 69–82.

Ghosh, T. S., Rampelli, S., Jeffery, I. B., Santoro, A., Neto, M., Capri, M., ... & O'Toole, P. W. (2020). Mediterranean diet intervention alters the gut microbiome in older people reducing frailty and improving health status: The NU-AGE 1-year dietary intervention across five European countries. *Gut*, 69(7), 1218–1228.

Global Nutrition Report. (2022). Country Nutrition Profile: India. https://globalnutritionreport.org/resources/nutrition-profiles/asia/southern-asia/india/

Grosso, G., Mateo, A., Rangelov, N., Buzeti, T., & Birt, C. (2020). Nutrition in the context of the sustainable development goals. *European Journal of Public Health*, *30*(Supplement_1), i19–i23.

Gupta, A., Gupta, S., & Nongkynrih, B. (2013). Integrated child development services (ICDS) scheme: A journey of 37 years. *Indian Journal of Community Health*, 25(1), 77–81.

Gupta, S., Pingali, P., & Pinstrup-Andersen, P. (2019). Women's empowerment and nutrition status: The case of iron deficiency in India. *Food Policy*, 88, 101763.

Heckert, J., Raghunathan, K., Myers, E., Ramani, G. V., Faas, S., Ferguson, N., ... & Shrestha, S. (2023). *Development of a Women's Empowerment Metric for Water, Sanitation, and Hygiene (WE-WASH)*. International Food Policy Research Institute.

Jose, S., Gulati, A., & Khurana, K. (2020). *Achieving Nutritional Security in India: Vision 2030*. Indian Council for Research on International Economic Relations.

Joshi, A., Arora, A., Amadi-Mgbenka, C., Mittal, N., Sharma, S., Malhotra, B., ... & Loomba, M. (2019). Burden of household food insecurity in urban slum settings. *PloS One*, 14(4), e0214461.

Kabeer, N. (2021). Three faces of agency in feminist economics: Capabilities, empowerment, and citizenship. In Berik, G. & Kongar, E (eds.), *The Routledge Handbook of Feminist Economics* (pp. 99–107). Routledge.

Kaluwa, C., Oduma, J., Abdirahman, F. A., Kitoga, B. K., Opondoh, A. A., Muchibi, J., ... & Amuguni, J. H. (2022). Using the Women empowerment in livestock index (WELI) to examine linkages between women smallholder livestock farmers' empowerment and access to livestock vaccines in Machakos County of Kenya: Insights and critiques. *Vaccines*, 10(11), 1868.

Kaur, R. (2021). Estimating the impact of school feeding programs: Evidence from mid day meal scheme of India. *Economics of Education Review*, 84, 102171.

Khandelwal, S., Dayal, R., Bhalla, S., & Paul, T. (2014). A review of Government programmes for women and children in India: Implications for nutrition during the thousand day period. *Indian Journal of Nutrition and Dietetics*, 51, 322–339.

Lentz, E., Bageant, E., & Narayanan, S. (2021). Empowerment and nutrition in Niger: Insights from the women's empowerment in nutrition grid. *Food Security*, 13(5), 1227–1244.

Lufuke, M., Bai, Y., Fan, S., & Tian, X. (2022). Women's empowerment, food security, and nutrition transition in Africa. *International Journal of Environmental Research and Public Health*, 20(1), 254.

Malapit, H. J. L., Sraboni, E., Quisumbing, A. R., & Ahmed, A. U. (2019). Intrahousehold empowerment gaps in agriculture and children's well-being in Bangladesh. *Development Policy Review*, 37(2), 176–203.

Malapit, H. J., Sproule, K., Kovarik, C., Meinzen-Dick, R. S., Quisumbing, A. R., Ramzan, F., ... & Alkire, S. (2014). *Measuring Progress Toward Empowerment: Women's Empowerment in Agriculture Index: Baseline Report*. International Food Policy Research Institute.

Manfredini, M. (2020). The effects of nutrition on maternal mortality: Evidence from 19th-20th century Italy. *SSM-Population Health*, 12, 100678.

Masa, R., Chowa, G., & Nyirenda, V. (2017). Prevalence and predictors of food insecurity among people living with HIV enrolled in antiretroviral therapy and livelihood programs in two rural Zambian hospitals. *Ecology of Food and Nutrition*, 56(3), 256–276.

McKay, F. H., Sims, A., & Van Der Pligt, P. (2023). Measuring food insecurity in India: A systematic review of the current evidence. *Current Nutrition Reports*, 12(2), 358–367.

Mishra, A. S., Lakhera, P. C., & Pandey, A. (2021). Assessment of nutritional anemia on the basis of dietary pattern estimation among the population of Garhwal Himalayan region. *Journal of Family Medicine and Primary Care*, 10(2), 669–674.

Mishra, A., Mishra, S. K., Baitharu, I., & Das, T. K. (2020). Food security and nutritional status among rural poor: Evaluating the impact of Rural Livelihood Mission in Odisha, India. *Journal of Reviews on Global Economics*, 9, 141–148.

Moser, C. (2012). *Gender Planning and Development: Theory, Practice and Training*. Routledge.

Naik, V., & Nethrayini, K. R. (2019). Impact assessment of National Food Security Mission (NFSM) on pulses production in Karnataka, India-An economic analysis. *Asian Journal of Agricultural Extension, Economics & Sociology*, 33(1), 1–12.

Narayanan, S., Lentz, E., Fontana, M., De, A., & Kulkarni, B. (2019). Developing the women's empowerment in nutrition index in two states of India. *Food Policy*, *89*, 101780.

National Nutrition Monitoring Bureau. (2017). *Diet and Nutritional Status of Urban Population in India and Prevalence of Obesity, Hypertension, Diabetes and Hyperlipidaemia in Urban Men and Women*. National Institute of Nutrition. www.nin.res.in/downloads/NNMB%20Urban%20Nutrition%20Report%20-Brief%20%20%20report.pdf

Njuki, J., Eissler, S., Malapit, H., Meinzen-Dick, R., Bryan, E., & Quisumbing, A. (2022). A review of evidence on gender equality, women's empowerment, and food systems. *Global Food Security*, 33, 100622.

Nutrition and Food Security. (n.d.). United Nations India. https://india.un.org/en/171969-nutrition-and-food-security

Park, J. H., Moon, J. H., Kim, H. J., Kong, M. H., & Oh, Y. H. (2020). Sedentary lifestyle: Overview of updated evidence of potential health risks. *Korean Journal of Family Medicine*, 41(6), 365–373. https://doi.org/10.4082/kjfm.20.0165

Paul, P. K., & Mondal, N. K. (2012). Impact of mid-day meal programme on academic performance of students: Evidence from few upper primary schools of Burdwan District in West Bengal. *International Journal of Research in Social Sciences*, 2(3), 391–406.

Pooja, M. (2022). National nutrition mission or Poshan Abhiyaan fighting with undernutrition among children, lactating mothers and pregnant women: An analysis. *Journal of the Asiatic Society of Mumbai National*, 96(10), 107–117.

Ramya, R. S. (2021). A demographic study of the multidimensional poverty of women in India. *European Journal of Marketing and Economics*, 4(2), 63–78.

Rao, K. M., Balakrishna, N., Arlappa, N., Laxmaiah, A., & Brahmam, G. N. V. (2010). Diet and nutritional status of women in India. *Journal of Human Ecology*, 29(3), 165–170.

Sachdev, Y., & Dasgupta, J. (2001). Integrated child development services (ICDS) scheme. *Medical Journal Armed Forces India*, 57(2), 139–143.

Saha, S., & Narayanan, S. (2022). A simplified measure of nutritional empowerment: Using machine learning to abbreviate the Women's Empowerment in Nutrition Index (WENI). *World Development*, 154, 105860.

Santhya, K. G., Ram, U., Acharya, R., Jejeebhoy, S. J., Ram, F., & Singh, A. (2010). Associations between early marriage and young women's marital and reproductive health outcomes: Evidence from India. *International Perspectives on Sexual and Reproductive Health*, 36(3), 132–139.

Shahid, S. M., & Bishop, K. S. (2019). Comprehensive approaches to improving nutrition: Future prospects. *Nutrients*, 11(8), 1760.

Shankar, B., Agrawal, S., Beaudreault, A. R., Avula, L., Martorell, R., Osendarp, S., ... & Mclean, M. S. (2017). Dietary and nutritional change in India: Implications for strategies, policies, and interventions. *Annals of the New York Academy of Sciences*, 1395(1), 49–59.

Shetty, P. (2013). Nutrition transition and its health outcomes. *The Indian Journal of Pediatrics*, 80, 21–27.

Sims, A., van der Pligt, P., John, P., Kaushal, J., Kaur, G., & McKay, F. H. (2021). Food insecurity and dietary intake among rural indian women: An exploratory study. *International Journal of Environmental Research and Public Health*, 18(9), 4851.

Sraboni, E., Malapit, H. J., Quisumbing, A. R., & Ahmed, A. U. (2014). Women's empowerment in agriculture: What role for food security in Bangladesh?. *World Development*, 61, 11–52.

Tadesse Tantu, A., Demissie Gamebo, T., Kuma Sheno, B., & Yohannis Kabalo, M. (2017). Household food insecurity and associated factors among households in Wolaita Sodo town, 2015. *Agriculture & Food Security*, 6, 1–8.

Tsiboe, F., Zereyesus, Y. A., Popp, J. S., & Osei, E. (2018). The effect of women's empowerment in agriculture on household nutrition and food poverty in Northern Ghana. *Social Indicators Research*, 138, 89–108.

UN Women. (n.d.). SDG 2: End Hunger, Achieve Food Security and Improved Nutrition and Promote Sustainable Agriculture. www.unwomen.org/en/news/in-focus/women-and-the-sdgs/sdg-2-zero-hunger

UNICEF. (2019). Nutritional Care of Pregnant Women in South Asia: Policy Environment and Programme Action. www.unicef.org/rosa/media/7836/file/Nutritional%20care%20of%20pregnant%20women%20in%20S.Asia_Policy%20environment%20and%20programme%20action_Final.pdf.pdf

Victora, C. G., Adair, L., Fall, C., Hallal, P. C., Martorell, R., Richter, L., & Sachdev, H. S. (2008). Maternal and child undernutrition: Consequences for adult health and human capital. *The Lancet*, 371(9609), 340–357.

Vir, S. C. (2023). Deendayal Antyodaya Yojana-National rural livelihood mission (DAY-NRLM): Potential of women collectives in improving maternal and child nutrition situation. In S. C. Vir (ed.), *Child, Adolescent and Woman Nutrition in India* (pp. 578–622). Routledge.

Visser, J., & Wangu, J. (2021). Women's dual centrality in food security solutions: The need for a stronger gender lens in food systems' transformation. *Current Research in Environmental Sustainability*, 3, 100094.

Wilunda, C., Wanjohi, M., Takahashi, R., Kimani-Murage, E., & Mutoro, A. (2023). Association of women's empowerment with anaemia and haemoglobin concentration in children in sub-Saharan Africa: A multilevel analysis. *Maternal & Child Nutrition*, 19(1), e13426.

World Economic Forum. (2020).The Global Gender Gap Report 2020. Retrieved from www3.weforum.org/docs/WEF_GGGR_2020.pdf

World Health Organisation. (1998). The World Health Report 1998 Life in the 21st Century: A Vision for All. Retrieved from https://apps.who.int/gb/archive/pdf_files/WHA51/ea3.pdf

World Health Organization. (2023). *The State of Food Security and Nutrition in the World 2023: Urbanization, Agrifood Systems Transformation and Healthy Diets Across the Rural–Urban Continuum* (Vol. 2023). Food & Agriculture Organization.

Yaya, S., Uthman, O. A., Okonofua, F., & Bishwajit, G. (2019). Decomposing the rural-urban gap in the factors of under-five mortality in sub-Saharan Africa? Evidence from 35 countries. *BMC Public Health*, 19, 1–10.

Yila, J. O., & Sylla, A. (2020). Women empowerment in addressing food security and nutrition. In Filho, W. L., Azul, A. M., Brandli, L., Özuvar, P. G., & Wall, T (eds.), *Zero Hunger* (pp. 980–990). Cham: Springer International Publishing.

Zheng, X. Y., Han, Y. L., Chao, G. U. O., Zhang, L., Yue, Q. I. U., & Gong, C. H. E. N. (2014). Progress in research of nutrition and life expectancy. *Biomedical and Environmental Sciences*, 27(3), 155–161.

5 Challenges in Capturing Child Nutrition Realities in India

The Role of Village-Level Data (Case Studies)

Prachi Bhasin and Shikha Saxena

5.1 INTRODUCTION

Growth and development in children are very compound and are influenced by various factors like environmental factors, socioeconomic status, genetic composition, medical history, and nutritional intake. This early phase of life lays the foundation of one's health for later life. Consumption of adequate nutrition during this period is crucial for proper development and growth (Mascarenhas et al., 1998; Singh, 2020). India is one of the fastest economically growing nations, with an increase of over 50% in its GDP since 1991. This expanding economy has coincided with the rapidly rising malnutrition rates among children (Chatterjee, 2021). According to the Global Hunger Index (GHI 2023, n.d.), out of 125 countries, India stands on the 111th rank, having 28.7 as a GHI, which is within the range of hunger classed as Serious. This GHI score of India consists of one sixth of child stunting, one third of undernourishment, one sixth of child wasting, and one third of child mortality. However, these data were obtained from a tiny sample size, and they also excluded the initiatives taken by the Indian government to ensure food security. Figure 5.1 illustrates the components of India's GHI score.

Contrary to the GHI, the data obtained from the National Family Health Survey NFHS-5 showed improved nutritional indicators for under-5 children compared to the NFHS-4 (NFHS-4, 2017). The NFHS-5 data are associated with the pre-pandemic period. As per the NFHS-5, wasting (low weight for height) decreased from 21% to 19.3%, stunting (low height for age) reduced from 38.4% to 35.5%, and the prevalence of underweight fell from 35.8% to 32.1%.

Regular evaluation of child nutritional status, such as NFHS and GHI, is essential. This ensures that the children grow and develop properly, with no malnutrition-related health issues, and have an enhanced overall well-being. The data of these evaluations are regularly and easily available to the public, communities, healthcare workers, and the government for a better understanding of where the nation stands in terms of child nutrition. This data act as a guide in planning, implementing, and regulating

DOI: 10.1201/9781003487227-5

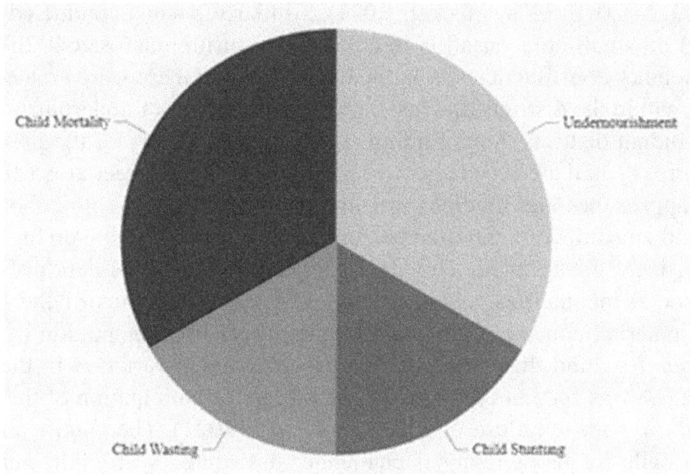

FIGURE 5.1 Components of the Global Hunger Index score for India.

nutrition-related policies and action plans for low- and middle-income nations along with high-income nations (Kim et al., 2021). The significant differences in the disease patterns along with the associated risk factors, in any country, have aided in acknowledging that the national averages are insufficient (Dowell et al., 2016), thus increasing the need to obtain, analyze, and make subnational-level data on the health and well-being of the population (i.e., villages, communities, and tribes). Regardless of the constant accentuation by newer studies on focusing more on variation at finer and smaller geographic levels (Kim et al., 2016, 2018) such as villages or communities, the majority of studies that investigate the subnational levels are somehow completely centered around macro geographic areas, for instance, Chinese provinces (Zhou et al., 2016), or states or districts located in India (Dandona et al., 2017; Kim et al., 2021; Menon et al., 2018).

The Indian districts function as Central Administrative Units (CAU). The Transformation of Aspirational Districts Initiative determines the importance of these districts in the Indian policy administration and has identified 115 districts as aspirational. The Indian government had elected and prioritized these districts for assigning the financial and human resources to boost progress in six developmental domains ((NITI Aayog & Government of India, 2019). Similarly, on the basis of the prevalence of child undernutrition at the district level, different phases of India's POSHAN Abhiyaan have been implemented (NITI Aayog & Government of India, 2018).

However, in recent times, it has been noted that at the district level, the conventional exercise of evaluating health indicators tends to conceal the variations across smaller geographic locations like different administrative blocks or various villages within a single district. Also, current studies have adopted a multilevel approach and have found that within a single district, there is significant small-area heterogeneity in various indicators associated with development and health like women's body mass index (BMI), child nutrition, child-sex ratio, and poverty (Kim et al., 2016, 2018;

Rodgers et al., 2020; Štorkánová et al., 2021). Similarly, a study conducted by Rajpal et al. (2021) on small-area variation in child undernutrition across 640 districts and 543 parliamentary constituencies in India discovered that there were greater levels of inequalities within the districts that had a greater prevalence of undernutrition among children in Indian districts. Such findings supported the theory of the prevalence of variations across small areas (villages) within a single much larger area (district).

Various approaches and methods are employed during data collection. The data collected by the health workers often get aggregated while focusing on higher levels, for instance, local government. This data aggregation limits the depth of data analysis. The social inequalities rooted in the socioeconomic status of the household along with maternal education also hamper the proper implementation of the nutritional interventions and their analysis. A total geographic variation in the range of 54.2% to 72.3% was accounted for in Indian villages in anticipation of the estimates of child anthropometric failure in 2021 (Kim et al., 2021). The significance of this village data calls for recognizing if challenges associated with child nutrition are to be explored and dealt with. Village-level data allows more precise, focused, and well-informed prioritization, which can radically shift the paradigm of Indian policymaking, hence actually aiding in preventing nutrition-associated complications in children. A more comprehensive understanding of child nutrition realities in India can be achieved by utilizing strategies such as precision mapping, ASHA workers' involvement, employing advanced technological tools, and collecting fine-grained data, which we will be discussing later in the chapter.

5.2 ANTHROPOMETRIC FAILURE IN CHILDREN

India stands in 111th position in the rankings given by the GHI (GHI 2023), which is alarming. About one third of the global stunting prevalence is accounted for by India (Menon et al., 2018), and malnutrition in children continues to be one of the primary public health challenges in India. The anthropometric measures or indicators used for assessing the nutritional status of children under 5 years of age are wasting, stunting, and underweight, and rely on the weight, height/length, age, and sex of the children. Wasting refers to the condition in which the child possesses low weight for height, which can be a result of inadequate food intake or a recent health issue that resulted in weight loss. When a child has a short height for his age, she/he is classified as stunted. Stunting can occur due to inadequate nutritional intake for a prolonged period of time influenced by recurring and chronic illness. Similarly, a child with low weight for his/her age is considered underweight (Ghosh, 2020).

WHO developed a set of standardized anthropometric Z-scores for nutritional status assessment of children under 5 years of age which includes a weight for height Z-score (WHZ), weight-for-age Z-score (WAZ), and height for age Z-score (HAZ) (World Health Organization, 2006). Table 5.1 represents the association between the nutritional status and Z-score.

Children with a Z-score less than −3SD of the median Z-score of the reference population come under the category of severe acute malnutrition (SAM) (Kumar et al., 2018). Comparing these three anthropometric indices against an international

TABLE 5.1
Relationship Between Nutritional Status and Z-Score

Nutritional Status	Z-Score
Wasting	WHZ < −2 SD of the median WHZ score of reference population
Stunting	HAZ < −2 SD of the median HAZ score of reference population
Underweight	WAZ < −2 SD of the median WAZ score of the reference population

Source: World Health Organization (2006).

Note: SD = standard deviation.

reference population gives three distinct patterns of child anthropometric failure and poor growth and development. Although these indices are extremely useful in child nutritional status assessment, there is one limitation: that they may overlap one another, resulting in the possibility of a child falling into two of the three categories, or even into all three categories, at the same time (Khan & Das, 2020). Child malnutrition is associated with increased vulnerability to infectious diseases and impaired cognitive development (Jain et al., 2021a), thus hindering the child's educational and economic outcomes in the long run. Moreover, moderate to mild undernutrition, such as MAM, is further linked with high risks of child mortality (Swaminathan et al., 2019a) as well as accounting for about 50% of child deaths (<5 years) globally every year (Verma & Prasad, 2021).

India has been working for decades to devise policies and launch and implement programs to combat the persistent complications associated with malnutrition. The Indian government approved the National Nutrition Strategy, 2017, which laid out measures in order to escape the vicious cycle of malnutrition through life (NITI; Aayog, 2020). Later, the Indian government released the National Nutrition Mission (NNM), which came to be known as the POSHAN (Prime Minister's Overarching Scheme for Holistic Nutrition) Abhiyaan in the initial months of 2018. The primary aim of NNM was to bring down malnutrition and its associated challenges prevailing in children and women of India (Ministry of Women and Child Development, 2018; Swaminathan et al., 2019b) by 2% annually.

5.3 SMALL-AREA VARIATIONS IN CHILD ANTHROPOMETRIC FAILURE

The nutritional status, growth, and development of a child depend largely on factors like household socioeconomic status, culture, beliefs, living conditions, surrounding environment, demography, climate, and food availability (KC et al., 2018; Striessnig & Bora, 2020). The availability and accessibility of foods are directly or indirectly controlled by agricultural yields and patterns, which means that geographic location plays a significant role in the distal determinants of nutrition (Khan & Mohanty, 2018). These factors vary extensively across regions.

Most of the studies for assessing the prevalence of malnutrition in India together with exploring social and demographic factors associated with malnutrition have been investigated at individual and household levels. However, Indian districts are geographically large, thus exhibiting wide variations or heterogeneity in social and demographic indicators, and ultimately there is great geographical heterogeneity in the less known malnutrition variation across districts (Khan & Mohanty, 2018) as it is considered that malnutrition and poverty are highly associated. The geographical heterogeneity of malnutrition among children in Indian districts is also demonstrated by the research conducted by Khan and Mohanty (2018). Planning for public health and addressing the underlying mesoscale variables linked to child nutrition in India may benefit from the findings. Additionally, the study recommends allocating health resources and putting child health-specific interventions into action in the areas with higher rates of malnutrition prevalence. Indicators of malnutrition also show considerable declines when compared to other proximate and distal determinants, which highlights the importance of intersectoral coordination in the battle against malnutrition in India. Another study breaks down the variation in child anthropometry and anthropometric failure in the country (Mejía-Guevara et al., 2015), showing that there is very little explanation for the variation, even though the majority of it remains at individual level. Most importantly, the distribution of individual-level variables is unable to account for a sizable portion of the variation that may still be attributed to the environmental level (i.e., communities and states). This presents a chance for contextual interventions, which, given the situation of persisting undernutrition among children in India, must immediately concentrate on developing a sufficient and high-quality basic public health infrastructure, which is crucial for the nutrition of children.

Planning intervention in a highly populated nation like India, with finite resources, massive developmental challenges, and geographical and sociocultural variations, requires the determination of the most suitable geographic policy units. The existing data, academic studies, and policy discussions on health and development in the country primarily depend on the average performances of the Indian districts (Rajpal et al., 2021), which overlooks the existence of crucial small-area heterogeneity and other significant policy units within districts. Rajpal et al. (2021) also observed high variation in undernutrition in children across villages/administrative blocks. Their multilevel model estimated a much higher contribution in the total child anthropometric failure variation by villages/administrative blocks. This study is subject to certain limitations as well:

1. It primarily focused on urban administrative blocks and rural villages to study small-area variations, but these cannot be compared directly based on their administrative role and size.
2. Its precisely weighted estimates of mean prevalence and inter-village/administrative block standard deviation (SD) across districts did not account for the socioeconomic and demographic factors which could be contributing to a higher child undernutrition burden for many districts.

All the studies and data collectively conclude variations in children's health and nutritional status across smaller areas. These areas like villages or administrative blocks demand more precise and targeted attention from the policymakers.

5.4 LOSS OF DATA GRANULARITY ON AGGREGATION

Fine-grained data can be referred to as detailed and specific information at the level that is vital for the identification of trends, patterns, and individual needs within a population. Capturing precise and fine data at a sufficiently granular level has persistently been a challenge. Researchers observed that fine-grained or disaggregated data gathered by Anganwadi workers are not available to everyone, since they are mostly found in registers or, if digitized, are aggregated upward and provided to authorities who oversee schemes (Kim et al., 2021). The regularly obtained field data under the Integrated Child Development Scheme (ICDS) are full of issues related to quality (Nambiar et al., 2022). Data of child nutritional status along with their correlates at the district level were initially made available by the NFHS in its fourth round. This information was also included in the most current round, which was conducted at a faster, 4-year interval which allowed for a more thorough analysis and gave researchers an excellent chance to investigate variations at the district level throughout India using a variety of geocoding and small-area estimation approaches (Kim et al., 2021; Srivastava et al., 2021). There is now a better understanding of the geographic variations in the patterns of child undernutrition along with its correlates, only because of the availability of district level data from NFHS-4 and NHFS-5. Research has also contributed to highlighting the importance of coordinated efforts and proactive measures in addressing the problem of undernourishment among children (Menon et al., 2018; Nambiar et al., 2022).

Data granularity is lost during the process of collecting individual data at the local government unit level and aggregating it to the national level, which is where most decision-making takes place. Averages at the state or district level conceal microlevel differences. To meet India's nutritional targets, microdata collection and additional analysis are essential. Focusing on local development issues in such areas will assist local and regional authorities that have the power to make decisions, such as the Block Development Officers and Members of Panchayats, in comprehending the many variations at granular levels and the success and failure of ground-level policies and interventions (Nambiar et al., 2022). The availability of such data would help highlight regional differences, analyze patterns and correlates of child undernutrition at a finer scale, and identify areas that require prioritization.

The lack of fine-grained data can impact the results of child malnutrition in several ways (Maitra et al., 2017), some of which are as follows:

1. *Inaccurate results:* It is difficult to determine the prevalence and severity of child malnutrition in particular communities without precise data. This may lead to over or underestimation of the issue, which will influence the allocation of resources and approaches.
2. *Limited understanding of causes:* Individual behaviors, healthcare accessibility, socioeconomic variables, and environmental influences are among the

primary causes of child malnutrition that require fine-grained data to fully comprehend. In the absence of this comprehensive data, our understanding of the fundamental root causes of malnutrition may remain limited.

3. *Ineffective targeting of intervention:* The lack of fine-grained data may result in general or all-encompassing interventions that are not able to adequately address the unique requirements of undernourished kids in various areas. Adapting interventions based on comprehensive data is essential to optimize results and impact.
4. *Policy formulation challenges:* At the government level, the absence of fine-grained data can hinder the formulation of evidence-based policies and programs to address child malnutrition. Without a clear understanding of the specific issues faced by different communities, policy formulation may lack nuance and effectiveness. To mitigate the impact of the lack of fine-grained data on child malnutrition, it is crucial to emphasize the collection of detailed and individual-level data through robust evaluation systems. This can involve the use of digital technologies, such as mobile data collection tools, to gather and analyze fine-grained data at scale.

Data collected by health workers often get aggregated upwards and may not be digitized at all points of delivery. Aggregated summaries or trends may lead to the loss of individual data and restrict the depth of analysis. Acquiring fine-grained data and performing precision mapping, which involves gathering data from a smaller geographic area, are crucial for determining priority target areas and evaluating the efficaciousness of local plans and policies. When individual local authorities are given access to fine-grained data, they may fully realize its utility by converting it into action on the ground (Kim et al., 2021). These measures would facilitate the accountability of gram panchayats and local health, sanitation, and nutrition committees for children's well-being and development.

There has always been a persistent significant disparity in the assessment of the prevalence of malnutrition among the states and union territories. These differences have indicated that, rather than sticking with a single national approach, interventions must be developed and guided following the specific issues of each region (Kapur & Suri, 2020) at the subnational levels.

5.5 VARIATIONS IN DATA COLLECTION APPROACHES FOR NUTRITIONAL SURVEILLANCE

As stated in the first set of guidelines on the topic, published in 1976, nutritional surveillance in low-income countries entails the routine and methodical collecting of data on nutritional outcomes and exposures: "Surveillance should provide ongoing information about the nutritional conditions of the population and the factors that influence them" (WHO, 1976). Globally, undernutrition is receiving a greater spotlight. Since the government has pledged to address this issue in their nations, longitudinal data are now required to address issues of accountability and equity. Hence, there is a new and significant potential function for nutrition surveillance (Tuffrey, 2016).

The data collected from nutritional surveillance are put to use in various manners, including tracking the progress made toward reaching nutrition goals, identifying risk factors for malnutrition, assessing the nutritional status, evaluating programs and interventions, assessing the delivery and coverage of services, assessing the impact of policy changes, and assessing the influence of changes in nutrition policies (Tuffrey & Hall, 2016).

Primary data for nutrition surveillance are obtained mainly through three methods: the sentinel monitoring system, repeated cross-sectional surveys, and data collection in schools. The three main sources for collecting secondary data for surveillance are feeding centers, anthropometry data from healthcare centers, and community-based anthropometric data.

5.6 PRIMARY DATA COLLECTION

Sentinel monitoring system

In sentinel monitoring systems, data are routinely provided from a predetermined sample of sites. These systems frequently use purposive sampling at one point or another. The reports may be used to identify patterns within the target population. The target group may be all citizens of the country, as in the case of Mozambique's system (Doledec, 2014), residents of a livelihood zone, a region that is particularly prone to malnutrition, or some other specifically designated geographic area. These systems, when put in place correctly, allow for the efficient use of scarce resources for surveillance purposes. They also facilitate quick, adaptable problem-solving and subsequent monitoring. In India, the system was specifically created to gather data on maternal nutrition status, Infant and Young Child Feeding (IYCF), and child anthropometry through the nation's current healthcare system. These data were intended to help identify national nutrition trends and to give early warning signs of any potential malnutrition issues that would need to be addressed (Chinjekure et al., 2018).

Repeated cross-sectional surveys

At the subnational level, repeated surveys are being conducted at regular intervals of 1, 3, 4, 6, or 12 months for nutrition surveillance reasons using probability sampling techniques. For the reasons mentioned above, cluster sampling is employed practically. New clusters can be created for every cycle of data gathering, or previously created clusters can be utilized in later rounds. The development of nutrition survey methods that require relatively small samples without significantly sacrificing precision has received attention recently, considering the high expense of high-quality surveys. Cross-sectional surveys are being used more frequently to track nutrition status since they are less expensive and yield more reliable results than they did decades ago (Tuffrey & Hall, 2016).

Rapid SMART, a less expensive rapid survey technique derived from the conventional SMART method, was recently created a few years ago for use in emergencies (SMART, 2014). The surveys can communicate significant findings within a day or two of data collection by collecting data on a limited number of variables and requiring a fixed sample size that allows for sufficient precision to be achieved.

Data collection in schools

In collecting data in schools, there is typically no sampling involved in the technique to gather data on schoolchildren; instead, all children at a certain stage or stages of schooling are involved. This sets the approach apart from other primary data collection approaches for nutrition surveillance. The limitations of this approach are related to potential sources of bias, but overall, it is less expensive than traditional surveys. For instance, children enrolled in school are unlikely to be representative of the broader community if the percentage of kids starting Class 1 in a few years after the official entry age is less than roughly 80%. Additionally, bias is created if the dataset is incomplete and if the missing children do not occur randomly, for instance if school attendance is less and the children most likely to miss school are those from lower socioeconomic backgrounds (Tuffrey & Hall, 2016).

5.7 SECONDARY DATA COLLECTION

Feeding centers

Admissions to feeding centers and community-based management of acute malnutrition (CMAM) help in the collection of secondary data. CMAM data reporting is mandatory in several countries, yet the individual national systems are often unable to sync with the new reporting package. This results in parallel reporting systems as well as different performance indicator calculations sometimes. The continuous reporting of categories and indicators might be promoted by using the recommended guidelines and the CMAM reporting software, which allows the comparison of the performance data across clinics, implementers, and nations.

Various other new methods for survey have been introduced, such as centric systematic area sampling (CSAS), simplified lot quality assurance sampling evaluation of access and coverage (SLEAC), semi-quantitative evaluation of access and coverage (SQUEAC), and simple spatial survey methods (S3M) (Tuffrey & Hall, 2016). These methods have made it possible to conduct coverage audits more efficiently, quickly, and regularly.

Anthropometric data from healthcare centers

The primary source of the anthropometric data that are regularly collected by the health systems is child-based growth monitoring in healthcare centers. These data are then utilized for surveillance and may contribute to providing an early warning of increasing food insecurity and declining health conditions in communities. By identifying susceptible geographic locations, such data may help with intervention targeting decisions. The data may be particularly helpful in emergency situations where physical insecurity precludes conducting surveys. Sentinel clinics are selected at sites based on factors such as community vulnerability or the clinic's typicality within a livelihood zone (Tuffrey & Hall, 2016). Resources are then allocated to these critical clinics to enhance data-gathering and analysis procedures.

Community-based anthropometric data

A variety of methods are used by community health systems to gather anthropometry data, such as screening children for malnutrition, screening children for community-based growth monitoring, and screening children for referral to feeding programs.

5.8 VARIABLES TO CONSIDER WHEN SELECTING METHODS FOR DATA COLLECTION

The five most important variables that are to be considered when selecting a method for data collection for a study are as follows (see also Table 5.2).

1. *Accuracy* of the data collected is extremely important for a data collection process which lays the foundation of any study. Data accuracy ensures that the results obtained and the study conclusions are correct.
2. *Time* consumed in data collection represents the importance and relevance of the data. However, too much time consumption can be somewhat inconvenient to the investigators.
3. *Costs* incurred during the process of data collection, similar to the time consumed, represent the importance of the data: the greater the cost, the higher

TABLE 5.2
Data Collection Methods

Data Collection Method	Accuracy	Time	Cost	Utility	Reliability and Validity
Primary Data Collection					
(a) Sentinel monitoring system	High	Moderate	Moderate	High	High
(b) Repeated cross-sectional surveys	High	Moderate	Moderate	High	High
(c) Data collection in schools	Moderate	Low	Low	Moderate	Moderate
Secondary Data Collection					
(a) Feeding center	Moderate	Low	Low	High	Moderate
(b) Anthropometric data from healthcare centers	High	Low	Low	High	High
(c) Community-based anthropometric data	Moderate	Low	Low	High	Moderate

the importance of the data and the conclusion. Higher costs also indicate the number of staff and volunteers employed and the type of technologies used.

4. *Utility* is the most crucial factor to consider while gathering data, since it indicates the value of the information regardless of whether the original goal is being achieved.
5. *Reliability and validity* of the data are another essential component of data collecting, because a result based on invalid or unreliable data will not be regarded as credible.

5.9 HOUSEHOLD SOCIOECONOMIC STATUS AND CHILD MALNUTRITION

Household wealth also affects the issue of malnutrition in children. In rural India, child malnutrition has been reported to mainly affect poor children. For example, limited access to maternal healthcare services, compromised newborn care due to parental illiteracy, and many other factors are responsible for the vulnerability of low-income children to malnutrition. In addition, according to a study by scholars Cashman et al. (2021), "economic resources, measured through ownership of household assets, are positively correlated with parental involvement in education." This implies that families with more assets can afford learning materials and activities, which may alter the role of malnutrition. Moreover, the decomposition analysis conducted in the study emphasizes the fact that variations in undernutrition among richer and poorer households have been accountable for household wealth. Thus, the researchers indicate that closing the gap between privileged and underprivileged households is possible if economic differences are addressed through increased availability of public services and educational campaigns regarding maternal and child health in poor communities (Alcott & Rose, 2017; Cashman et al., 2021).

One important issue in understanding the extent of undernutrition among children in India, especially in the states that make up the Empowered Action Group (EAG) is the correlation between household wealth and malnutrition. Research has repeatedly demonstrated that compared to children from wealthier homes, those from poorer households are more likely to experience malnutrition. The availability of wholesome food, access to sufficient healthcare, clean water, and sanitary facilities are all closely related to this connection (Chowdhury et al., 2023). The ability of families to pay for medical bills and make investments in their children's well-being is also influenced by family wealth. To create successful interventions to reduce child malnutrition in India, particularly in the EAG states, the discrepancy in household income must be addressed. The socioeconomic condition of the household has a significant influence on how common child malnutrition is in India. Research suggests that having a wealthier home is linked to having more access to different types of social capital, which can have a big impact on how well children do in school. Richer households tend to gain from social capital networks, which include linkages to formal institutions like government, healthcare, and education, as well as from bonding and bridging groups. They also profit from easier access to resources. Improved child health outcomes can result from these types of social capital, especially when it comes to lowering the likelihood of underweight children. The distribution of social capital is emphasized as a critical component in resolving health disparities among children in rural India, coupled with its differential value and geographic location (Story & Carpiano, 2017). Through an awareness of how socioeconomic variables influence access to various types of social capital, interventions to address health inequalities and malnutrition in children may be successfully adapted for vulnerable communities.

Child malnutrition is significantly influenced by socioeconomic disparity in India. Child malnutrition is still a serious problem in the country, even with its impressive economic progress. Many children suffer from stunting, being underweight, and wasting. This discrepancy is frequently associated with economic disparities that exist within India across various areas and socioeconomic categories. The distribution of childhood malnutrition reveals the socioeconomic gap, with poor regions having greater rates of malnourishment. There is an unequal distribution of child malnutrition due to several factors, including poverty, restricted educational opportunities, poor sanitary facilities, and lack of access to safe drinking water (Singh et al., 2019). Furthermore, a mother's height, education, and health-seeking habits are important factors that impact her child's nutritional condition. To effectively combat child malnutrition in India, socioeconomic inequality must be addressed. Specific interventions that improve marginalized communities' capacity to access essential resources, improve educational opportunities, and improve their access to basic amenities can all help reduce the quantity of malnourished children in the country.

It is impossible to exaggerate the significance of families in explaining variations in child malnutrition in India. Analysis of data from the National Family Health Survey of India found that households, not communities, districts, or states, had the highest amount of variance in child malnutrition outcomes. This highlights how important it is to address socioeconomic factors at the household level, such as asset and social deprivation, to avoid poor child development outcomes in those households that are already at risk (Jain et al., 2021b). Policymakers may successfully tackle child malnutrition in India by identifying families as a significant source of variation and implementing targeted household-level interventions that are in line with the objectives of the National Nutrition Strategy (NNS). India's urban population's disparity in child undernutrition is a complex problem with many underlying causes. Even with India's notable economic progress, a considerable proportion of children living in metropolitan areas still experience undernourishment. Health-related issues, demographics, and socioeconomic differences all have an impact on this undernutrition. According to a National Family Health Survey analysis of 640 districts, there is an adverse relationship between district economic development and children underweight and stunting. There are considerable regional variations in the frequency of stunting and underweight children, with larger percentages seen in areas such as central, east, and west India. Open defecation, mother's height and education, and availability of clean drinking water are important factors that contribute to the disparity in undernutrition that affects children living in urban areas. Furthermore, the research emphasizes that maternal, environmental, and health-seeking variables account for over 85% of the disparity in stunting, underweight, and wasting in urban children. The results highlight the critical need for focused legislative initiatives to combat poverty, provide access to nutrition-specific treatments for children under 2 years, promote good hygiene, and educate the public on nutrition and health (Singh et al., 2020).

5.10 CASE STUDIES

Maharashtra

In two districts of the Indian state of Maharashtra, namely Pune District and Sangli District, a community-based cross-sectional study was carried out in 16 randomly chosen clusters in 2019. Mothers of children under the age of 5 years were interviewed as a part of a household-to-household survey to gather data. The coverage included 2929 mothers in total, along with 3671 children under 5 years. The differences found in the information gathered from the two areas in the Indian state of Maharashtra might offer important new perspectives on the frequency and contributing variables of undernourishment in children. Researchers can find differences in socioeconomic characteristics, healthcare availability, malnutrition rates, and nutritional behaviors by examining the data for each district independently. These variations might be caused by several things, including regional variations in healthcare facilities, educational attainment, economic growth, and cultural norms (Gothankar et al., 2018; Murarkar et al., 2020). Comprehending these variances is crucial in customizing treatments and policies to suit the unique requirements of individual communities.

Researchers might further improve their understanding of localized variables impacting child malnutrition by using village-level data in the study. With this fine-grained approach, specific interventions may be made at the village level, guaranteeing that resources are distributed effectively to tackle the distinct problems that each community faces.

Chakradharpur, Jharkhand

The malnutrition research conducted in Chakradharpur, Jharkhand, offers a thorough grasp of the community's knowledge, attitudes, and caregiving practices (KAP analysis) concerning health and nutrition, as well as how these factors affect the behavior of those seeking healthcare. The study's findings indicate that traditional and cultural practices offer a significant role in the healthcare and nutrition of newborns, infants, and young children. The research involved in-depth interviews and group discussions with a variety of stakeholders, including mothers/caregivers, frontline health workers, community representatives, and social leaders. The study also emphasized the lack of social safety nets, seasonal male migration, and restricted access to local health facilities as additional variables that put mothers and caregivers at risk and ultimately impacted appropriate infant care and feeding habits (Chaand et al., 2019). This study emphasizes the importance of collecting data at the village level because it allows for a more detailed and personalized understanding of the issues and attitudes related to malnutrition. This helps to create programs and interventions specifically tailored to the needs and circumstances of the villages.

West Bengal

The purpose of the West Bengal study in India was to determine the prevalence of malnutrition among rural teenagers in the age range of 10 to 17 years, as well as the relationship between this condition and sociodemographic variables. The results showed that undernutrition impacted a sizable fraction of adolescents, with around 54% being stunted and 49% being considered thin (Pal et al., 2017). Numerous sociodemographic characteristics, including lower social class, parental education levels, economic position, home cleanliness, and the employment status of the mother, have been associated with this high frequency of undernutrition. It was noted that teenagers with working mothers were more likely to be thin and stunted and that adolescents from economically poor homes were more likely to experience undernourishment.

The study also underlined the critical link between adolescent undernutrition and poverty, emphasizing the necessity of focused initiatives to reduce poverty and health and nutrition education programs. It was also emphasized how crucial village-level data are to the study of malnutrition in India. To successfully address this urgent public health issue, village-level data collection offers a thorough understanding of the socioeconomic and environmental elements impacting undernutrition. This understanding enables personalized treatments and policy actions. The study showed that undernutrition in teenagers living in rural West Bengal is mostly caused by poverty (Pal et al., 2017). The findings point to the necessity of comprehensive initiatives that include health and nutrition-focused education in addition to tactics for reducing poverty. The study also highlights how important village-level data are as a starting point for comprehending and treating undernutrition among Indian adolescent populations.

Village-level data collection provides important insights into the intricate interactions between socioeconomic and environmental elements that contribute to undernutrition, allowing for the creation of targeted interventions and policies. Overall, the results of this study offer important support for the creation of thorough and effective plans to fight undernutrition among West Bengali rural teenagers and, maybe, in other comparable situations throughout India.

5.11 SIGNIFICANCE OF VILLAGE-LEVEL DATA

Village-level data collection offers a more grainy and nuanced understanding of malnutrition in India compared to district-level data collection. India's different sociocultural geography results in significant variations in malnutrition frequency within sections, making village-level data essential for targeted interventions. By collecting data at the village level, policymakers gain a perception of localized factors impacting malnutrition, such as access to healthcare, sanitation, and nutritive resources. Also, village-level data collection facilitates the identification of marginalized communities and vulnerable populations within sections. It enables the identification of specific villages or administrative blocks with disproportionately high malnutrition rates, allowing for effective interventions and allocation of resources.

Village-level data allow the investigators to capture intra-village differences, pressing pockets of extreme deprivation or neglect that may go unnoticed in broader quarter-position assessments. Likewise, village-level data collection promotes community engagement and power in addressing malnutrition. By involving original stakeholders in data collection processes, similar to community health workers and village leaders, there is a greater likelihood of generating accurate and practicable data. This participatory approach fosters community-led enterprise and results, empowering townlets to take the power of their health issues and drive sustainable change. Overall, village-level data collection is a pivotal tool for policymakers and interpreters in designing targeted interventions, addressing original differences, and fostering community-led approaches to combat malnutrition in India. Village-level data collection also facilitates the perpetration of contextually applicable interventions acclimatized to the unique requirements of each community. Unlike the superficial district-level data, which may mask variations in malnutrition frequency across small geographical areas, village-level data allow for the design of interventions that address specific challenges and influence community coffers. For example, a village with limited access to clean water may bear interventions concentrated on improving water and sanitation structures to help waterborne conditions contribute to malnutrition. It enhances the effectiveness of monitoring and evaluation by furnishing real-time feedback on the impact of interventions. Regular data collection at the village level enables stakeholders to track progress, identify arising trends, and acclimate strategies consequently. This iterative process of data-driven decision-making fosters adaptive and responsive approaches to addressing malnutrition, ensuring that resources are allocated efficiently, and interventions remain applicable and effective over time.

Therefore, village-level data collection is necessary to comprehensively understand malnutrition in India, allowing for targeted interventions, community engagement, and substantiation-ground policymaking. By landing the complications of original surroundings and empowering communities to be active actors in the result, village-level data collection holds immense potential to drive meaningful change and ameliorate health issues for vulnerable populations across the country.

5.12 CONCLUSION

This chapter explores the difficulties in documenting the realities of child malnutrition in India, emphasizing the significance of village-level statistics in comprehending and mitigating malnutrition. The various elements impacting a child's growth and development are highlighted at the beginning of the chapter, with a focus on the need for early-stage sufficient nutrition. India continues to have high rates of child malnutrition despite its economic prosperity, as the GHI rankings show, which continues to be a topic for debate due to the lack of in-depth and proper data collection practices conducted for its evaluation. Though nutritional indicators fluctuate among data sources, policymakers and intervention planners need regular reviews to make well-informed decisions.

The main topic of discussion is the necessity of capturing variances at lower geographic levels, such as villages, by moving beyond district-level evaluations. India's many administrative divisions make it difficult to properly address child nutrition and result in a loss of data granularity. Key markers of child malnutrition include wasting, stunting, and being underweight, with severe acute malnutrition presenting a serious risk to a child's health. To effectively diagnose and treat child malnutrition on an individual basis, fine-grained data must be available. Planning for nutrition interventions and surveillance requires using various data-gathering techniques, such as sentinel monitoring systems, recurrent cross-sectional surveys, and data collection in schools.

The chapter also highlights the differences in health outcomes depending on economic circumstances by delving more into the relationship between family socioeconomic status and child malnutrition. Case studies from West Bengal, Jharkhand, and Maharashtra highlight the connection between hunger and poverty and provide insight into regional differences. Data collected at the village level prove to be an invaluable resource for comprehending the regional elements that impact malnutrition and for creating focused treatments for underprivileged populations. The gathering of village-level data is crucial for providing a sophisticated understanding of malnutrition, focused treatments, community involvement, and evidence-based policymaking. Village-level data have great potential to drive meaningful change and improve health outcomes for vulnerable people in India by capturing intra-village disparities, addressing specific obstacles, and empowering communities. The main topic of debate is the necessity of capturing variances at lower geographic levels, such as villages, by moving beyond district-level evaluations. India's many administrative divisions make it difficult to properly address child nutrition. To comprehend the incidence and causes of malnutrition, the chapter also emphasizes the relevance of programs like the National Nutrition Mission (POSHAN Abhiyaan) and the value of data granularity.

REFERENCES

Alcott, B., & Rose, P. (2017). Learning in India's primary schools: How do disparities widen across the grades? *International Journal of Educational Development*, *56*, 42–51. https://doi.org/10.1016/j.ijedudev.2017.05.002

Cashman, L., Sabates, R., & Alcott, B. (2021). Parental involvement in low-achieving children's learning: The role of household wealth in rural India. *International Journal of Educational Research*, *105*, 101701. https://doi.org/10.1016/j.ijer.2020.101701

Chaand, I., Horo, M., Nair, M., Harshana, A., Mahajan, R., Kashyap, V., Falero, F., Escruela, M., Burza, S., & Dasgupta, R. (2019). Malnutrition in Chakradharpur, Jharkhand: An anthropological study of perceptions and care practices from India. *BMC Nutrition*, *5*(1), 35. https://doi.org/10.1186/s40795-019-0299-2

Chatterjee, P. (2021). India's child malnutrition story worsens. *The Lancet Child & Adolescent Health*, *5*, 319–320. https://doi.org/10.1016/S2352-4642(21)00064-X

Chinjekure, A., Shams, Dr. M. Q., Qureshi, Dr. A. B., Safi, Dr. S., & Noor, Dr. R. N. (2018). *Screening for maternal and child malnutrition using sentinel-based national nutrition surveillance in Afghanistan*. ENN.

Chowdhury, S., Kasemi, N., Singh, A., Chakrabarty, M., & Singh, S. (2023). Decomposing the gap in undernutrition among under-five children between EAG and non-EAG states of India. *Children and Youth Services Review*, *145*, 106796. https://doi.org/10.1016/j.childyouth.2022.106796

Dandona, L., Dandona, R., Kumar, G. A., Shukla, D. K., Paul, V. K., Balakrishnan, K., Prabhakaran, D., Tandon, N., Salvi, S., Dash, A. P., Nandakumar, A., Patel, V., Agarwal, S. K., Gupta, P. C., Dhaliwal, R. S., Mathur, P., Laxmaiah, A., Dhillon, P. K., Dey, S., … Swaminathan, S. (2017). Nations within a nation: Variations in epidemiological transition across the states of India, 1990–2016 in the Global Burden of Disease Study. *The Lancet*, *390*(10111), 2437–2460. https://doi.org/10.1016/S0140-6736(17)32804-0

Doledec, D. (2014). *Analysis of the sentinel site nutrition surveillance system in Mozambique*. Washington, DC: USAID Food and Nutrition Technical Assistance.

Dowell, S. F., Blazes, D., & Desmond-Hellmann, S. (2016). Four steps to precision public health. *Nature*, *540*(7632), 189–191. https://doi.org/10.1038/540189a

GHI 2023. (n.d.). www.globalhungerindex.org

Ghosh, S. (2020). Factors responsible for childhood malnutrition: A review of the literature. *Current Research in Nutrition and Food Science Journal*, *8*(2), 360–370. https://doi.org/10.12944/CRNFSJ.8.2.01

Gothankar, J., Doke, P., Dhumale, G., Pore, P., Lalwani, S., Quraishi, S., Murarkar, S., Patil, R., Waghachavare, V., Dhobale, R., Rasote, K., Palkar, S., & Malshe, N. (2018). Reported incidence and risk factors of childhood pneumonia in India: A community-based cross-sectional study. *BMC Public Health*, *18*(1), 1111. https://doi.org/10.1186/s12889-018-5996-2

Jain, A., Rodgers, J., Kim, R., & Subramanian, S. (2021a). The relative importance of households as a source of variation in child malnutrition: A multilevel analysis in India. *International Journal for Equity in Health, 20*. Article 225. https://doi.org/10.1186/s12939-021-01563-7

Jain, A., Rodgers, J., Kim, R., & Subramanian, S. V. (2021b). The relative importance of households as a source of variation in child malnutrition: A multilevel analysis in India. *International Journal for Equity in Health*, *20*(1), 225. https://doi.org/10.1186/s12939-021-01563-7

Kapur, K., & Suri, S. (2020). *Towards a malnutrition-free India: Best practices and innovations from POSHAN Abhiyaan*. New Delhi: Observer Research Foundation.

KC, S., Wurzer, M., Speringer, M., & Lutz, W. (2018). Future population and human capital in heterogeneous India. *Proceedings of the National Academy of Sciences*, *115*(33), 8328–8333. https://doi.org/10.1073/pnas.1722359115

Khan, J., & Das, S. K. (2020). The burden of anthropometric failure and child mortality in India. *Scientific Reports*, *10*(1), 20991. https://doi.org/10.1038/s41598-020-76884-8

Khan, J., & Mohanty, S. K. (2018). Spatial heterogeneity and correlates of child malnutrition in districts of India. *BMC Public Health*, *18*(1), 1027. https://doi.org/10.1186/s12889-018-5873-z

Kim, J., Liu, Y., Wang, W., Blossom, J. C., Dwivedi, L. K., James, K. S., Sarwal, R., Kim, R., & Subramanian, S. V. (2021). Estimating the Burden of Child Undernutrition for Smaller Electoral Units in India. *JAMA Network Open*, *4*(10), e2129416. https://doi.org/10.1001/jamanetworkopen.2021.29416

Kim, R., Bijral, A. S., Xu, Y., Zhang, X., Blossom, J. C., Swaminathan, A., King, G., Kumar, A., Sarwal, R., Lavista Ferres, J. M., & Subramanian, S. V. (2021). Precision mapping child undernutrition for nearly 600,000 inhabited census villages in India. Proceedings of the National Academy of Sciences, 118(18). https://doi.org/10.1073/pnas.2025865118

Kim, R., Kawachi, I., Coull, B. A., & Subramanian, S. V. (2018). Contribution of socioeconomic factors to the variation in body-mass index in 58 low-income and middle-income countries: An econometric analysis of multilevel data. *The Lancet Global Health*, *6*(7), e777–e786. https://doi.org/10.1016/S2214-109X(18)30232-8

Kim, R., Mohanty, S. K., & Subramanian, S. V. (2016). Multilevel geographies of poverty in India. *World Development*, *87*, 349–359. https://doi.org/10.1016/j.worlddev.2016.07.001

Kumar, P., Bijalwan, V., Patil, N., Daniel, A., Sinha, R., Dua, R., & Seth, A. (2018). Comparison between weight-for-height Z-score and mid upper arm circumference to diagnose children with acute malnutrition in five districts in India. *Indian Journal of Community Medicine*, *43*(3), 190–194. https://doi.org/https://doi.org/10.4103%2Fijcm.IJCM_310_17

Maitra, A., Rote, R. E., & Kuntagod, N. (2017). Managing child malnutrition via digital enablement: Insights from a field trial. In *2017 IEEE Global Humanitarian Technology Conference (GHTC)*, 1–7. New York: IEEE. https://doi.org/10.1109/GHTC.2017.8239273

Mejía-Guevara, I., Krishna, A., Corsi, D. J., & Subramanian, S. V. (2015). Individual and ecological variation in child undernutrition in India. *Journal of South Asian Development*, *10*(2), 168–198. https://doi.org/10.1177/0973174115588841

Menon, P., Headey, D., Avula, R., & Nguyen, P. H. (2018). Understanding the geographical burden of stunting in India: A regression-decomposition analysis of district-level data from 2015–16. *Maternal & Child Nutrition*, *14*(4). https://doi.org/10.1111/mcn.12620

Mascarenhas, M. R., Zemel, B., & Stallings, V. A. (1998). Nutritional assessment in pediatrics. *Nutrition*, *14*(1), 105–115. DOI: https://doi.org/10.1016/S0899-9007(97)00226-8

Ministry of Women and Child Development. (2018). *PM launches National Nutrition Mission, and pan India expansion of Beti Bachao Beti Padhao, at Jhunjhunu in Rajasthan*. New Delhi: Press Information Bureau.

Murarkar, S., Gothankar, J., Doke, P., Pore, P., Lalwani, S., Dhumale, G., Quraishi, S., Patil, R., Waghachavare, V., Dhobale, R., Rasote, K., Palkar, S., & Malshe, N. (2020). Prevalence and determinants of undernutrition among under-five children residing in urban slums and rural area, Maharashtra, India: A community-based cross-sectional study. *BMC Public Health*, *20*(1), 1559. https://doi.org/10.1186/s12889-020-09642-0

Nambiar, A., Agnihotri, S. B., Singh, A., & Arunachalam, D. (2022). Region matters: Mapping the contours of undernourishment among children in Odisha, India. *PloS One*, *17*(6), e0268600. https://doi.org/10.1371/journal.pone.0268600

NFHS-4. (2017). International Institute for Population Sciences (IIPS) and ICF. IIPS: Mumbai. https://dhsprogram.com/pubs/pdf/fr339/fr339.pdf

NITI Aayog. (2020). *Accelerating progress on nutrition in* India: What *w*ill *i*t *t*ake? Third *p*rogress *r*ep*ort*. New Delhi: NITI Aayog.

NITI Aayog, & Government of India. (2018). *Transforming nutrition in* India: POSHAN Abhiyaan. New Delhi: NITI Aayog.

NITI Aayog, & Government of India. (2019). *Transformation of aspirational districts*. New Delhi: NITI Aayog.

Pal, A., Pari, A. K., Sinha, A., & Dhara, P. C. (2017). Prevalence of undernutrition and associated factors. *International Journal of Pediatrics and Adolescent Medicine*, *4*(1), 9–18. https://doi.org/10.1016/j.ijpam.2016.08.009

Rajpal, S., Kim, J., Joe, W., Kim, R., & Subramanian, S. V. (2021). Small area variation in child undernutrition across 640 districts and 543 parliamentary constituencies in India. *Scientific Reports*, *11*(1), 4558. https://doi.org/10.1038/s41598-021-83992-6

Rodgers, J., Kim, R., & Subramanian, S. V. (2020). Explaining within- vs between-population variation in child anthropometry and hemoglobin measures in India: A multilevel analysis of the national family health survey 2015–2016. *Journal of Epidemiology*, *30*(11), 485–496. https://doi.org/10.2188/jea.JE20190064

Singh, S. K., Srivastava, S., & Chauhan, S. (2020). Inequality in child undernutrition among urban population in India: A decomposition analysis. *BMC Public Health*, *20*(1), 1852. https://doi.org/10.1186/s12889-020-09864-2

Singh, S., Srivastava, S., & Upadhyay, A. K. (2019). Socio-economic inequality in malnutrition among children in India: An analysis of 640 districts from National Family Health Survey (2015–16). *International Journal for Equity in Health*, *18*(1), 203. https://doi.org/10.1186/s12939-019-1093-0

SMART. (2014). *Guidelines: Rapid SMART surveys for emergencies*. New York: ACF International.

Srivastava, S., Chandra, H., Singh, S. K., & Upadhyay, A. K. (2021). Mapping changes in district level prevalence of childhood stunting in India 1998-2016: An application of small area estimation techniques. *SSM – Population Health*, *14*, 100748. https://doi.org/10.1016/j.ssmph.2021.100748

Štorkánová, H., Oreská, S., Špiritović, M., Heřmánková, B., Bubová, K., Komarc, M., Pavelka, K., Vencovský, J., Distler, J. H. W., Šenolt, L., Bečvář, R., & Tomčík, M. (2021). Plasma Hsp90 levels in patients with systemic sclerosis and relation to lung and skin involvement: A cross-sectional and longitudinal study. *Scientific Reports*, *11*(1), 1. https://doi.org/10.1038/s41598-020-79139-8

Story, W. T., & Carpiano, R. M. (2017). Household social capital and socioeconomic inequalities in child undernutrition in rural India. *Social Science & Medicine*, *181*, 112–121. https://doi.org/10.1016/j.socscimed.2017.03.043

Striessnig, E., & Bora, J. K. (2020). Under-five child growth and nutrition status: Spatial clustering of Indian districts. *Spatial Demography*, *8*(1), 63–84. https://doi.org/10.1007/s40980-020-00058-3

Swaminathan, S., Hemalatha, R., Pandey, A., Kassebaum, N. J., Laxmaiah, A., Longvah, T., Lodha, R., Ramji, S., Kumar, G. A., Afshin, A., Gupta, S. S., Kar, A., Khera, A. K., Mathai, M., Awasthi, S., Rasaily, R., Varghese, C. M., Millear, A. I., Manguerra, H., … Dandona, L. (2019a). The burden of child and maternal malnutrition and trends in its indicators in the states of India: The Global Burden of Disease Study 1990–2017. *The Lancet Child & Adolescent Health*, *3*(12), 855–870. https://doi.org/10.1016/S2352-4642(19)30273-1

Swaminathan, S., Hemalatha, R., Pandey, A., Kassebaum, N. J., Laxmaiah, A., Longvah, T., Lodha, R., Ramji, S., Kumar, G. A., Afshin, A., Gupta, S. S., Kar, A., Khera, A. K., Mathai, M., Awasthi, S., Rasaily, R., Varghese, C. M., Millear, A. I., Manguerra, H., … Dandona, L. (2019b). The burden of child and maternal malnutrition and trends in its indicators in the states of India: The Global Burden of Disease Study 1990–2017. *The Lancet Child & Adolescent Health*, *3*(12), 855–870. https://doi.org/10.1016/S2352-4642(19)30273-1

Tuffrey, V. (2016). A perspective on the development and sustainability of nutrition surveillance in low-income countries. *BMC Nutrition*, *2*(1), 15. https://doi.org/10.1186/s40795-016-0054-x

Tuffrey, V., & Hall, A. (2016). Methods of nutrition surveillance in low-income countries. *Emerging Themes in Epidemiology*, *13*(1), 4. https://doi.org/10.1186/s12982-016-0045-z

Verma, P., & Prasad, J. B. (2021). Stunting, wasting and underweight as indicators of undernutrition in under five children from developing Countries: A systematic review. *Diabetes & Metabolic Syndrome: Clinical Research & Reviews*, *15*(5), 102243. https://doi.org/10.1016/j.dsx.2021.102243

WHO. (1976). *Methodology of nutritional surveillance. Report of a joint FAO/UNICEF/WHO expert committee*. Geneva: WHO.

World Health Organization. (2006). *WHO child growth standards: Length/height-for-age, weight-for-age, weight-for-length, weight-for-height and body mass index-for-age: Methods and development.* WHO.

Zhou, M., Wang, H., Zhu, J., Chen, W., Wang, L., Liu, S., Li, Y., Wang, L., Liu, Y., Yin, P., Liu, J., Yu, S., Tan, F., Barber, R., Coates, M., Dicker, D., Fraser, M., Gonzalez-Medina, D., Hamavid, H., … Liang, X. (2016). Cause-specific mortality for 240 causes in China during 1990–2013: A systematic subnational analysis for the Global Burden of Disease Study 2013. *The Lancet*, 387(10015), 251–272.

6 Evaluating the Advantages and Disadvantages of Rice Fortification for Improved Food and Nutrition Security

Shireesha Mukka, Harika Vasa, and Maheshwar Mekam

6.1 INTRODUCTION

Widespread hunger and malnutrition affect 65 million people, including refugees and displaced individuals. Providing people with a healthy and nourishing diet helps reduce the risk of long-term health issues, reduces poverty, and enhances their ability to withstand future challenges (Thakur et al., 2023). Malnutrition is characterized by an imbalance of nutrients within the human body, resulting in detrimental effects on health. Hunger is commonly known as the distress caused by insufficient food intake. The 1996 World Food Summit stated that every individual should be able to access safe and nourishing food without experiencing hunger. The declaration highlights the importance of addressing food security globally and promoting equal access to food. It emphasizes the role of sustainable agriculture and responsible resource management in creating a better world for future generations. It is a call to action for all stakeholders to prioritize eradicating hunger and promoting social justice worldwide.

The United Nations Sustainable Development Goals (SDGs) and the 2030 Agenda aim to establish a worldwide setting where hunger and malnutrition are eliminated in every form (Olson et al., 2021). Hidden hunger refers to a type of malnutrition that arises when the consumption and assimilation of essential vitamins and minerals fall below the necessary levels for maintaining optimal health and growth. Various factors contribute to micronutrient deficiencies, including inadequate dietary intake and increased need for micronutrients during certain life stages such as pregnancy and breastfeeding, in addition to dealing with health conditions like illnesses and infections (Gani et al., 2018). Micronutrient deficiencies have the potential to result in a decline of approximately 4% to 5% in gross domestic product (GDP) (Food Fortification | World Food Programme, 2024).

 DOI: 10.1201/9781003487227-6

The World Health Organization (WHO) and the United Nations Food and Agriculture Organization (FAO) are at the forefront of global efforts to tackle nutritional deficiencies. They are implementing four key approaches to improve dietary intake: fortifying food products with essential nutrients, providing micronutrient supplements, educating about nutrition, and implementing disease control measures (Olson et al., 2021). Enhancing diets by incorporating various foods with essential nutrients is the most effective way to address deficiencies and diseases. However, the cost, availability, and accessibility needed to achieve a diverse diet can be barriers to reaching this goal solely through dietary diversification. As a result, food fortification, micronutrient supplements, and biofortification are regarded as valuable and cost-effective complementary methods (WFP-Food Fortification, 2022).

6.2 FOOD FORTIFICATION

Food fortification has been defined as the addition of one or more essential nutrients to a food, whether or not it is normally contained in the food, to prevent or correct a demonstrated deficiency of one or more nutrients in the population or specific population groups (Food Fortification, n.d.). The Food Safety and Standards Authority of India (FSSAI) defines fortification as the addition of key vitamins and minerals such as iron, iodine, zinc, and vitamins A and D to staple foods such as rice, wheat, oil, milk, and salt. It is done to improve nutritional value and provide a public health benefit with minimal risk to health (Kunal Khureja, 2022).

Food fortification is an effective strategy focused on reducing the occurrence of micronutrient deficiencies and improving the general health of the population. According to CODEX, fortification or enrichment refers to the process of incorporating vital nutrients into food products with the objective of preventing or rectifying documented nutrient deficiencies within the population or specific demographic groups (Efficacy and Safety of Iron Fortified Rice in India: A White Paper NITI Aayog ICMR-NIN, 2023). Nevertheless, the ingredient incorporated into food to enhance its nutritional content must not disrupt the absorption of other nutrients. It should be consumed in a quantity that poses no adverse health risks. Many studies have proved that fortifying food is generally a more economical and profitable approach than supplementing in tackling specific public health issues (Alfthan et al., 2015). Food fortification is an essential strategy for combating hidden hunger and effectively addressing nutritional deficiencies (Olson et al., 2021). Food fortification programs strive to narrow the gap between the existing consumption levels and the recommended intake (Estimated Average Requirement, EAR) for the population (Whitfield et al., 2021). Achieving the desired impact on nutritional status through fortification programs necessitates robust support, which can be attained by implementing food regulation, quality assurance measures, and rigorous monitoring (Mannar & Wesley, 2023).

Food fortification can be implemented either through government-enforced mandatory regulations or voluntarily by food manufacturers. Mandatory fortification involves legally requiring specific nutrients to be added to certain food products to address deficiencies in the general population's diet. However, voluntary fortification grants food manufacturers the autonomy to choose whether to enrich their products with extra vitamins and minerals. This is typically done to gain a competitive edge in the market or cater to consumers' specific preferences. Both approaches play a vital role in improving public health by ensuring that people have access to essential nutrients, even if these are not naturally present in their diets at adequate levels. While mandatory fortification aims to reach a broader population and address widespread nutrient deficiencies, voluntary fortification offers flexibility and innovation in product development.

Regardless of whether fortification is mandatory or voluntary, the goal remains the same: to promote better nutrition and reduce the risk of health issues related to nutrient deficiencies in the community. The implementation of mandatory food fortification is the sole means by which the Food and Drug Administration (FDA) ensures compliance with its established standards of identity. These standards specify the specific type and quantity of nutrients that must be incorporated into a specific food product (Datta & Vitolins, 2016).

Principles of food fortification programs

- A considerable number of individuals have diets that do not meet the recommended intake of essential nutrients.
- The food(s) utilized to provide the nutrient(s) are expected to be consumed in amounts that will have a substantial impact on the dietary needs of the population in need.
- The inclusion of the nutrient is unlikely to disrupt the balance of vital nutrients.
- The added nutrient remains stable when stored and used correctly.
- The food provides the nutrient in a physiologically accessible form.
- There is a credible assurance that intake will not lead to toxicity (Datta & Vitolins, 2016).

6.3 WHY RICE FORTIFICATION?

More than half of the global population relies on rice as a crucial staple, providing vital nutrients and calories. This essential food not only offers a diverse array of vitamins, minerals, and nutritional values but also surpasses maize, wheat, and potatoes in terms of its content. Moreover, rice is an abundant source of vitamin E and B5, carbohydrates, thiamine, calcium, folate, and iron. Its antioxidant properties are further enhanced by the presence of beneficial compounds like phenols, phytic acid, flavonoids, sterols, and anthocyanins, potentially aiding in the prevention of cardiovascular disease and diabetes (Mohidem et al., 2022). Its adaptability to different climates has allowed it to be grown in numerous regions across the globe. Rice is grown in over 100 countries, predominantly in Asia, contributing to 90% of the world's total rice production (Fukagawa & Ziska, 2019). By 2030, it is projected that global rice production will increase significantly, ranging from 58 to 567 million tonnes (Mohidem et al., 2022). Remarkably, India emerged as the second-largest rice producer in 2020, making an outstanding contribution of 178.3 million tonnes to the global output (FAOSTAT, n.d.).

Rice stands as a highly popular grain globally, being consumed extensively. China, the most populous nation, surpasses all other countries in rice consumption, with a staggering 150 million metric tons consumed during the period 2023–24. In the same timeframe, India consumed 118 million metric tons of rice, securing its position as the second-largest consumer (Shahbandeh, 2024). As a result of the significant global demand for rice, the fortification process plays a crucial role in addressing hidden hunger, reducing the risk of deficiencies, and promoting overall well-being. Several nations have been enriching rice with vital nutrients and minerals for a significant amount of time. This custom is especially common in areas where rice is a primary food source and is regularly incorporated into traditional recipes (Fortification of Rice, 2023). In India, rice is commonly fortified with vitamin B12, folic acid, and iron. Additionally, some other micronutrients like vitamin B1, niacin, zinc, selenium, and vitamins A and E are also used for fortification (Ghosh & Pundir, 2018).

Rice, being a staple food for over 3.5 billion individuals worldwide, plays a crucial role in providing essential calories. The increasing demand for and consumption of processed rice types have resulted in a notable decline in their nutritional content. This decrease in nutrient content has contributed to the widespread occurrence of micronutrient deficiencies, posing significant health challenges in the modern era. Therefore, enhancing rice through fortification with vital nutrients presents a promising way to bridge the nutritional gap among populations and address the prevailing health concerns associated with inadequate micronutrient intake (Senguttuvel et al., 2023).

Importance of rice fortification

Fortifying rice is becoming more widely acknowledged as a crucial approach to combating prevalent nutritional deficiencies, particularly in communities where rice is a primary dietary staple. Enriching it with vital nutrients like vitamins, proteins, minerals, and antioxidants can play a crucial role in addressing food insecurity, battling diseases, and enhancing people's general health and wellness (Figure 6.1).

- *Combating hidden hunger:* Despite appearing healthy, some individuals may experience malnutrition due to inadequate nutrients in their diet. This lack of micronutrients, referred to as hidden hunger, can have detrimental effects on one's health. Multiple elements contribute to the occurrence of micronutrient deficiencies. These factors encompass inadequate consumption of essential nutrients, heightened requirements for micronutrients during specific life phases like pregnancy and breastfeeding, and the presence of health conditions such as infections and diseases (Gani et al., 2018).
- *Restoration of depleted nutrients:* During food processing, a significant amount of nutrients is lost. For instance, in the process of milling rice, the husk, bran, and germ are removed to produce white rice, which is commonly consumed. This process also results in the loss of fat and micronutrient-rich bran layers. Additionally, the grain polishing leads to an even more significant depletion of essential vitamins (Kunal Khurana, 2022).
- *Poor health statistics:* The most recent National Family Health Survey, NFHS-5 (2019–21), indicates that approximately 90% of children aged around 6 to

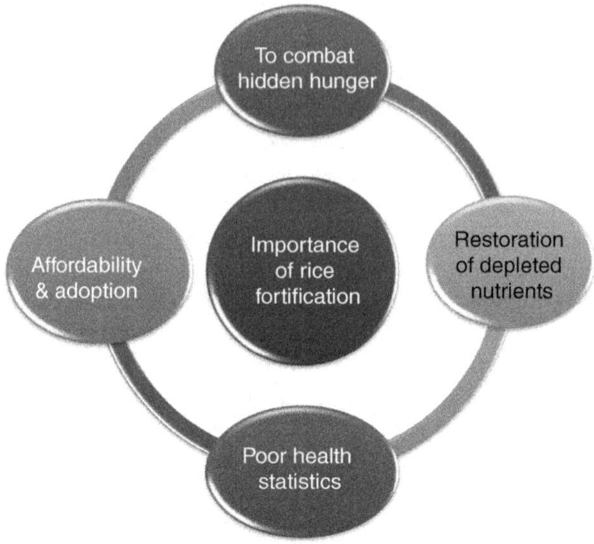
To combat hidden hunger
Affordability & adoption
Importance of rice fortification
Restoration of depleted nutrients
Poor health statistics

FIGURE 6.1 Importance of rice fortification.

23 months in India failed to receive enough nutritious food. Furthermore, in the survey, more than two thirds (67.1%) of children aged 6 to 59 months were found to have anemia based on the diagnosis; 25% of men aged 5 to 49 were found to be anemic; that percentage increased to 57% for women in the same age bracket; 52.2% of pregnant women aged 15 to 49 were found to be anemic; and in the case of adolescent boys and girls the ratio of anemia prevalence was found to be 31.1% and 59.1% (Kunal Khurana, 2022; Press Information Bureau, 2022).

- *Affordability and adoption:* Fortification is an incredibly cost-effective method of addressing nutrient deficiencies. Additionally, it offers easy adoption as it generally does not necessitate significant adjustments in the fortified food's taste, appearance, or texture. However, it is crucial to highlight that there may be a few exceptions where this does not apply (Kunal Khurana, 2022).

6.4 WHAT IS FORTIFIED RICE?

Fortified rice is a mixture of fortified kernels and non-fortified rice (also called traditional or polished rice) in a specific ratio (often 1:100) as per the regulatory and market requirements (PATH, 2015).

Global scenario of rice fortification

Many countries have been fortifying foods since the 1920s, nearly eliminating nutrition-related diseases like rickets, goiter, pellagra, and beriberi (Table 6.1). Although mineral and vitamin deficiencies impact countries globally, the most significant rates are observed in Asia, Latin Africa, and America (Food Fortification,

TABLE 6.1
Countries with Mandatory and Voluntary Rice Fortification with Iron

No.	Country	Year	Legislation Status
1	India	2018	Voluntary
2	Belize	2015	Voluntary
3	Bangladesh	2015	Voluntary
4	Bahrain	2012	Voluntary
5	USA	2017	Mandatory
6	Solomon Islands	2018	Mandatory
7	Philippines	2000	Mandatory
8	Peru	2018	Mandatory
9	Papua New Guinea	2007	Mandatory
10	Panama	2009	Mandatory
11	Nicaragua	2014	Mandatory
12	Venezuela	1993	Voluntary
13	Myanmar	2019	Voluntary
14	Canada	2021	Voluntary

Source: Efficacy and Safety of Iron Fortified Rice in India - A White Paper NITI Aayog ICMR-NIN (2023).

n.d.). In a concerted global initiative to combat nutritional deficiencies, six countries have made it mandatory to enrich rice with vital nutrients such as iron and folic acid. These countries are Nicaragua, Costa Rica, Panama, the Philippines, Papua New Guinea, and the USA. The progress in implementing these mandates varied among the nations by 2016. Costa Rica had successfully achieved full compliance, while Papua New Guinea had reached an 80% fortification rate. The USA stood at 70%, whereas the Philippines lagged at 1%, with varying rates in Panama and Nicaragua. Apart from these six countries, an additional group of six nations, namely Brazil, Peru, Colombia, Indonesia, Mali, and Myanmar, had adopted voluntary fortification programs in response to market demand. The collective objective of these fortification efforts is to enhance the levels of essential micronutrients in rice, thereby improving the health and well-being of populations in these regions (Guideline: Fortification of Rice with Vitamins and Minerals as a Public Health Strategy, 2018). In addition to the six countries that have mandatory rice fortification legislations, the Solomon Islands also adheres to mandatory rice fortification, which includes essential micronutrients such as zinc, iron, niacin, thiamine, and folic acid (Solomon Islands Receives First Shipment of Fortified Rice, 2019; Rohner et al., 2023). Around 31% of the global population is affected by a lack of zinc. As a result, over 400 million children die each year. Approximately 80% of people worldwide suffer from inadequate iron levels, with 30% of the individuals experiencing anemia because of insufficient iron levels. Every year, 800,000 deaths are caused by iron deficiency. There has been substantial advancement worldwide in rice to improve the levels of grain zinc, iron, and protein. Currently, there exist a total of 37 biofortified rice varieties that have been specifically bred to be rich sources of provitamin A, zinc, iron, and protein. Among these varieties, 21 originate from other countries, while 16 are native to India. A noteworthy feature of these biofortified rice strains is that they exhibit high levels of key nutrients, with iron content exceeding 10 mg/kg, zinc content surpassing 24 mg/kg, and protein content of over 10% in polished rice for the Indian varieties, meeting global standards. Additionally, the non-Indian varieties have zinc content higher than 28 mg/kg in polished rice. Such biofortified rice strains have been identified as ideal for commercial farming due to their exceptional nutritional profile and suitability for cultivation (Senguttuvel et al., 2023).

The Copenhagen Consensus suggests that investing Rs.1 in fortification yields economic benefits worth Rs. 9 (Explainer / Benefits of Rice Fortification, 2022). During the Nutrition for Growth Summit in Tokyo in 2021, the World Food Programme (WFP) pledged to improve the distribution of fortified rice, wheat flour, and maize meal in its programs. The goal is to increase the proportion from 60% in 2020 to 80% by 2025. Additionally, the WFP will collaborate with at least 40 countries to strengthen their national systems and ensure the provision of fortified foods to the most vulnerable families (Food Fortification, n.d.). Rolling out rice fortification initiatives on a broader scope has the potential to significantly improve public health by decreasing micronutrient deficiencies and related health problems. Government agencies, NGOs, and food industry stakeholders are working together to promote the benefits of rice fortification and ensure its successful integration into food supply chains. Collaboration and investment in research and infrastructure are essential to overcome challenges and ensure the sustainability and effectiveness of rice fortification efforts. By prioritizing the fortification of rice, we can make a tangible difference in combating malnutrition and improving the nutritional status of communities worldwide.

Rice fortification in India

The FSSAI is the regulatory authority responsible for ensuring food safety in India. It plays a crucial role in promoting the consumption of fortified foods across the country (Efficacy and Safety of Iron Fortified Rice in India - A White Paper NITI Aayog ICMR-NIN, 2023). To achieve this, the FSSAI has implemented the Food Safety and Standards (Fortification of Foods) Regulations, 2018. These regulations establish guidelines for fortifying five essential food items, namely double-fortified salt, rice, wheat flour, edible oil, and milk. Currently, the fortification of the first three food items is encouraged on a voluntary basis (Qureshy et al., 2023). Micronutrient deficiencies are a widespread problem among women and children in India. To tackle this issue, the Prime Minister's office launched the National Nutrition Mission in early 2018. This initiative emphasizes the fortification of staple foods as a cost-effective solution to combat vitamin and mineral deficiencies. Among the primary staples in India, rice is considered the most effective medium to reach the underprivileged population. When fortified properly, rice can provide a wide range of essential minerals and vitamins. The fortified rice is then distributed to individuals at high risk of nutritional deficiencies through government food supplementation programs, including the Mid-Day Meal (MDM) scheme, Integrated Child Development Scheme (ICDS), and Public Distribution System (PDS) (Ghosh & Pundhir 2018). In the rice fortification program, all 269 districts across 27 states in India have successfully initiated the Targeted Public Distribution System (TPDS) to supply fortified rice to the public (269 Districts in 27 States Distributing Fortified Rice under Targeted Public Distribution System, 2023).

WHO recommendations for rice fortification

The WHO makes the following recommendations for rice fortification (Guideline: Fortification of Rice with Vitamins and Minerals as a Public Health Strategy, 2018).

- Enhancing iron levels in populations can be achieved through fortifying rice with iron, particularly in areas where rice is a staple food.
- Implementing rice fortification with vitamin A can help increase iron and vitamin A intake in populations as a public health intervention.
- Using rice fortification with folic acid is a viable public health strategy to improve the folate status of populations.

Standards for rice fortification

The Food Safety Standards (Fortification of Foods) Regulation, 2018, and the Food Safety and Standards (Food Products Standards and Food Additives) Regulations, 2011 have established the guidelines for fortified food, including rice. Following these regulations, rice fortification includes adding folic acid, vitamin B12, and iron. Additionally, specific quantities of micronutrients such as vitamins B1, B2, B3, B6, A and zinc are also incorporated (Kunal Khureja, 2022).

Recommended levels of micronutrients in fortified rice

The number of micronutrients added to fortified rice is determined by factors like the nutritional needs of the specific population, local eating habits, and regulations established by the national government or international food authorities and the WHO. The boundaries for incorporating micronutrients into rice during fortification have been established, specifically for individuals who consume 75 g to 149 g of rice daily (Saha & Roy, 2020; see Table 6.2).

TABLE 6.2
Recommended Levels of Micronutrients in Fortified Rice for Individuals Consuming 75 g to 149 g Daily

Micronutrient	Recommended Level in ppm
Folic acid	2.6
Vitamin A	3
Thiamine	10
Iron	120
Vitamin B6	12
Niacin	130
Zinc	80
Vitamin B12	0.02

Source: Saha & Roy (2020).

6.5 METHODS OF RICE FORTIFICATION

Various approaches have been utilized to create fortified rice containing vital micronutrients (see Figure 6.2). These methods encompass post-harvest fortification and pre-harvest fortification (Saha & Roy, 2020).

Post-harvest rice fortification methods

Enhancing rice with crucial nutrients and minerals through post-harvest fortification is essential for combating micronutrient deficiencies and enhancing public health. This process is a critical component of food security efforts, guaranteeing that people can enjoy a balanced diet. Thorough planning and execution are crucial to ensure the fortified rice's efficacy and safety. The following are the post-harvest rice fortification strategies.

In *dusting*, the rice kernels are delicately coated with a micronutrient powder using a precise and careful dusting process that utilizes the power of electrostatic forces. This unique method ensures that the essential micronutrients adhere evenly and effectively to each grain of rice. This results in a consistent and uniform distribution of these vital nutrients throughout the entire batch. As a result, the nutritional value of the rice is significantly enhanced. This meticulous application process guarantees thorough coverage of the rice grains with micronutrients, providing a reliable and efficient way to fortify the rice with these essential elements. Ultimately, customers receive a product that is not only delicious but also provides a wealth of vital vitamins

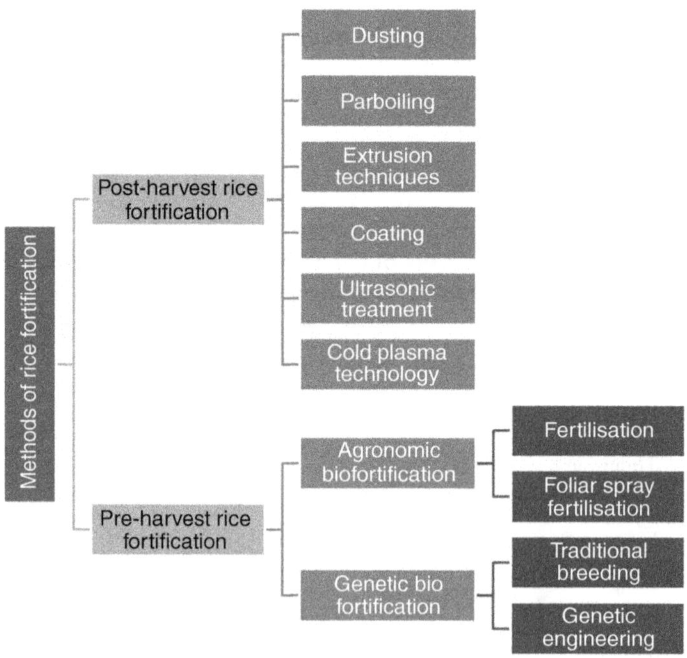

FIGURE 6.2 Methods of rice fortification.

and minerals for a nutritious diet. It is crucial to remember that washing the rice before cooking or using too much water can lead to the loss of vitamins and minerals (The Role of Rice Fortification in Improving Public Health Executive Summary, 2018; Saha & Roy, 2020).

Rice fortification through *parboiling* is an effective method employed to enhance the nutritional content of rice by incorporating either an individual nutrient or a combination of various essential nutrients for producing fortified rice (Jannasch et al., 2020). It involves a hydrothermal method that includes soaking, steaming, and drying. The soaking process raises the humidity level of the paddy, while the steam aids in starch gelatinization. This parboiling step allows micronutrients to transfer from the bran to the endosperm, which would typically be lost during milling and whitening. Soaking water with increased micronutrient levels is used to further enrich the endosperm. This ensures that the micronutrients penetrate the kernel and remain intact throughout processing and milling (Thiruselvam, 2014; Saha & Roy, 2020). Parboiling can seal any cracks in rice, leading to a firmer texture and ultimately increasing the milling yield while reducing breakage and enhancing the organoleptic characteristics of rice. This approach demonstrated exceptional preservation of nutrients following the procedures of cleansing and cooking, owing to the inward movement of nutrients towards the endosperm (Samaddar et al., 2017). This technique can be utilized to incorporate a range of micronutrients such as zinc (Wahengbam, Green, et al., 2019), calcium, iodine (Saha & Roy, 2020), iron (Patindol et al., 2017), β-carotene, and folic acid (Thiruselvam, 2014) to produce fortified rice. The primary producers of parboiled rice include India, Bangladesh, West Asia, Sri Lanka, and Thailand. These countries collectively account for approximately 90% of parboiled rice's total production and consumption. Parboiling is a widely utilized fortification technique at both industrial and domestic levels, with a long history as a traditional method and a rich historical background as a conventional technique. The fortification of rice through the parboiling method has demonstrated a notable enhancement in iron levels, reaching as high as 140 mg/kg of dry weight (Junaid-ur-Rahman et al., 2022).

Food *extrusion* is a process that utilizes high temperatures for a short amount of time, and it has been widely adopted for the continuous production of new and classic food items (Samyor et al., 2018; Das & Bhattacharya 2019; Saha & Roy, 2020). Extrusion processes, characterized by the temperature levels employed, are segmented into hot, cold, and warm extrusion techniques. Hot extrusion surpasses the starch melting thresholds, contrasting with cold extrusion, which operates at temperatures lower than the starch melting point. In the realm of extrusion methods, warm extrusion serves as an intermediate option, inducing partial melting of amylopectin through its operational temperatures (Saha & Roy, 2020). This method finds widespread usage in the food sector, especially in the fabrication of breakfast cereals, textured vegetable proteins, and various snacks. Notably, it stands out for its proficiency in enhancing rice, emerging as a prevalent and widely embraced technology. This specific extrusion technique focuses on producing rice analogues using rice flour, deviating from traditional methods of fortifying rice. The process entails blending rice flour with water, pivotal micronutrients, and a diverse range of additives. Subsequently, this mixture is shaped into a cohesive dough consistency and allowed to stabilize under controlled moisture conditions, setting the stage for subsequent processing and enhancements (Bajaj & Singhal, 2019). The processed dough undergoes a meticulous process where it is meticulously extruded through a specialized apparatus designed to generate a texture that closely resembles individual grains of rice. This extrusion process occurs within a controlled environment, with the option to adjust the temperature settings to either heightened or diminished levels, depending on the desired outcome. The resulting structure mimics the size and shape of rice grains, contributing to the overall quality and appearance of the final product. This systematic approach ensures consistency and precision in the creation of the dough, guaranteeing that each piece maintains its distinctive rice-like form. Whether subjected to increased heat or lowered temperatures, the dough is carefully handled through every stage of the process to achieve the optimal texture, flavor, and appearance that align with the intended culinary application. This carefully orchestrated procedure transforms the dough into a versatile ingredient that can seamlessly integrate into various recipes, enhancing the overall culinary experience for consumers (Steiger et al., 2014).

In *coating*, micronutrients are infused in significant amounts into a portion of the rice; subsequently, a water-resistant edible coating is applied to the rice kernels. These coated kernels are then blended with unfortified rice in varying ratios, which can range from 1 in 50 to 1 in 200. However, coating technologies face significant challenges, such as issues with taste and color, and some of the nutrients are lost during cleansing and other food processing. Moreover, there is a considerable variation among coating technologies, and consumers can quickly identify the fortified kernels, leading to their probable removal during rice cleaning (Guideline: Fortification of Rice with Vitamins and Minerals as a Public Health Strategy, 2018). The application of various edible coating materials to iron-fortified rice premix has proven to be effective in minimizing the loss of iron even after undergoing two rounds of washing with water (Mridula & Pooja, 2014).

Ultrasonic treatment and absorption enhances the nutritional value of milled rice by modifying its surface and promoting adsorption. By subjecting white long-grain rice to ultrasonic waves, the surface is transformed from smooth to porous. The sonication process leads to the breakdown of the surface shell, creating micropores, exposing cell walls, and breaking down the starchy endosperm into individual starch granules. Submerging the sonicated rice in a micronutrient solution enables the absorption of vitamins into the rice grains, resulting in fortified rice. Pantothenic acid (Bonto et al., 2018) and folic acid (Tiozon Jr. et al., 2021) can be effectively integrated into the milled rice using this technique, which allows for the efficient incorporation of essential nutrients that are beneficial for overall health and well-being.

Cold plasma technology is an innovative approach for producing fortified rice. White rice specimens were subjected to plasma treatment at a fixed voltage. The duration of plasma exposure was chosen based on the surface attributes, hydrophobicity, and thermal features. The plasma-treated rice was enhanced with optimal concentrations of iron and ascorbic acid solution using the central composite design of response surface methodology. The iron bioavailability is greater in plasma-treated rice than in other treatments. Moreover, the rice was blended with untreated rice in ratios of 1:100 and 1:200 before being packaged. This state-of-the-art approach demonstrates the potential to significantly boost the iron levels in rice, tackling the widespread issue of micronutrient deficiencies. Using cold plasma, this method presents a distinctive and efficient means of enhancing rice with crucial iron, ultimately supporting global nutrition and health efforts. This method for rice fortification marks a notable progression in the food sector, paving the way for novel opportunities to enhance the nutritional quality of staple food items. Embracing this innovative tactic can substantially impact addressing iron deficiency and associated health concerns while meeting the dietary needs of diverse populations worldwide (Akasapu et al., 2020).

Pre-harvest rice fortification methods

Pre-harvest rice fortification refers to the process of increasing the nutrient levels in rice prior to its harvest. Various techniques exist to enrich rice with vital nutrients before it is made available to consumers.

Biofortification, also known as biological fortification, pertains to the development and cultivation of nutritionally enriched food crops. These crops are specifically designed to have increased bioavailability for the human population. This is achieved through the utilization of modern biotechnology techniques, conventional plant breeding, and agronomic practices (Garg et al., 2018; Biofortification | International Rice Research Institute, 2018; Jena et al., 2018). Agronomic biofortification can be achieved by applying micronutrient fertilizers to the soil or directly to the leaves of the crop, and genetic biofortification involves the use of either traditional breeding or genetic engineering (Das et al., 2023). This groundbreaking strategy consists of the integration of agricultural and nutritional sciences to address malnutrition by elevating the concentrations of crucial nutrients such as provitamin A, zinc, and iron in staple foods without imposing any additional costs on consumers. It is crucial to recognize that numerous staple crops are deficient in key nutrients essential for promoting healthy growth and development in individuals. Thus, biofortification emerges as a forward-thinking solution to tackle these nutritional deficiencies head-on and enhance global food security for a healthier, more nourished population (Yadav et al., 2020).

In the field of agronomy, *fertilization* plays a crucial role in improving soil nutrient levels by incorporating key micronutrient salts using fertilizers. Historically, farming methods focused on utilizing nitrogen, phosphorus, and potassium fertilizers to boost soil quality prior to planting rice seedlings. Applying micronutrients as fertilizer during the fertilization process of rice can enhance the levels of these nutrients in the grain. Additionally, the effectiveness of micronutrients like iron in the fertilizer diminishes when applied to the soil, as soluble iron quickly converts into insoluble $Fe+3$ forms that are unavailable to plants. This process is unsuitable for immobile minerals; excess micronutrients are required, and the popularity of this process is limited due to the restricted uptake of salts during fertilization. Therefore, the adoption of foliar spray fertilization was implemented to address these issues (Saha & Roy, 2020).

Foliar spray fertilization is an effective technique used in agriculture, which involves the precise application of a specialized micronutrient-rich solution onto the surface of the plant's leaves. The micronutrients in the solution are essential for the plant's overall health, growth, and development. By spraying this solution directly onto the foliage, the plant can quickly absorb and utilize these nutrients, bypassing the need for them to travel through the soil. This targeted approach ensures that the plant receives the necessary nutrients promptly, promoting optimal growth and vitality. In addition, foliar spray fertilization is particularly beneficial for correcting and preventing nutrient deficiencies, as it responds promptly to specific plant needs. Overall, this method provides a convenient and efficient way to enhance the nutrient levels of plants, ultimately leading to improved yields, better quality crops, and healthier, more resilient plants (Niu et al., 2021). This method can be applied to incorporate zinc to produce fortified rice (Phuphong et al., 2018; Biswas et al., 2018; Khampuang et al., 2021).

Traditional breeding involves selectively mating plants with desired traits to create offspring with improved characteristics. This technique is utilized to fortify rice before harvesting to cultivate varieties with increased nutrient levels. By choosing rice strains with elevated nutrient content, combining two varieties with complementary traits, utilizing hybridization, backcrossing, marker-aided selection (MAS), and involving participatory plant breeding, breeders can enhance the nutrient profiles, yield, and overall performance of rice varieties. Despite the time-consuming process of developing and introducing new strains, they are well-received and seamlessly incorporated into current agricultural practices (Senguttuvel et al., 2023).

Genetic engineering is a technique employed to alter the genetic composition of organisms, such as rice crops, to introduce favorable characteristics. It enables the introduction of genes responsible for specific nutrients, thereby facilitating preharvest rice fortification. Various methods, including gene insertion, gene silencing, gene editing, promoter engineering, and stacked traits, can be utilized to enhance the nutritional value of rice grains. Nevertheless, genetic engineering gives rise to apprehensions regarding safety, regulation, and public acceptance. Regulatory authorities diligently oversee genetically modified crops to guarantee their safety for human consumption and the environment before commercial cultivation (Senguttuvel et al., 2023). Varieties of crops exhibit higher resistance towards various biotic and abiotic stresses (Ansari et al., 2015). Agronomic practices and traditional breeding methods can meet the necessary goals; however, if there is limited genetic variation for a particular nutrient, traditional breeding may fall short. In such cases, genetic modification can help boost the micronutrient levels in essential crops, as its effectiveness has been proven (Wakeel et al., 2018).

Currently, there are 37 unique biofortified rice strains accessible globally, which have been developed using advanced breeding methods to boost their nutritional content and health advantages. These biofortified rice varieties play a crucial role in advocating for improved nutrition and supporting sustainable agriculture and food security efforts. The ongoing progress in biofortification technology and the sharing of information regarding these enhanced rice types show great potential in enriching dietary variety, reducing micronutrient deficiencies, and ultimately enhancing the welfare of communities, especially in developing nations where rice serves as a primary food source. The biofortified rice varieties are listed in Table 6.3.

TABLE 6.3
Biofortified Rice Varieties in the World

No.	Country	Name of Variety	Year of Release	Parameter (Zn, Fe, Protein, and Vit A)
1	Bangladesh	BRRI Dhan 62	2013	Zn 19.6 mg/kg
2	Philippines	NSIC Rc172 (MS 13)	2003	Fe 13 to 21 mg/kg (brown rice)
3	Bangladesh	BRRI Dhan 64	2014	Zn 25 mg/kg
4	India	Chhattisgarh Zinc Rice 1	2015	Zn 22 to 24 mg/kg
5	Bangladesh	BRRI Dhan 72	2015	Zn 25 mg/kg
6	Bangladesh	BRRI Dhan 74	2016	Zn 24.2 mg/kg
7	Philippines	NSICRc460	2016	Zn 19.6 mg/kg
8	Bangladesh	BRRI Dhan 69	2016	Provitamin A and low GI 54.9
9	India	DRR Dhan 45	2016	Zn 22.3 mg/kg
10	India	CR Dhan 310	2016	Protein 10.3%
11	Indonesia	INPARI IR Nutri Zinc	2016	Zn 26 mg/kg
12	Bangladesh	BU Aromatic Dhan-2	2016	Zn 22 mg/kg; Fe 10 mg/kg
13	Bangladesh	BU Aromatic Hybrid Dhan-1	2016	Zn 21.8 mg/kg; Fe 10 mg/Kg
14	India	Surabhi	2017	Zn 22.84 mg/kg
15	India	GR-15	2017	Zn 21.58 mg/kg
16	India	Surabhi	2017	Zn 22.84 mg/kg
17	India	DRR Dhan 48	2017	Zn 20.91 mg/kg
18	India	DRR Dhan 49	2017	Zn 26.13 mg/kg
19	Bangladesh	BRRI Dhan 84	2017	Zinc 27.6 mg/kg; Fe 10.1mg/kg; protein 9.7%
20	Bangladesh	Binadhan 20	2017	Zn 26.5 mg/kg; Fe 20 to 31 mg/kg
21	India	Chhattisgarh Zinc Rice-2	2018	Zn 22 to 24 mg/kg
22	India	ZincoRice-MS(R-RHZ-LI-23)	2018	Zn 27.4 mg/kg
23	India	CR Dhan 315	2018	Zn 24.9 mg/kg
24	India	CR Dhan 311	2019	Protein 10.1% and Zn 20.1 mg/kg
25	Bolivia	CIAT BIO-44 +Zinc	2019	Zn 25 mg/kg
26	Indonesia	INPARI 47 Nutri Zn	2019	Zn 29.54 mg/kg
27	Bangladesh	BRRI Dhan 96	2019	Protein 10.8%
28	El Salvador	CENTA A-Nutremas	2019	Zn 22.86 mg/kg; Fe 6.9mg/kg
29	Nicaragua	INTA Las Minas	2020	Zn 25.0 mg/kg
30	India	CR Dhan 411	2021	Protein 9.88%
31	Colombia	Fedearroz BIO Zn 035	2021	Zn 26 mg/kg
32	Bangladesh	BRRI Dhan 100	2021	Zn 25.7 mg/kg
33	India	DRR Dhan 63	2021	Zn 24.2 mg/kg
34	Bangladesh	BRRI Dhan 102	2022	Zn 25.5 mg/kg
35	India	DRR Dhan 69 (BRRI Dhan 100)	2022	Zn 25.7 mg/kg
36	India	DRR Dhan 67 (BRRI Dhan 84)	2022	Zn 27.6 mg/kg
37	Philippines	NSIC Rc648	2022	Zn 23.2 mg/kg

Source: Senguttuvel et al. (2023).

6.6 LABELING CRITERIA FOR FORTIFIED RICE

Fortified rice labels are required to include detailed information about the added nutrients, their quantities, nutritional facts, daily value percentages, ingredients, allergen details, storage instructions, manufacturer information, country-specific regulations, and certifications. These criteria are designed to ensure that consumers have access to transparent information regarding the nutritional content and quality of fortified rice enabling them to make well-informed choices about their food. Common fortification ingredients found in fortified rice include iron, folic acid, vitamin A, zinc, vitamin B12, and vitamin D. Additionally, the label should provide standard nutritional information such as calories, carbohydrates, protein, fat, fiber, and other essential micronutrients. Some labels may also indicate the percentage of the recommended daily intake for each fortified nutrient. Different countries and regions have different symbols for labeling fortified rice. These symbols often take the form of icons or logos that represent the added nutrients. Some examples of these symbols include F+ , nutrient icons, government endorsements, global fortification logos, and symbols for national fortification programs. These symbols can consist of letters, numbers, or images and may be accompanied by additional letters or icons representing specific nutrients. Government endorsements may also be used to indicate that the fortification standards have been met. Consumers can find information about fortification on the packaging of the product, including details about the specific nutrients that have been added and their respective amounts. The design and use of these symbols can vary greatly depending on the local regulations and practices within the industry (Food Safety and Standards (Fortification of Foods) Regulations, 2018).

6.7 BIOAVAILABILITY

Bioavailability refers to the portion of vitamins or nutrients that can be absorbed in a metabolically active form from the total amount (Bhatnagar & Padilla-Zakour, 2021). The bioavailability of essential nutrients in fortified rice is a critical factor in ensuring its effectiveness in combating nutritional deficiencies. In the study conducted by Jyrwa et al. (2020), the extrusion technology was used to fortify rice with micronutrients, such as folic acid, vitamin B12, and iron. The research focused on assessing fortified rice retention, stability, bioavailability, and sensory evaluation. The findings revealed that the bioavailable iron content in the fortified rice was higher than in unfortified rice. Additionally, the inclusion of vegetables and fruits further enhanced the bioavailability of iron. Overages were included in the premixes to make up for the loss of B complex vitamins that occurred during the rinsing of rice. However, it was observed that there was poor retention of nutrients when cooking rice with excess water and decanting. Therefore, it is crucial to educate the target population and school kitchen personnel on proper cooking methods to minimize nutrient losses.

Consuming fortified rice can help bridge the gaps in dietary iron intake and meet the required dietary requirements (Jyrwa et al., 2020). The study of (Wahengbam, Das, et al., 2019) revealed iron and folic acid-enriched parboiled rice, through the innovative application of the brown rice parboiling method, resulted in a product that not only demonstrated a notable increase in the bioavailability and bioaccessibility of essential micronutrients in in-vitro techniques but also exhibited a reduced rate of starch hydrolysis, highlighting its potential as a nutritionally beneficial option. Furthermore, the fortified rice showcased a noteworthy characteristic of having slightly to moderately lower glycemic index (GI) values when compared to its unfortified counterpart, indicating a positive impact on blood sugar levels and overall health outcomes (Wahengbam, Das, et al., 2019).

6.8 TOXICITY

In the realm of fortification, managing the potential hazards resulting from excessive intake of fortificants is a critical concern that must not be overlooked. Hence, implementing strict regulations governing the production of fortified goods is imperative to safeguard consumers' health and well-being. The guidelines established by international bodies for setting maximum levels of micronutrients must be considered. The factors include the daily recommended intake of nutrients, the source of the micronutrient, and the age of the population (Saha & Roy, 2020). It is crucial to consider that an excessive intake of certain nutrients can lead to toxicity; therefore, the risks should not outweigh the benefits for a specific group of people. The tolerable upper limit (TUL) indicates the intake level where the risk of toxicity becomes unacceptable. Ideally, the TUL should be set significantly higher than the nutrient requirement value to ensure safety even if intake levels are higher than usual. However, when the TUL value is low and close to the distribution of requirement values, caution must be exercised when increasing the intake of that particular nutrient (Muralidharan et al., 2024).

Safety of fortified rice

Ensuring the safety of fortified rice is of utmost importance for consumers. This requires a meticulous selection of fortificants that prioritize safety, bioavailability, and compatibility with rice processing methods. Compliance with regulatory standards, such as those established by the FSSAI, is crucial. Implementing quality control measures is necessary to monitor fortificant concentration and distribution, prevent contamination, and uphold product integrity. Managing allergens is also crucial, and offering allergen-free products and providing appropriate labeling is an important parameter. Continuous monitoring and surveillance play a key role in identifying any safety concerns. Educating consumers about the benefits and safety of fortified rice can foster trust and confidence. Additionally, further research is imperative to evaluate the long-term health impacts (Efficacy and Safety of Iron Fortified Rice in India - A White Paper NITI Aayog ICMR-NIN, 2023).

6.9 FACTORS AFFECTING RICE FORTIFICATION

Various factors can significantly impact the successful fortification of rice to enhance its nutritional value (Figure 6.3). The process of fortifying rice involves several considerations, such as the type and amount of fortificant added, the technology used for fortification, and the regulations in place to ensure compliance with quality standards.

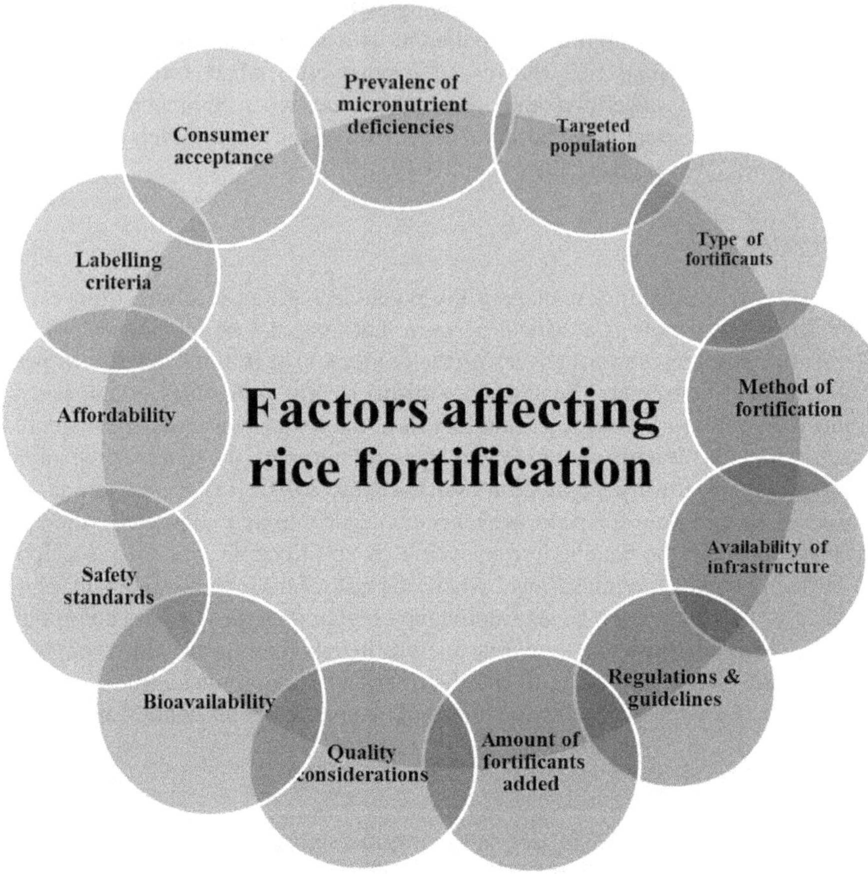

FIGURE 6.3 Factors affecting rice fortification.

Additionally, factors like the availability of fortification facilities, infrastructure for distribution, and public acceptance of fortified rice products play crucial roles in the effectiveness of rice fortification initiatives. Furthermore, understanding consumer preferences, cultural attitudes towards fortified foods, and the economic feasibility of fortification programs are essential aspects to consider when implementing rice fortification strategies. Overall, a comprehensive analysis of the factors affecting rice fortification is necessary to develop sustainable and successful fortification programs that can effectively address malnutrition and promote public health (Olson et al., 2021).

6.10 ADVANTAGES OF RICE FORTIFICATION

Rice fortification offers numerous advantages for enhancing food security and improving nutritional outcomes on a broader scale. By incorporating essential vitamins and minerals into rice, this process not only contributes to addressing malnutrition but also helps in safeguarding the population against various health deficiencies. The fortification of rice plays a crucial role in ensuring that individuals receive a more balanced and complete diet, thereby promoting overall well-being and reducing the risk of developing nutrient-related diseases. Furthermore, the enhanced nutritional profile of fortified rice can have far-reaching effects on public health, especially in regions where access to diverse and nutrient-rich foods may be limited. Overall, the practice of fortifying rice represents a strategic and sustainable approach to bolstering food and nutritional security, ultimately leading to healthier communities and a more resilient population.

Combating micronutrient deficiencies

Adding vital micronutrients like vitamin A, zinc, and iron to rice can effectively address the issue of micronutrient deficiencies commonly found in populations that heavily depend on rice as their main source of sustenance. These deficiencies are responsible for various health complications, including anemia, weakened immune system, and visual impairments (Mahapatra et al., 2021; Efficacy and Safety of Iron Fortified Rice in India - A White Paper NITI Aayog ICMR-NIN, 2023).

Enhancing overall well-being

The consistent intake of enriched rice by students aged 6 to 12 years in Gujarat state, India, as a part of the Mid-Day Meal Scheme, proved to be successful in enhancing hemoglobin levels and cognitive performance while also reducing the prevalence of anemia. The enriched rice provided a significant portion of the children's daily nutritional requirements, offering approximately 10% of the RDA for iron, 25% to 33% for vitamin A, thiamine, vitamin B6, and niacin, meeting 100% of the requirements for folic acid and vitamin B12. These results highlight the potential benefits of incorporating fortified rice into widespread school feeding schemes to enhance the well-being of at-risk school children (Mahapatra et al., 2021). The Large-Scale Food Fortification (LSFF) program has significantly improved functional health indicators, including reduced rates of goiter, anemia, and neural tube defects. It also enhanced micronutrient biomarker levels, improved reserves of iron, and reduced the onset of iron deficiency in children and women. The program led to a 34% decrease in anemia, a 41% reduction in neural tube defects, and a 74% reduction in goiter, highlighting the effectiveness of fortification programs in addressing health concerns (Keats et al., 2019).

Combating anemia

In the comprehensive analysis of the Cochrane Review on Rice Fortification, 1634 individuals were carefully considered across seven randomized controlled trials (RCTs). These trials specifically targeted school children within the age bracket of 5 to 18 years and women who are not pregnant or breastfeeding and fall within the age range of 18 to 49 years. The research findings revealed that the prevalence of anemia stood at 388 cases per 1000 individuals who consumed unfortified rice. Remarkably, upon switching to fortified rice, which included iron either alone or in conjunction with other vital micronutrients, the prevalence of anemia reduced to 279 cases per

1000 individuals. This substantial decline translated to an absolute reduction of 109 cases per 1000 individuals. Furthermore, the relative risk associated with this positive outcome was determined to be 0.72 with a confidence interval of 0.54 to 0.97, underscoring the significant impact of fortified rice consumption on combating anemia in vulnerable population (Efficacy and Safety of Iron Fortified Rice in India - A White Paper NITI Aayog ICMR-NIN, 2023). Iron-fortified rice enhances both hemoglobin levels and cognitive abilities in children (Mahapatra et al., 2021).

Types of fortificants added

Iron fortification of rice with ferric pyrophosphate (FePP) has been proposed due to its favorable sensory properties. Enhancing the bioavailability of FePP can be achieved through micronization or by incorporating tri-sodium citrate (TSC) and citric acid (CA) into ferric pyrophosphate (Ward et al., 2019). The FSSAI mandates the incorporation of ferric pyrophosphate (28 to 42.5 mg/kg) or sodium iron ethylene-di-amine-tetra-acetate-trihydrate (14 to 21.25 mg/kg) into rice to fortify it with essential iron. This fortification process ensures that rice becomes a more nutritious food source, helping to combat iron deficiency and promote better public health outcomes in India (Efficacy and Safety of Iron Fortified Rice in India - A White Paper NITI Aayog ICMR-NIN, 2023).

Bioavailability and bioaccessibility

Enriched rice boosts the intake and accessibility of essential nutrients, offering a well-rounded dietary choice with increased levels of vitamins and minerals. This elevates the nutritional content of the rice, helping address malnutrition and deficiencies in communities. Fortifying rice is a pragmatic and effective method to encourage healthier eating habits and enhance overall public health (Wahengbam, Das, et al., 2019; Jyrwa et al., 2020).

Agricultural sustainability

Rice biofortification has the potential to positively impact agricultural sustainability, as it promotes the cultivation of more nutrient-rich varieties that require fewer chemical fertilizers and pesticides. Embracing rice fortification through biofortification represents a promising strategy for addressing public health challenges related to malnutrition and ensuring a more resilient food system in the long term. This approach not only improves the overall health outcomes of consumers but also contributes to food security by ensuring that individuals have access to a more balanced diet (Das et al., 2023).

Cost-effectiveness

The process of fortifying rice is not only cost-effective but also highly impactful, presenting a promising solution to the ongoing global malnutrition crisis. This approach holds significant potential to effectively tackle nutritional deficiencies on a large scale, offering a sustainable strategy that can substantially enhance overall dietary intake and combat various nutrient deficiencies worldwide (Olson et al., 2021).

Economic benefits

Food fortification is a method employed to combat nutrient deficiencies by incorporating vital vitamins and minerals into food items. It improves health outcomes and offers economic benefits by preventing malnutrition and illnesses, reducing healthcare costs and productivity losses. Fortified foods also support national growth by creating a healthier workforce. Investment in food fortification programs is a proactive approach to public health and a strategic decision with significant social and economic implications (Olson et al., 2021).

Remedy for malnutrition

Fortified rice serves as a remedy for malnutrition in underprivileged communities, particularly children and those experiencing financial constraints. By providing necessary nutrients, it fills the nutritional void and contributes to sustainable progress. This initiative supports global health targets and enhances nutritional security, paving the way for a healthier future through wider access to fortified rice (Olson et al., 2021; Senguttuvel et al., 2023).

Benefits to farmers and consumers

Initiatives to fortify rice can boost agricultural development by increasing the demand for rice varieties rich in nutrients. This promotes investments in the research and enhancement of rice varieties with enhanced nutritional content, which is advantageous for both farmers and consumers (Das et al., 2023).

High yields

Genetically engineered rice has the potential to greatly enhance agricultural practices through its ability to achieve high yields, boost nutritional content, and introduce bioactive components. This innovative approach not only tackles food security concerns but also contributes to human well-being by creating nourishing and functional food products. The unique combination of its high yield potential, improved nutritional value, and abundant bioactive components positions genetically modified rice as a valuable resource in promoting agricultural sustainability and global health (Kobayashi et al., 2023).

Enhancing food security

The promotion of food security involves a range of strategies, including fortification, to enhance the nutritional content of staple foods. Fortification not only enhances the dietary requirements met by these foods but also reduces reliance on external sources for essential nutrients. By fortifying rice, communities can ensure their dietary needs are met, strengthening overall food security. This approach helps to build more sustainable and resilient local food systems, addressing food insecurity and crises. Fortification also empowers communities to navigate challenges related to food availability, promoting self-reliance and a stable foundation for nutritional well-being. Ultimately, fortification plays a crucial role in combating malnutrition and hunger, improving the health and resilience of communities in the face of food-related uncertainties (Olson et al., 2021).

Stress-resistant plants

Genetic engineering has improved the resistance of biofortified rice crops to various stress factors, including pests, diseases, and environmental conditions. These modified varieties are designed to withstand pests, diseases, and extreme temperatures, resulting in improved yields and quality of grains. This not only contributes to food security but also addresses malnutrition by providing essential nutrients (Ansari et al., 2015).

Rice varieties with high nutritional value

Enhancing the nutritional content of rice through biofortification shows great potential in addressing the issue of micronutrient deficiencies, also known as hidden hunger, which is a global issue affecting vulnerable populations. By breeding rice varieties rich in micronutrients like iron and zinc, this sustainable solution eliminates the need for chemical food additives. Prioritizing research and investment in rice biofortification is crucial for improving public health outcomes and combating nutrient deficiencies, particularly in countries heavily reliant on rice as a staple food (Das et al., 2023).

6.11 DISADVANTAGES OF RICE FORTIFICATION

Disadvantages of rice fortification include the potential risks associated with excessive intake of fortified nutrients, such as vitamin toxicity or mineral overload. Additionally, there may be challenges related to the acceptability and taste of fortified rice, which could impact consumer preferences and adoption rates. Another drawback is the need for careful regulation and monitoring to ensure that fortification levels are consistent and meet safety standards, which can be resource-intensive and require strong governance mechanisms. Furthermore, incorporating fortification processes into existing rice production systems may require substantial investments in infrastructure and technology, posing economic barriers for some producers. While rice fortification shows potential in addressing nutrient deficiencies and improving public health outcomes, these drawbacks emphasize the significance of thorough planning, involving stakeholders, and continuous evaluation to minimize potential disadvantages and maximize the advantages of this intervention.

Availability

Accessing fortified rice poses a significant hurdle for people in economically disadvantaged areas due to inadequate distribution and storage infrastructure. This obstacle can impede the effectiveness of fortification initiatives designed to enhance nutritional results. Overcoming logistical challenges is essential to guarantee fair access to vital fortified food items, fostering improved nutrition for those in need (Dasher et al., 2023).

Taste preferences

Fortifying a product can alter its flavor and consistency, potentially leading to a decrease in consumer satisfaction (Bambridge-Sutton, 2023). Despite efforts to promote brown rice over white polished rice, many still prefer the latter due to taste preferences, convenience, and cultural traditions. There is a significant gap between knowledge and practice, and it is crucial to continue advocating for brown rice's nutritional value and health benefits. Initiatives should focus on educating the public about brown rice's higher fiber content and micronutrient profile (Das et al., 2023).

Types of fortificants added

Fortifying rice with iron presents additional challenges when it comes to incorporating easily absorbable and water-soluble forms such as ferrous sulfate and ferrous fumarate. These forms have unappealing sensory attributes that could potentially negatively affect consumer acceptance. On the other hand, ferric pyrophosphate (FePP), although not as readily absorbed, is recommended for fortifying rice due to its more favorable taste profile. The appealing flavor of ferric pyrophosphate makes consumers more likely to embrace iron-fortified rice, even though its bioavailability is lower compared to other forms of iron. This trade-off is worth considering in enhancing the palatability and overall acceptance of the product. Therefore, the use of ferric pyrophosphate in fortifying rice offers a promising solution to maintain a balance between nutritional benefits and sensory appeal, ensuring that iron-fortified rice remains a viable and appealing option for consumers who want to increase their iron intake through staple foods like rice (Hennigar & Hamaker, 2022).

Hazards associated with consuming too much

Certain types of fortified rice might include additional ingredients or fortifying agents that could present health hazards if consumed excessively or by susceptible groups like expectant mothers or young children (Hennigar & Hamaker, 2022). Studies examining the potential negative impacts of soluble iron compounds, such as $FeSO_4$ or ferric fumarate, when administered in large quantities exceeding 1mg/kg body weight per day, must not be indiscriminately extrapolated to iron-fortified rice containing FPP. The reason behind this cautionary approach lies in the distinct variations observed in the ways these compounds interact with the human body. For example, while studies may indicate adverse effects of $FeSO_4$ or ferric fumarate at high doses, it cannot be conclusively assumed that similar outcomes would occur with iron-fortified rice supplemented with FPP due to the differing bioavailability and metabolic pathways of these iron sources. Hence, any generalizations drawn from studies focusing on soluble iron compounds should be interpreted with care in relation to the specific context of iron-fortified rice with FPP, considering factors like absorption rates, distribution mechanisms, and biochemical reactions unique to each form of iron supplement (Efficacy and Safety of Iron Fortified Rice in India - A White Paper NITI Aayog ICMR-NIN, 2023).

Loss of essential nutrients during food processing

In developing nations where washing rice is a common practice, dusting is not advised to fortify rice. Excessive washing and cooking with excess water can lead to significant nutrient loss, which is a concern in regions with limited access to diverse and nutrient-rich foods. In the USA, the significance of minimizing nutrient loss during rice preparation is acknowledged to the extent that rice packaging labels include a caution against rinsing the rice or using excessive water. This labeling requirement aims to educate consumers about the potential impact of improper rice preparation on its nutrient content. It highlights the importance of preserving the nutritional value of rice, which serves as an important source of energy and vital nutrients for people of every age. This reminder acts as a powerful tool in promoting healthier cooking practices and safeguarding valuable nutrients for overall well-being (Steiger et al., 2014).

Reduced consumer acceptance

One of the drawbacks often linked with fortifying rice using the extrusion method is the likelihood of disrupting its inherent composition, potentially leading to changes that could influence its traditional flavor and texture profile. This alteration may extend to the deprivation of certain nutrients that are sensitive to heat and the oxidation of iron, particularly evident in instances where steaming is involved. Such modifications can not only impact the sensory experience of consuming the fortified rice but also pose concerns regarding the nutritional value and overall quality of the end product. The transformation of its natural state through extrusion carries the risk of compromising the authenticity of the rice (Akasapu et al., 2020), potentially diminishing its appeal to consumers who value traditional taste and texture characteristics. Therefore, while fortification through this method offers enhanced nutritional benefits, it is crucial to carefully consider and mitigate the factors that may alter the rice's original properties to ensure that the final product remains well-balanced and appealing to the target audience (Akasapu et al., 2020). Hot extrusion is a common method for manufacturing iron-fortified rice; however, the process of heating can lead to an increase in resistant starch content, ultimately reducing the availability for absorption of iron in the body. However, on the other side, cold-extruded iron-fortified rice may offer better iron bioavailability, but it is also associated with higher iron losses when cooked (de Pee et al., 2018).

Presence of anti-nutrients

In zinc- and iron-fortified rice, the presence of phytic acid, a natural compound found in many grains and seeds can have an impact on the absorption of essential minerals. Phytic acid binds to iron and zinc, forming complexes that make it challenging for the body to access and utilize these nutrients effectively. As a result, consuming foods rich in phytic acid alongside iron and zinc sources may hinder the body's ability to fully benefit from these vital minerals (Senguttuvel et al., 2023). To address this problem various strategies can be employed during food preparation, such as soaking, fermentation, or sprouting, which can help reduce the phytic acid content of rice and other grains, thereby enhancing the absorption of iron and zinc (Saha & Roy, 2020; Bhatnagar & Padilla-Zakour, 2021). An alternative approach involved in the development of transgenic crops is through the manipulation of the phytic acid biosynthetic pathway using RNA interference (RNAi) to silence its key enzymes (Majumder et al., 2019). Additionally, incorporating vitamin C-rich foods in meals containing iron-fortified rice can promote better iron absorption and enhance bioavailability counteracting the potential inhibitory effects of phytic acid (Jyrwa et al., 2020). Understanding the interplay between phytic acid and mineral absorption is crucial for maximizing the nutritional benefits of iron- and zinc-fortified rice, ensuring optimal health outcomes for individuals seeking to improve their nutrient intake (Majumder et al., 2019).

A myth

A myth about fortified rice kernels (FRK), synthetic rice, was circulated, claiming it was made from "plastic". FRK grains float during cooking, leading to misinterpretations and confusion. This led to consumers discarding FRK in the garbage, perpetuating the misconception. Despite clarifications, the confusion persisted, highlighting the dangers of superficial observations and the need for critical thinking in today's interconnected world (Panchami & Rao 2023).

Illnesses

During certain health complications like sickle cell anemia or thalassemia, the incorporation of iron-fortified rice may have adverse effects by building the individual's iron storage, leading to further illnesses (Panchami & Rao 2023).

6.12 CONCLUSION

Rice fortification is an efficient and far-reaching method to enhance food security; fortifying rice with essential nutrients represents a positive step in the global effort to eliminate malnutrition and achieve Zero Hunger, which is a crucial component of SDG 2. The widespread consumption of fortified rice holds promise in reaching a significant portion of the population, thereby making a substantial impact in the fight against hunger. This approach is particularly beneficial in regions where rice is a staple, as it helps combat nutrient deficiencies. Additionally, fortifying rice helps to preserve cultural dietary traditions and fights against hidden hunger, which refers to unnoticed micronutrient deficiencies. Rice fortification is a crucial initiative aimed at improving food security and addressing malnutrition through various strategies like education, community engagement, media campaigns, policy advocacy, and monitoring. It can work hand in hand with existing public health initiatives, ensuring sustainability in the long term and seamless integration into current supply chains. Governments have taken steps to support rice fortification by implementing regulations that establish fortification standards, quality control measures, and monitoring systems. However, it is imperative to exercise caution and implement necessary safeguards to prevent any potential adverse effects on health and well-being.

Looking ahead, with the projected 25% increase in the world's population by 2050, there will be a heightened demand for rice production and consumption in traditional regions to combat food insecurity effectively. It is essential to recognize that just providing energy through food may not be sufficient to address the complex challenges of food security in the contemporary era. Considering this, integrating targeted nutrition into existing and upcoming rice varieties emerges as a sustainable and impactful solution to address food insecurity and combat deficiencies in essential micronutrients. This strategic approach advocates for the development of rice strains that not only cater to energy needs but also offer a comprehensive and balanced nutritional profile, fostering a healthier and more secure global food landscape to support sustainable development goals. Rice fortification presents a practical and scalable solution to tackle malnutrition and enhance food security.

REFERENCES

269 Districts in 27 States Distributing Fortified Rice under Targeted Public Distribution System. (2023, April 6). Press Information Bureau. https://pib.gov.in/PressReleaseIframePage.aspx?PRID=1914231

Akasapu, K., Ojah, N., Gupta, A. K., Choudhury, A. J., & Mishra, P. (2020). An innovative approach for iron fortification of rice using cold plasma. *Food Research International*, 136, 109599. https://doi.org/10.1016/j.foodres.2020.109599

Alfthan, G., Eurola, M., Ekholm, P., Venäläinen, E.-R., Root, T., Korkalainen, K., Hartikainen, H., Salminen, P., Hietaniemi, V., Aspila, P., & Aro, A. (2015). Effects of nationwide addition of selenium to fertilizers on foods, and animal and human health in Finland: From deficiency to optimal selenium status of the population. *Journal of Trace Elements in Medicine and Biology*, 31, 142–147. https://doi.org/10.1016/j.jtemb.2014.04.009

Ansari, M. ur R., Shaheen, T., Bukhari, S. A., & Husnain, T. (2015). Genetic improvement of rice for biotic and abiotic stress tolerance. In *Turkish Journal of Botany* (Vol. 39, Issue 6, pp. 911–919). TurkiyeKlinikleri Journal of Medical Sciences. https://doi.org/10.3906/bot-1503-47

Augustus Bambridge-Sutton. (2023, December 12). What are consumer attitudes to fortification? Consumers often care about taste over health. *Food Navigator-Europe*. www.foodnavigator.com/Article/2023/12/12/fortification-consumer-attitudes-to-taste-and-texture-of-fortified-products

Bajaj, S. R., & Singhal, R. S. (2019). Effect of extrusion processing and hydrocolloids on the stability of added vitamin B12 and physico-functional properties of the fortified puffed extrudates. *LWT*, 101, 32–39. https://doi.org/10.1016/j.lwt.2018.11.011

Bhatnagar, R. S., & Padilla-Zakour, O. I. (2021). Plant-based dietary practices and socioeconomic factors that influence anemia in India. In *Nutrients* (Vol. 13, Issue 10). MDPI. https://doi.org/10.3390/nu13103538

Biofortification | International Rice Research Institute. (2018). www.irri.org/biofortification

Biswas, J. C., Haque, M. M., Khan, F. H., Islam, M. R., Dipti, S. S., Akter, M., & Ahmed, H. U. (2018). Zinc fortification: Effect of polishing on parboiled and unparboiled rice. *Current Plant Biology*, 16, 22–26. https://doi.org/10.1016/j.cpb.2018.11.002

Bonto, A. P., Camacho, K. S. I., & Camacho, D. H. (2018). Increased vitamin B5 uptake capacity of ultrasonic treated milled rice: A new method for rice fortification. *LWT*, 95, 32–39. https://doi.org/10.1016/j.lwt.2018.04.062

Das, A. B., & Bhattacharya, S. (2019). Characterization of the batter and gluten-free cake from extruded red rice flour. *LWT*, 102, 197–204. https://doi.org/10.1016/j.lwt.2018.12.026

Das, K., Roy, P., Kumar, R., & Tiwari, S. (2023). *Biofortification of Rice, An Impactful Strategy for Nutritional Security: Current Perspectives and Future Prospect*. London: IntechOpen. www.intechopen.com

Dasher, R. K. A. A. M. (2023). *Rice Fortification in India: Progression and Insights*. Gurugram: Institute for Competitiveness.

Datta, M., & Vitolins, M. Z. (2016). Food fortification and supplement use—Are there health implications? *Critical Reviews in Food Science and Nutrition*, 56(13), 2149–2159. https://doi.org/10.1080/10408398.2013.818527

de Pee, S., Tsang, B. L., Zimmerman, S., & Montgomery, S. J. (2018). Rice fortification. In M.G. Venkatesh-Mannar & R.F. Hurrell (eds.), *Food Fortification in a Globalized World* (pp. 131–141). Elsevier. https://doi.org/10.1016/B978-0-12-802861-2.00013-4

DSM. (2018, May). The Role of Rice Fortification in Improving Public Health The Role of Rice Fortification in Improving Public Health Executive summary. DSM. www.dsm.com/content/dam/dsm/human-nutrition/pdfs/DSM_Rice_Fortification_and_Public_Health_Whitepaper_HighRes.pdf

Hemalatha, R., Samarasimha Reddy, N., Challa, S., Venkatesh, K., Pullakhandam, R., Nandeep, E. R., Teena, D., Mahesh Kumar, M., & Raghavendra, P. (2023). Efficacy and Safety of Iron Fortified Rice in India - A White Paper. ICMR-National Institute of Nutrition, Hyderabad.

Explainer / Benefits of Rice Fortification. (2022, April). *Manorama Yearbook.* www.manoramayearbook.in/current-affairs/india/2022/04/09/upsc-rice-fortification-benefits.html

FAOSTAT. (n.d.). *Crops and Livestock Products.* Retrieved May 17, 2024, from www.fao.org/faostat/en/#data/QCL

Food Fortification. (n.d.). UN World Food Programme (WFP). Retrieved May 17, 2024, from www.wfp.org/

Food Fortification Initiative. (2019, July 31). Solomon Islands Receives First Shipment of Fortified Rice. FFI. www.ffinetwork.org/ffimedia/solomon-islands-receives-first-shipment-of-fortified-rice

FSSAI. (2018). Food Safety and Standards (Fortification of Foods) Regulations. FSSAI India. www.fao.org/faolex/results/details/en/c/LEX-FAOC180268/

Fukagawa, N. K., & Ziska, L. H. (2019). Rice: Importance for global nutrition. In *Journal of Nutrition Science Vitaminology*, 65. www.riceassociation.org.uk/content/1/18/types-

Gani, G., Gulzar, B., Bashir, O., & Bhat, T. A. (2018). Hidden hunger and its prevention by food processing: A review. *International Journal of Unani and Integrative Medicine*, 2(3), 1–10. www.researchgate.net/publication/330535249

Garg, M., Sharma, N., Sharma, S., Kapoor, P., Kumar, A., Chunduri, V., & Arora, P. (2018). Biofortified crops generated by breeding, agronomy, and transgenic approaches are improving lives of millions of people around the world. In *Frontiers in Nutrition,* 5. Frontiers Media S.A. https://doi.org/10.3389/fnut.2018.00012

Ghosh, S., & Pundhir, A. (2018). Food Fortification: A Nutritional Management Strategy in India. www.researchgate.net/publication/328723532

Hennigar, S. R., & Hamaker, B. R. (2022). Optimizing fortification of rice with micronutrients to improve public health. *Journal of Nutrition*, 152(5), 1179–1180. https://doi.org/10.1093/jn/nxac023

Jannasch, A., Brownmiller, C., Lee, S.-O., Mauromoustakos, A., & Wang, Y.-J. (2020). Simultaneous fortification of rice with folic acid and β-carotene or vitamin A by limited-water parboiling. *Journal of Cereal Science*, 96, 103096. https://doi.org/10.1016/j.jcs.2020.103096

Jena, J., Sethy, P., Jena, T., Ranjan Misra, S., Kumar Sahoo, S., Kumar Dash, G., Jagadish Jena, C., & Palai, J. (2018). Rice biofortification: A brief review. ~ 2644 ~. *Journal of Pharmacognosy and Phytochemistry*, 7(1), 2644–2647.

Junaid-ur-Rahman, S., Chughtai, M. F. J., Khaliq, A., Liaqat, A., Pasha, I., Ahsan, S., Tanweer, S., Saeed, K., Siddiqa, A., Mehmood, T., Ali, A., Aziz, S., & Sameed, N. (2022). Rice: A potential vehicle for micronutrient fortification. *Clinical Phytoscience*, 8(1), 14. https://doi.org/10.1186/s40816-022-00342-3

Jyrwa, Y. W., Palika, R., Boddula, S., Boiroju, N. K., Madhari, R., Pullakhandam, R., & Thingnganing, L. (2020). Retention, stability, iron bioavailability and sensory evaluation of extruded rice fortified with iron, folic acid and vitamin B12. *Maternal and Child Nutrition*, 16(S3). https://doi.org/10.1111/mcn.12932

Keats, E. C., Neufeld, L. M., Garrett, G. S., Mbuya, M. N. N., & Bhutta, Z. A. (2019). Improved micronutrient status and health outcomes in low- and middle-income countries following large-scale fortification: Evidence from a systematic review and meta-analysis. *The American Journal of Clinical Nutrition*, 109(6), 1696–1708. https://doi.org/10.1093/ajcn/nqz023

Khampuang, K., Lordkaew, S., Dell, B., & Prom-u-thai, C. (2021). Foliar zinc application improved grain zinc accumulation and bioavailable zinc in unpolished and polished rice. *Plant Production Science*, 24(1), 94–102. https://doi.org/10.1080/1343943X.2020.1797512

Kobayashi, K., Wang, X., & Wang, W. (2023). Genetically modified rice is associated with hunger, health, and climate resilience. In *Foods* (Vol. 12, Issue 14). Multidisciplinary Digital Publishing Institute (MDPI). https://doi.org/10.3390/foods12142776

Kunal Khureja. (2022). Rice Fortification: Benefits, Concerns-Explained, Pointwise-ForumIAS Blog. https://forumias.com/blog/rice-fortification-benefits-concerns-and-guidelines/

Panchami, L. R., & Rao, P. (2023, April 5). Understanding Barriers and Facilitators for Rice Fortification in India – FFOODS Spectrum. https://nuffoodsspectrum.in/2023/04/05/understanding-barriers-and-facilitators-for-rice-fortification-in-india.html

Mahapatra, S., Parker, M. E., Dave, N., Zobrist, S. C., Shajie Arul, D., King, A., Betigeri, A., & Sachdeva, R. (2021). Micronutrient-fortified rice improves haemoglobin, anaemia prevalence and cognitive performance among schoolchildren in Gujarat, India: A case-control study. *International Journal of Food Sciences and Nutrition*, 72(5), 690–703. https://doi.org/10.1080/09637486.2020.1855126

Majumder, S., Datta, K., & Datta, S. K. (2019). Rice biofortification: High iron, zinc, and Vitamin-A to fight against "hidden hunger". In *Agronomy* (Vol. 9, Issue 12). MDPI AG. https://doi.org/10.3390/agronomy9120803

Mannar, M. G. V., & Wesley, A. S. (2023). Food fortification. In SR Quah (ed.), *Reference Module in Biomedical Sciences*. Elsevier. https://doi.org/10.1016/B978-0-323-99967-0.00022-3

Mohidem, N. A., Hashim, N., Shamsudin, R., & Che Man, H. (2022). Rice for food security: Revisiting its production, diversity. *Rice Milling Process and Nutrient Content. Agriculture*, 12(6), 741. https://doi.org/10.3390/agriculture12060741

Mridula, D., & Pooja, J. (2014). Preparation of iron-fortified rice using edible coating materials. *International Journal of Food Science and Technology*, 49(1), 246–252. https://doi.org/10.1111/ijfs.12305

Muralidharan, J., Hegde, S. G., Ghosh, S., Mondal, A., Arjun, M., Thomas, T., Kurpad, S. S., Davis, C., Sachdev, H. S., & Kurpad, A. V. (2024). Mandatory fortification of rice in the public distribution system in India: An ethics perspective. In *Indian Journal of Medical Ethics* (Vol. 9, Issue 1, pp. 26–30). Forum for Medical Ethics Society. https://doi.org/10.20529/IJME.2023.064

Niu, J., Liu, C., Huang, M., Liu, K., & Yan, D. (2021). Effects of foliar fertilization: A review of current status and future perspectives. In *Journal of Soil Science and Plant Nutrition* (Vol. 21, Issue 1, pp. 104–118). Springer Science and Business Media Deutschland GmbH. https://doi.org/10.1007/s42729-020-00346-3

Olson, R., Gavin-Smith, B., Ferraboschi, C., & Kraemer, K. (2021). Food fortification: The advantages, disadvantages and lessons from sight and life programs. In *Nutrients* (Vol. 13, Issue 4). MDPI AG. https://doi.org/10.3390/nu13041118

PATH, G. A. for I. N. (GAIN). (2015). Rice Fortification Toolkit Technical Manual. www.micronutrient.org/CMFiles/PubLib/Report-67-VMD-A-Global-Damage-Assessment-Report1

Patindol, J., Fragallo, L., Wang, Y., & Durand-Morat, A. (2017). Impact of feedstock, parboiling condition, and nutrient concentration on simultaneous fortification of two U.S. long-grain rice cultivars with iron and zinc. *Cereal Chemistry*, 94(6), 984–990. https://doi.org/10.1094/CCHEM-05-17-0115-R

Phuphong, P., Cakmak, I., Dell, B., & Prom-u-thai, C. (2018). Effects of foliar application of zinc on grain yield and zinc concentration of rice in farmers' fields. *Chiang Mai University Journal of Natural Sciences*, 17(3). https://doi.org/10.12982/CMUJNS.2018.0013

Press Information Bureau. (2022, February 4). https://pib.gov.in/PressReleasePage.aspx?PRID=1795421

Qureshy, L. F., Alderman, H., & Manchanda, N. (2023). Benefit-cost analysis of iron fortification of rice in India: Modelling potential economic gains from improving haemoglobin and averting anaemia. *Journal of Development Effectiveness*, 15(1), 91–110. https://doi.org/10.1080/19439342.2023.2168728

Rohner, F., Wirth, J. P., Zeng, W., Petry, N., Donkor, W. E. S., Neufeld, L. M., Mkambula, P., Groll, S., Mbuya, M. N., & Friesen, V. M. (2023). Global coverage of mandatory large-scale food fortification programs: A systematic review and meta-analysis. *Advances in Nutrition*, 14(5), 1197–1210. https://doi.org/10.1016/j.advnut.2023.07.004

Saha, S., & Roy, A. (2020). Whole grain rice fortification as a solution to micronutrient deficiency: Technologies and need for more viable alternatives. *Food Chemistry*, 326, 127049. https://doi.org/10.1016/j.foodchem.2020.127049

Samaddar, A., Mohibbe Azam, M., Singaravadivel, K., Venkatachalapathy, N., Swain, B. B., & Mishra, P. (2017). Postharvest management and value addition of rice and its by-products. In S. Mohanty, P.G. Chengappa, Mruthyunjaya, J.K. Ladha, S. Baruah, E. Kannan, & A.V. Manjunatha (eds.), *The Future Rice Strategy for India* (pp. 301–334). Elsevier. https://doi.org/10.1016/B978-0-12-805374-4.00011-7

Samyor, D., Deka, S. C., & Das, A. B. (2018). Effect of extrusion conditions on the physicochemical and phytochemical properties of red rice and passion fruit powder based extrudates. *Journal of Food Science and Technology*, 55(12), 5003–5013. https://doi.org/10.1007/s13197-018-3439-9

Senguttuvel, P., Padmavathi, G., Jasmine, C., Sanjeeva Rao, D., Neeraja, C. N., Jaldhani, V., Beulah, P., Gobinath, R., Aravind Kumar, J., Sai Prasad, S. V., Subba Rao, L. V., Hariprasad, A. S., Sruthi, K., Shivani, D., Sundaram, R. M., & Govindaraj, M. (2023). Rice biofortification: Breeding and genomic approaches for genetic enhancement of grain zinc and iron contents. In *Frontiers in Plant Science* (Vol. 14). Frontiers Media S.A. https://doi.org/10.3389/fpls.2023.1138408

Shahbandeh, M. (2024). Rice Consumption by Country 2023/24 | Statista. www.statista.com/statistics/255971/top-countries-based-on-rice-consumption-2012-2013/

Steiger, G., Müller-Fischer, N., Cori, H., & Conde-Petit, B. (2014). Fortification of rice: Technologies and nutrients. *Annals of the New York Academy of Sciences*, 1324(1), 29–39. https://doi.org/10.1111/nyas.12418

Thakur, S., Singh, A., Insa, B., & Sharma, S. (2023). Food fortification in India as malnutrition concern: A global approach. In *Sustainable Food Technology* (Vol. 1, Issue 5, pp. 681–695). Royal Society of Chemistry. https://doi.org/10.1039/d3fb00079f

Thiruselvam, N. (2014). Micronutrients fortification of rice by parboiling: Lab scale and Pilot scale studies. *Journal of Nutrition & Food Sciences*, 4(4). https://doi.org/10.4172/2155-9600.1000281

Tiozon Jr., R. N., Camacho, D. H., Bonto, A. P., Oyong, G. G., & Sreenivasulu, N. (2021). Efficient fortification of folic acid in rice through ultrasonic treatment and absorption. *Food Chemistry*, 335, 127629. https://doi.org/10.1016/j.foodchem.2020.127629

Wahengbam, E. D., Das, A. J., Green, B. D., Shooter, J., & Hazarika, M. K. (2019). Effect of iron and folic acid fortification on in vitro bioavailability and starch hydrolysis in ready-to-eat parboiled rice. *Food Chemistry*, 292, 39–46. https://doi.org/10.1016/j.foodchem.2019.04.044

Wahengbam, E. D., Green, B. D., & Hazarika, M. K. (2019). Fortification of zinc in a parboiled low-amylose rice: Effects of milling and cooking. *Journal of the Science of Food and Agriculture*, 99(7), 3434–3442. https://doi.org/10.1002/jsfa.9561

Wakeel, A., Farooq, M., Bashir, K., & Ozturk, L. (2018). Micronutrient malnutrition and biofortification: Recent advances and future perspectives. In M.A. Hossain, T. Kamiya, D.J. Burritt, L.-S. Phan Tran, & T. Fujiwara (eds.), *Plant Micronutrient Use Efficiency: Molecular and Genomic Perspectives in Crop Plants* (pp. 225–243). Elsevier. https://doi.org/10.1016/B978-0-12-812104-7.00017-4

Ward, E., Suleria, H., Joseph, M., Alavi, S., & Lindshield, B. (2019). Ferric pyrophosphate in extruded, fortified rice leads to better iron outcomes than ferric phosphate in rats (P24-014-19). *Current Developments in Nutrition*, 3, nzz044.P24-014-19. https://doi.org/10.1093/cdn/nzz044.P24-014-19

WFP. (2024). Food Fortification | World Food Programme. WFP. www.wfp.org/food-fortification

WFP-Food Fortification. (2022). *Food Fortification: An Effective and Safe Way to Fight Micronutrient Malnutrition and Its Consequences.* https://docs.wfp.org/api/documents/WFP-0000139908/download/?_ga=2.90642136.375232078.1716187634-1083957579.1714937073

Whitfield, K. C., Smith, T. J., Rohner, F., Wieringa, F. T., & Green, T. J. (2021). Thiamine fortification strategies in low- and middle-income settings: A review. *Annals of the New York Academy of Sciences*, 1498(1), 29–45. https://doi.org/10.1111/nyas.14565

WHO. (2018). Guideline: Fortification of Rice with Vitamins and Minerals as a Public Health Strategy. Geneva: WHO. https://iris.who.int/bitstream/handle/10665/272535/9789241550291-eng.pdf

WHO. (2023, August 9). Fortification of Rice. E-Library of Evidence for Nutrition Actions. Geneva: WHO. www.who.int/tools/elena/interventions/rice-fortification

WHO. (2024). *Food Fortification.* WHO. www.who.int/health-topics/food-fortification#tab=tab_1

Yadav, D. N., Bansal, S., Tushir, S., Kaur, J., & Sharma, K. (2020). Advantage of biofortification over fortification technologies. In Op. Gupta, V. Pandey, S. Narwal, P. Sharma, S. Ram, & G.P. Singh (eds.), *Wheat and Barley Grain Biofortification* (pp. 257–273). Elsevier. https://doi.org/10.1016/B978-0-12-818444-8.00010-9

7 Role of Nutrigenomics in Improving Nutritional Status

Jharna Puppala, Naga Jyothi Ala, and Maheshwar Mekam

7.1 INTRODUCTION

The Human Genome Project and the powerful tools of molecular biology paved the way for an era of "nutrigenomics" or nutritional genomics, a concept that came into being in 2001. The field of nutrigenomics is concerned with understanding the relationship between nutrition, genetics, and diseases or simply the interplay of risk factors responsible for diet-related chronic health issues, which in turn may help resolve the underlying genetic mechanisms and aid in therapeutics.

Nutrigenomics has been described as the impact of genetic diversity on nutrition by linking single-nucleotide polymorphisms or gene expression to a nutrient's physiological effects, metabolism, absorption, and excretion. That has to do with the concept of genotype-based individualized nutrition. Though nutrigenomics is still in its infancy, its contribution to human wellness will become clear over the next ten years as foods and the ways in which food affects our genes will be more fully understood. Hopefully, this will allow for such tailored dietary guidance.

At a genetic level, nutritional genomics will enable a better understanding of people's reactions to food compounds based on post-genomics, genomics, transcriptomics, proteomics, metabolomics, and more (Meiliana & Wijaya, 2020). Its main aim is to understand the response of the human body to diet via an integrated approach known as systems biology, as shown in Figure 7.1. The goal is to facilitate the prevention and management of diseases with the strategy of targeted nutrition. Hippocrates (460–360 BC), the father of medicine, once said, "Leave your drugs in the chemist's pot if you can heal the patient with food."

Advances in clinical genetics have already assisted in developing an in-depth knowledge of patterns of genetic variants and gene expression, to develop treatment strategies for managing chronic degenerative diseases that impact public health. With nutrigenomics, we can further evaluate nutrients and their interaction with genes that play a role in health and disease and help in understanding the processes of regulation of metabolism (Vyas, 2022).

DOI: 10.1201/9781003487227-7

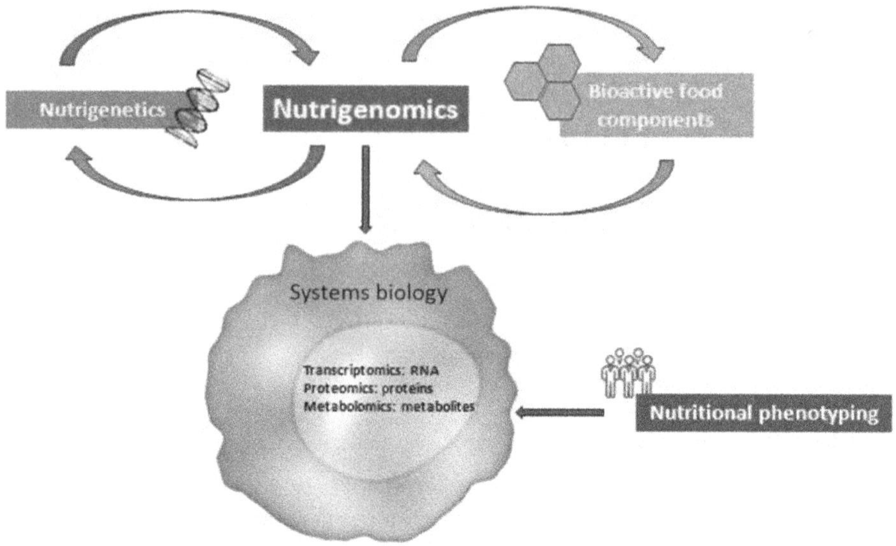

FIGURE 7.1 Effect of bioactive food components on systems biology. (Adapted from Munshi & Duvvuri, 2008.)

7.2 ARCHITECTURE OF THE GENOME

The architecture of the entire genome, as opposed to individual genes, provides the greatest understanding of the crucial roles that genes play in an individual's existence.

The majority of our cells' nuclei contain two copies of the human genome (one from each parent), which is made up of more than 3 billion deoxyribonucleic acid (DNA) base pairs arranged into chromosomes. About 21,000 genes, which are linear information units, are used to encode the proteins that our bodies require (Mullins et al., 2020). Only a small portion (<1%) of the genome is made up of genes; the remainder is made up of huge sections with unclear functions, repetitive sequences, and so-called regulatory machinery—regions crucial for regulating the transcription of different genes (Salzberg, 2018). The DNA code is "read" by transcriptional machinery, which then generates mRNA. Subsequently, this mRNA travels to ribosomes, where it joins amino acids to form the encoded proteins by interaction with translational machinery. A typical gene's organization, which is made up of several parts known as exons and introns, is shown in Figure 7.2. Spliceosomes eliminate intronic sections from both of the original transcriptions, leaving just exons in the mature mRNA transcripts. Furthermore, different transcripts containing only specific exons can be produced by a single gene, meaning that a single gene can encode multiple protein isoforms (Larochelle, 2016).

7.3 OVERVIEW OF NUTRIGENOMICS AND NUTRIGENETICS

Nutritional genomics comprises two important branches: nutrigenomics and nutrigenetics. Nutrigenomics is the study of the interaction between the genes

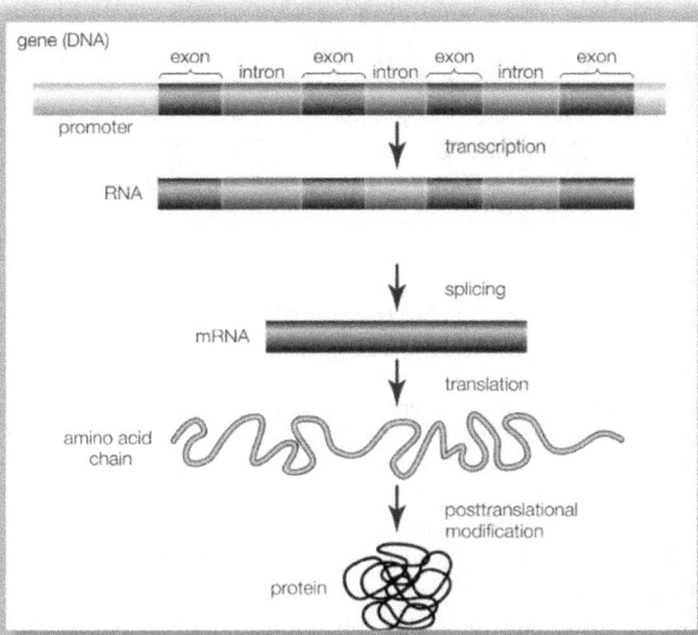

FIGURE 7.2 A typical structure of gene organization. (Adapted from Encyclopedia Britannica, 2008.)

and dietary components and associated regulations that control dietary metabolism. Nutrigenetics is the subject which identifies genetic responses and variations related to dietary components. In 1975, Richard Brennan coined the term nutrigenetics in his book *Nutrigenetics: New Concepts for Relieving Hypoglycemia* (Simopoulos, 2010).

Nature has gifted us food sources containing various nutrients that we consume in our diet, and these dietary factors acting as co-factors in the metabolic pathways constantly interact with DNA. There are two levels of interaction of nutrients and genomes:

- Nutrients and their derivatives can regulate gene expression by inducing or repressing gene expression in turn affecting individuals' phenotype.
- The metabolic pathways and bioactivity of their mediators can be altered by single-nucleotide polymorphisms, which also affect the ability to interact with the nutrients, as shown in Figure 7.3.

Nutrigenomics links genetics to different areas of human beings, namely physiology, biochemistry, bioinformatics, proteomics, metabolomics, and transcriptomics (Kiani, 2022). The principles of nutrigenomics are based on the following:

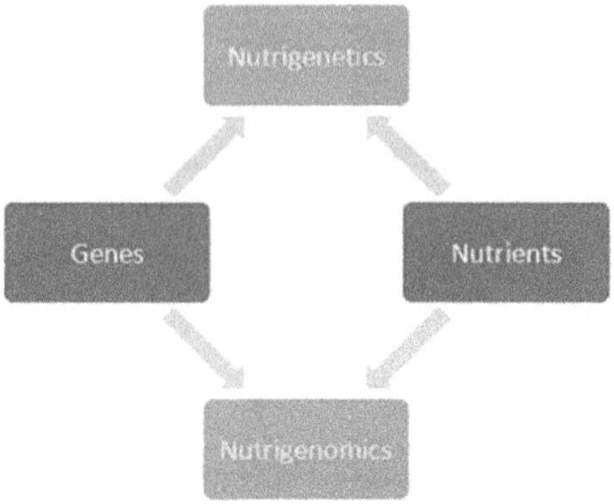

FIGURE 7.3 Interaction of genes and nutrients. (Adapted from Farhud et al., 2010.)

- the effects of genetic diversity prevalent in various ethnicities and nutrients' bioavailability and metabolism;
- cultural, geographical, and socioeconomic factors influencing types of food and their availability;
- the role of malnutrition in gene functioning, which can alter genome stability leading to alterations in the coding sequence and chromosomal aberrations, which eventually results in disturbed dosage of genes and phenotypes (Naureen et al., 2020).

Nutrigenomics is an evolving subject that is based on the application of molecular biology approaches to explore, analyze, and realize the physio-biochemical reactions of individuals or group of people to specific diets.

Nutrigenetics is the genetic composition of an individual that evolves because of their nutrient intake (i.e., gene–nutrient interaction), and studies on gene–nutrient interaction are still in their infancy. Both polygenetic and monogenetic diseases are susceptible to influence by individual genotypes of food. Many metabolic illnesses such as phenylketonuria (PKU), inherited conditions such as hemochromatosis, and abnormality of oxidation of fatty acids could be managed with dietary restrictions based on the patient's genetic makeup. Knowledge is being gained on interactions between nutrients which can occur based on the pattern of meal consumption, leading to the onset of some illnesses and disorders.

Nutrigenomics and nutrigenetics are likely to play a significant role in treating chronic diseases and in promoting health and wellness via both basic and clinical research, which is critical for the future of personalized nutrition and precision healthcare (Marcum, 2020).

7.4 ROLE OF GENETIC VARIANTS

Genetic polymorphism is another genetic concept that is responsible partly for variations in an individual's response to bioactive food components. The variability induced by single-nucleotide polymorphisms (SNPs) in the genes associated with the inflammatory process sensitizes people to make changes in their dietary pattern. For instance, the efficacy of fish oil in reducing the production of proinflammatory cytokine tumor necrosis factor is modulated by polymorphisms in specific genes.

By enabling our understanding of personal uniqueness and by the role of SNPs, doors have been opened for managing and optimizing human wellness through tailored nutrition. An example of nutrigenomics involving the relationship is between an intake of non-alcoholic caffeinated beverages and the gene for the enzyme cytochrome P450 1A2. According to Caterina and Sohemy (2016), this specific gene is essential for about 95% of caffeine metabolism and exhibits significant interindividual variation in its function. It is believed that caffeine stimulates the central nervous system and enters the gastrointestinal tract quickly. As per reports, 227 mg of caffeine is ingested daily by about 90% of adults, mostly through regular beverages including tea, coffee, energy drinks, and soft drinks. Genetic variations affecting the enzyme methylxanthine, which metabolizes caffeine in the liver, are the cause of the significant variation in the effects of caffeine on individuals (Mullins et al., 2020).

The two known variants of the CYP1A2 are the CYP1A2*1A variant, which is associated with rapid caffeine metabolism, and the CYP1A2*IF variant, which is associated with slow caffeine metabolism. Prior studies have revealed an association between having the variant gene (i.e., CYP1A2*IF), consumption of caffeine, and myocardial infarction of the non-fatal type. In contrast, the CYP1A2*1A variant conferred a protective effect due to a four times quicker metabolism of caffeine (Nehlig, 2018).

Another significant aspect to discuss in this chapter is the genetics of non-alcoholic fatty liver disease (NAFLD) which is considered as an "epidemic of the new millennium". The most prevalent liver disease in the world today is NAFLD (Puppala et al., 2014). With a prevalence of roughly 30% in Western countries and 5–18% in Asian regions, its incidence in adults and children is quickly increasing due to the ongoing obesity and type 2 diabetes epidemics (Benedict & Zhang, 2017). It is now a global public health concern as a result. Particularly in genetically predisposed populations, environmental variables have been shown to be important in the etiology of NAFLD. Junk food, particularly the standard "Western-style" diet heavy in simple carbs, saturated fat, and highly processed foods, is one of the most significant contributing factors among these.

Triglycerides and free fatty acids build up in the liver's hepatocytes, causing NAFLD. Although there is a hereditary tendency to NAFLD, the exact characterization of the genetic variables causing NAFLD is still lacking. It has been demonstrated that some gene variations increase the likelihood of developing NAFLD. The disease starts with simple fatty liver and progresses to non-alcoholic steatohepatitis (NASH), hepatic steatosis, more severe and irreversible liver cirrhosis, and finally hepatocellular carcinoma (Chen et al., 2015). NAFLD will undoubtedly be the main cause of liver transplantation in the next few years, along with liver-related morbidity and mortality (Bertot & Adams, 2016).

The patatin-like phospholipase domain containing the PNPLA3 gene, which is found on chromosome 22(22q13.31), codes for a lipase-active protein that affects triglycerides in hepatocytes and retinyl esters in liver stellate cells. The PNPLA3 gene polymorphism (rs738409) gives rise to three genotypes: C/C, G/G, and C/G. The G/G and C/G genotypes are associated with the development of NAFLD (Mazo et al., 2019). Studies on adults and children have demonstrated the relationship between food and PNPLA3 gene polymorphism. Methionine is changed to isoleucine at position 148 in G allele carriers, increasing lipogenic activity and encouraging hepatocyte triglyceride synthesis and storage (Trepo et al., 2016). Sterol regulatory element binding protein 1c (SREBP-1c) regulates glucose and insulin in mouse liver and human hepatocytes, while PNPLA3 is mostly impacted by dietary status (Chen et al., 2015). Additionally, it was found that in obese and insulin-dependent mice, fasting had an impact on the mRNA transcript levels of the PNPLA3 gene.

Previous research indicates that NAFLD, a lifestyle condition, may be prevented by taking PUFA supplements, consuming less sugar, and eating more fruits, vegetables, and whole grains (Meroni et al., 2020). Determining the precise function of particular SNPs is challenging, though, as the majority of SNPs have no functional effects, while others may have disastrous implications due to their appearance in a variety of uncommon genetic illnesses. Furthermore, a lot of disorders linked to nutrition are complicated and have several hereditary variations. Finding SNPs that affect food–gene interactions and figuring out which people and groups are most likely to react to particular dietary treatments are the difficult tasks at hand. These genetic studies might be helpful in the management of the disease by developing novel treatment strategies based on an individual's genotype and a well-planned low-calorie dietary regime. Table 7.1 displays examples of well-researched SNPs and their impacts on diet and health to date.

7.5 OMICS TECHNOLOGY IN NUTRITION SCIENCE

The use of omics applications is expected to change food science and nutrition research in the near future due to the diversity and rapid advancements of potential analytical platforms and computer-based analysis (Alfaro & Young, 2018). The methods used to analyze the structure, function, and intermolecular interactions

TABLE 7.1
Role of Polymorphisms in Nutrition and Health

No.	Gene	SNP	Nutrition and Health Condition
1	ADH1B	rs1229984, rs2066702	Alcohol metabolism
2	CYP1A2	rs762551	Caffeine metabolism
3	FTO	rs9939609	Obesity and appetite
4	PNPLA3	rs738409	Non-alcoholic fatty liver disease
5	APOE	rs7412, rs429358	Cardiovascular and Alzheimer's disease
6	GC	rs7041, rs4588	Vitamin D transport
7	MTHFR	rs1801133	Folate metabolism
8	FADS1	rs174537	Long-chain fatty acid biosynthesis

Source: Mullins et al. (2020).

TABLE 7.2
Techniques at Omics Level to Establish the Impact of Nutrients on Human Health

Area	Techniques	Applications
DNA	Next generation sequencing (NGS), microarray, pyrosequencing, nanostring, polymerase chain reaction (PCR) based methods	To determine genotype patterns caused by the indirect interaction of genes with certain nutrient
RNA	NGS, microarray, pyrosequencing, PCR-based methods	To determine levels of RNA from tissues sources to study the effects of nutrients on transcriptomic profile
Proteins	Mass spectrometry (MS), high-performance liquid chromatography (HPLC), HPLC- tandem mass spectrometry (HPLC/MS)	Validation of mRNA expression protein levels
Metabolites	Nuclear magnetic resonance, (NMR) spectroscopy	Quantification of metabolites Predicting the effect of nutrients and for validation of omics

Source: Irimie et al. (2019).

of different biomolecules in biological samples are generally referred to as omics (Coughlin, 2014). With the use of these high-throughput technologies, it is possible to identify a global collection of gene products, or expressed genes, proteins, and metabolites in the examined sample(s), and to perform several measurements at once.

High-throughput omics measures that are frequently employed include proteomics, metabolomics, transcriptomics, and genomes. External stimuli, such as the individual's genetic composition, the settings of the experiment, the macro and micro environments, and nutritional status, among others, have an impact on the results of these measurements. As a result, the advancements in the aforementioned high-throughput omics technology offer a wealth of possibilities for comprehending the molecular effects of nutrition and the enormous variety in responses. Technological innovation is needed to improve the ability and efficacy of immunology, nutritional formulation, and disease diagnosis, as well as to assess the safety and quality of food (Chaudhary et al., 2021). Current advanced technologies/techniques applied in the areas of nutrigenetics and nutrigenomics are as shown in Table 7.2 (Irimie et al., 2019).

7.6 DIET AND GENE EXPRESSION PROFILE

Nutrients influence gene activity both directly and indirectly. They do so by regulation of the signaling pathways and/or by their role as a ligand for transcription factors. With genomics of nutrition, one can understand how the factors of diet or nutrients affect the expression of gene, affecting the quantities in production of proteins and their metabolites. Several studies have been undertaken to evaluate the impact of various dietary factors on gene functioning that are associated with the susceptibility of the disease. Communities and people following a high-calorie diet pattern, having highly refined grains, desserts after their meals, and meat that is processed may have developed a gene expression profile related to cancer signaling and inflammation (Bouchard-Mercier et al., 2013). In a similar vein, those who consume high amounts of fat, especially saturated fat, may have evolved gene expression patterns linked to inflammation, glucose intolerance, hepatic lipid buildup, and increased neuropeptide production (Vo et al., 2013). Moreover, diets low in choline and folate cause deregulation of the lipid metabolism gene, which raises the risk of NAFLD (Tryndyak et al., 2016).

Conversely, some research on the modulation of essential gene expression by nutritional and bioactive dietary molecules has also shown beneficial effects. Increased consumption of monounsaturated fatty acids (MUFAs) has been linked to aberrant lipid storage and decreased expression of a gene implicated in inflammation. According to Huerta et al. (2015), polyunsaturated fatty acids (PUFAs) control the expression of the neuropeptide gene implicated in energy balance. Bioactive food ingredients, including genistein (found in soybeans), curcumin (found in turmeric), resveratrol (found in red wine and grapes), and theaflavin (found in black tea), have anti-cancer effects. According to Cao et al. (2015), they accomplish this by upregulating and downregulating the genes that promote and prevent tumor growth, respectively.

Atypical metabolism is developed by cancer cells to maintain their unchecked development. PUFAs omega-3 and omega-6 have an impact on the expression of genes related to inflammation (TNF-alpha, IL-1 beta, IL-6, IL-18), angiogenesis (VEGF, PDGF, IGF-1, MMP-2), and proliferation (cyclin, P53, Wnt, PTEN, etc.), which means they can regulate the development of tumors. A change in the exposure to a certain food can have a negative interaction of dietary genes with environmental, biological, and genetic components, which can result in multiple unfavorable effects. This was noted when consumption of PUFAs was substituted for saturated fatty acids (SFA) in an effort to reduce LDL and total cholesterol. Additionally, a changed ratio of dietary omega-6 to omega-3 resulted from increased exposure to linoleic acid LA (omega-6), whereas omega-3 and alpha-linoleic acid (ALA) remained static. From 2:1 to more than 10:1, there was a fivefold rise. The rate of inflammation and illnesses linked to LA increased as a result of this increase.

The term epigenetics refers to a heritable but reversible mechanism that controls gene expression without also causing a permanent alteration to the DNA coding sequence. Epigenetic modifications are also significant. Diet–gene interactions have negative impacts, which is why these happen. The methylation of DNA in and around the promoter region, which inhibits gene production, is a significant epigenetic modification. Nutritional factors and DNA methylation, covalent histone modification, and noncoding RNA, including micro-RNA, interact intricately to cause obesity, dyslipidemia, Type 2 diabetes mellitus (T2DM), NAFLD, cancer, and cardiovascular disease (CVD). Eating a low-protein diet may cause changes in protein and glucose levels through modifications in NRIH-3 acetylation, which may result in a histone modification and raise the risk of T2DM. Once more raising the possibility of T2DM, deficiencies in calcium, magnesium, and vitamin D can alter the methylation patterns of the NFKB1A, HSD 11B1, and HSD 11B2 genes (Takaya et al., 2013).

One possible course of action is to reverse these epigenetic modifications by nutritional treatments. Particularly, a diet high in fish and low in red meat in the Nordic and Mediterranean regions causes the hypermethylation of proinflammatory genes, which has important anti-inflammatory effects on health. Through altering different metabolic profiles, dietary-based epigenetic alteration has been demonstrated to aid in the nutritional treatment of a number of disorders (Bahinipati et al., 2021).

7.7 INTERACTION OF NUTRIENTS AND GENES IN HEALTH

Omics techniques have the ability to identify new factors linked to a variety of complicated illnesses in addition to enabling the description of a vast number of molecular platforms (Ludhiadch et al., 2020). A database of functionally important SNPs would enable a clinical nutritionist to use SNP profiling to provide practical recommendations as part of their everyday clinical practice. Identifying genes which contribute to chronic disease initiation or progression along with understanding their regulation by dietary variables is a useful early step in this process. Several specific gene–disease–diet association studies have shown the promise of this approach in certain diseases.

Nutrition and genes in cancer

Cancer is a multifactorial and comprehensive disease, characterized by many gene mutations and alterations affecting many vital pathways, functions, and mechanisms. It is the second leading cause of death globally. It is a heterogeneous manifestation of uncontrolled division of cells with limited treatment potential. The dietary compounds available naturally can target many of these altered pathways, thus interfering not only in early tumorigenesis but also during late carcinogenesis. It is a well-established fact that dietary natural compounds can influence cancer risk and tumor behavior (Braicu et al., 2017). Studies on cancer prevention have found that specific dietary consumption of certain components affects important signaling pathways that are disrupted in causing certain malignancies (Vyas, 2022).

Nutrigenomics in cancer management will be of paramount importance in the future. Based on scientific data, intake of proper diet and nutrition can help prevent many malignancies and reduce cancer risk. It is noted through several studies that nearly 70% of cases of cancer and 35% of all human malignancies are associated with an imperfect dietary habit. Some examples are as follows.

- By examining sensitive biomarkers, deficiencies in certain nutrients that function as co-factors of enzymes that repair DNA and prevent DNA oxidation can be linked to specific genome and epigenome damage.

- Carcinogen metabolism gene polymorphism may also change the likelihood that a carcinogen would interact with particular cells to trigger the start of cancer activation.
- Eating a lot of red meat raises the risk of colorectal cancer in people because it contains the enzyme N-acetyltransferase (NAT), which acetylates heterocyclic aromatic amines, which can cause cancer.

Research has shown that dietary food components can have a synergistic effect with anti-cancer drugs leading to management of cancer (Kaushik et al., 2016).

Nutrition and genes in diabetes

A global pandemic and a chronic disorder, diabetes mellitus (DM) is showing a steady rise in its incidence across the globe from 387 million to a projected 592 million by 2035, as reported by the International Diabetes Federation (IDF) (Aguirreiree, 2013). Type 1 diabetes (T1DM) (previously known as insulin-dependent, juvenile, or childhood-onset) is caused by an infiltration of T lymphocytes into pancreatic islets, and their destruction is characterized by deficiency in production of insulin and requires daily administration of insulin. Type 2 diabetes (T2DM) is a common yet complex condition accounting for more than 90% of diabetes cases that occur due to insulin resistance and a relative lack of insulin along with increased demand for insulin.

Good eating practices and dietary supplements are important for the prevention and treatment of diabetes, as well as for effective management of the illness. Although the complete pathophysiology of DM is not so clear, it is evident that dietary variables, genetic predisposition, and interactions between nutrients and genes play a part in the development of this lifestyle illness. Nutritional genomics research focuses on how genetic variants affect dietary patterns, the function of gene–nutrient interactions, the relationship between gene–diet and phenotype, and epigenetic changes brought about by food ingredients. These investigations will help identify biomarkers for diagnosis and advance our knowledge of the early molecular processes that underlie DM. These tactics will support the creation of customized diet plans that optimize the consumption of nutrients and other useful food ingredients, which can both postpone and prevent the onset of DM and lessen its specific problems (Berna et al., 2014).

In an effort to identify the molecular events implicated in the development of disease, advanced genetics platforms have been widely employed. Although it is now increasingly practical to apply omics technologies, doing so produces a lot of complex data that might theoretically indicate how a particular nutrient interacts with every gene in the human genome. Over 70 genes have been found to be involved with T2DM thus far via association analysis. Furthermore, more than 100 SNPs have been found with T2DM using technologies such as genome-wide association study (GWAS) arrays (Hindorff et al., 2014). More than 40 of the previously discovered 50 new loci have been linked to T2DM and its associated characteristics, including fasting proinsulin, insulin, and glucose. We already know that nutrients, through their modulation of signaling molecules in intricate metabolic processes, can control the pattern of gene expression. Research on genomes has revealed that 65 gene polymorphisms are connected to the etiology of T2DM. Thanks to developments in human genome decoding and genome sequencing in the contemporary era of genomics, it is now possible to screen for mutations, especially SNPs that correlate with T2DM. This has given us insight into the role that genetic predisposition plays in the development of DM (Vorderstrasse, 2013).

Nutrition and genes in cardiovascular disease

The main cause of death in the USA and around the world is cardiovascular disease (CVD). According to a 2012 World Health Organization (WHO) report, CVD is a contributing factor in 17.5 million deaths worldwide. Lipid buildup, blood, pus, fibrosis, inflammation, and artery cell death all contribute to the development of intimal lesions in CVD. CVD must be prevented and treated with a balanced diet. Significant impacts of gene–diet interactions on CVD biomarkers and the onset and course of the disease have been demonstrated by recent studies. Studies conducted on a range of age groups and demographics have consistently demonstrated the effects of macronutrient and gene combinations, including those related to the fat mass and obesity-associated gene FTO, angiotensin-converting enzyme (ACE), peroxisome proliferator activated receptor gamma (PPARG), apolipoproteins (APOAs), and fatty acid desaturase (FADS), on the cardiovascular system. However, additional research is required to test and confirm the effects of gene–nutrient interactions for other genes that have been reported to be restricted to particular populations, ages, or genders (Voruganti, 2018).

Nutrition and genes in obesity

According to Karczewski et al. (2018), obesity is a newly recognized lifestyle condition that is linked to the development of numerous diseases, including cancer, T2DM, and CVD, as well as chronic low-grade inflammation. Various variables, including poor sleeping habits, physical inactivity, and unhealthy food patterns, are thought to be important in the development and progression of obesity as well as its co-morbidities. Obesity is a complex condition. An intriguing area of application for novel nutritional therapies at this time may be the evaluation of gene–diet interactions in regard to obesity and CVD, as evidence for this theory is mounting (Barrea et al., 2020).

Peripheral signaling peptides, including cholecystokinin, leptin, insulin, and ghrelin, as well as those linked to encoding taste receptors, affect how humans regulate how much food they eat and how much weight they gain because of certain genetic variations. Genes that encode modulators of energy expenditure control adipocyte development and differentiation, and uncoupling proteins are also known to exhibit polymorphic traits. Examples of polymorphic central regulators of energy intake are hypothalamic neuropeptides, neuropeptides Y, and melanocortin pathway components.

The science of nutrigenomics may have the potential to manage and treat the chronic inflammation of obesity. The bioactive chemicals such as green tea, which has tocopherol, can suppress the expression of certain genes and mitigate inflammatory activities, as it is an antioxidant and thus protects one from obesity (Shamim et al., 2017). To promote nutrigenetic studies, it is mandated to have deep insight into the subject of personalized nutrition and to develop dietary and lifestyle recommendations to manage weight and obesity complications and reduce the risk of CVD.

Nutrition and genes in metabolic syndrome

The term metabolic syndrome (MetS) refers to a group of characteristics that include central obesity, dyslipidemia, insulin resistance, fatty liver, hyperglycemia, and insulin resistance. These disorders can result in T2DM and CVD (Reddy et al., 2018). Fanning and Shea's (2018) research demonstrated the important impact that genetic susceptibility plays in the development of MetS. The human genome has not changed much throughout time, but the growing MetS incidence suggests that environmental influences are having an effect on the genome. There have been reports of certain genetic loci/genes linked to MetS, highlighting the greater significance of environmental variables. About 50 loci were found by the GWAS, many of which are unique and linked to obesity and DM (Grarup et al., 2014).

Disrupted postprandial lipid metabolism is a characteristic of MetS, and genes regulating fatty acid binding proteins, apolipoprotein B, apolipoprotein E, lipid metabolism, transcription factor 7-like 2, and perilipin have been linked to this. Moreover, an increasing risk for central obesity, DM, and MetS has been linked to genetic variations associated with inflammation, including those related to interleukin (IL)-1, IL-6, tumor necrosis factor-alpha (TNFα), and lymphotoxin.

Numerous additional genetic variants in genes, including acetyl-CoA carboxylase β and FTO (fat mass and obesity-associated protein), have been linked to an elevated risk of MetS. Claussnitzer et al. (2015) were able to restore brown adipose from white adipose tissue by converting FTO dangerous alleles into non-risky alleles using patient-derived primary adipocytes, thanks to the use of contemporary genome editing tools like CRISPR-CAS9. These findings showed that genetic polymorphisms had a part in the development of MetS. By modifying the variant SNPs (risky alleles of the gene) that cause diseases, genome editing techniques are currently being used to treat lifestyle CVDs like hypertension based on genotype data (Chadwick & Musunuru, 2017).

Nutrition and genes in inflammation

When living tissues are damaged, the body responds by creating inflammation, which can be either acute (a short-term, self-healing reaction) or chronic. It is generally recognized that the makeup of food systems affects inflammation, changing gene expression and interfering with communication cascades to regulate the immune response. According to Garg et al., this inflammation may linger for several years into later life and cause a variety of conditions, including gut allergies, cancer, atherosclerosis, and other conditions (Garg et al., 2022). Numerous immunological mediators have important functions in the regulation of inflammation by the immune system.

Curcuma longa, also known as turmeric, is a widely used and valuable spice. It has long been used in Ayurvedic medicine to cure inflammation. There are several bioactive compounds in turmeric, the most significant of which is curcumin, which is responsible for many of the plant's pharmacological properties, such as its antibacterial, anti-inflammatory, and antioxidant properties. There is proof that curcumin is a pleiotropic substance with the ability to interact with targets in the inflammatory pathway. This was found to be a promising treatment for certain cancers as well as inflammatory illnesses. The activity of H+, K+ -ATPase is significantly influenced by curcumin, which is also known to reduce histone H3 acetylation, which prevents the production of the gene (H+, K+ -ATPase). It controls the synthesis of p38 MAPK suppressors and cytokine signaling-1 (SOCS-1 and 3), which inhibit the expression of LPS-induced inflammatory mediators in macrophages, including IL-6, TNF-α, and COX-2 mRNAs. When nuclear translocation is further modified, LPS-induced SOCS-1 and -3 expression as well as p38 MAPK kinase activation are decreased.

Several bioavailability and safety studies have shown that oral administration of curcumin (diferuloylmethane) reduced TNF-α production and its activity in vitro, in vivo, and in people. Vitamin supplements have been demonstrated to be beneficial for a range of inflammatory conditions, such as skin diseases and precancerous and cancerous conditions. A derivative of vitamin A called retinol has been demonstrated to strengthen the immune system and stop the formation of tumors.

7.8 EMERGING CONCEPT OF PRECISION NUTRITION

Nutrients interact with and modify the molecular pathways underpinning the physiological functioning of living things, just like customized medications do. Individuals respond differently to lifestyle changes in terms of how dietary components are absorbed, digested, and utilized because of differences in their genetic composition. Therefore, it is better to follow genotype-specific dietary recommendations rather than broad ones. Precision nutrition is making personalized dietary recommendations based on genetics to maximize well-being (Meliani, 2020).

The emerging discipline of nutrigenetics will be used to tailor diets based on individual genetic variability (Kiani et al., 2022). Precision nutrition and precision medicine are built on the foundation of developing dietary recommendations for subgroups of individuals with various conditions. For example, disorders such as lactose intolerance, phenylketonuria, or celiac disease are treated with dietary instructions according to the individual's genetic background (Toro-Martin et al., 2017).

SNPs may be linked to chronic illnesses as a result of their interactions with specific meals or diets, as well as the consumption of micro- and macronutrients. For example, individuals from a Mexican study who consumed high amounts of fats and carbohydrates were found to have polymorphisms in taste perception genes, such as the CD36 gene and the sweet taste receptor TAS1R2 (Taste 1 Receptor Member 2) gene, which have been linked to dyslipidemia (Ramos-Lopez et al., 2017). Conversely, in people with low intakes of vitamin B6, vitamin B12, and folate, common variants of homocysteine metabolism-regulating genes, such as MTHFR (methylenetetrahydrofolate reductase) and MTR (methionine synthase), have been linked to an increased risk of breast cancer (Jiang-Hua et al., 2014).

In order to identify the precise genes involved in detoxification, oxidative stress defense, and the uptake and metabolism of nutrients, nutrigenetics is increasingly frequently used in clinical practice. It is interesting to note that SNPs in the vitamin D receptor (VDR) gene impact vitamin D availability and are linked to a higher

TABLE 7.3
Aspects of Personalized Nutrition

No.	Aspect
1	Genetic makeup
2	Diverse dietary conditions
3	Economic conditions
4	Health status
5	Individual variability

Source: Vyas (2022).

risk of osteoporosis in postmenopausal women who consumed less calcium (Barry et al., 2014).

Nutrigenetics is being used more and more in clinical practice to pinpoint the exact genes involved in detoxification, oxidative stress defense, and the uptake and metabolism of nutrients. In nutrigenetic research, polymorphisms in these genes are analyzed to determine how they affect eating habits. For example, diets based on certain ACE genotypes may propose a higher intake of sodium in comparison to the standard population-based dietary guidelines. A customized diet may also consider several other parameters, as indicated in Table 7.3 (Vyas, 2022).

7.9 INFLUENCE OF GENETIC POLYMORPHISM ON PHYSICAL ACTIVITY

Research suggests that genetic factors might contribute to some of the variation in physical activity. The discovery of genetic variants connected to physical activity may shed light on several elements of physical activity research. It is well known that maintaining a healthy weight involves both diet and activity. Physical activity levels may be impacted by genetic variants linked to obesity; on the other hand, living an active lifestyle may lower the risk of obesity.

On physical activity, 16 cross-sectional and interventional research investigations have been conducted. All of these investigations, which included adults and children from Europe and Africa, showed a noticeably strong association between FTO intron1 and physical activity (Claussnitzer et al., 2015). Furthermore, a recent meta-analysis comprising 111,421 people of European ancestry found a strong correlation between genetic risk scores for 12 obesity-related polymorphisms and physical activity. The impact of FTO variations was found to be mitigated by higher levels of physical activity during leisure time in a later meta-analysis that included 218,166 adults and 19,268 children. On the other hand, the hereditary tendency toward greater adiposity was aggravated by more sedentary lifestyle variables, such as watching TV.

With regard to the subcutaneous fat area, the Diabetes Prevention Program in the USA, which had 869 participants, found a high correlation between FTO genetic variations and 12-month lifestyle intervention approaches that included physical activity, food, and weight reduction. They found that the minor allele of an FTO variant was linked to increased subcutaneous fat formation in the control group as compared to the lifestyle intervention group. However, a recent study found that a vegetarian diet and regular exercise may help reduce the high body mass index brought on by the FTO gene mutation's rs3751812 minor allele. Moreover, it is widely recognized that dietary patterns influence other genes associated with physical activity, which influences the strength and form of muscles (Cassidy et al., 2016).

Research has further elucidated the protective effect of exercise on genetic variants associated with obesity, as demonstrated by a composite genetic risk score. In such studies it was reported that among people with higher genetic risk scores, high amounts of physical activity can reduce an individual's genetic vulnerability to obesity (Kiani et al., 2022).

7.10 FUNCTIONAL FOODS AND NUTRIGENOMICS

Natural foods high in antioxidants, fatty acids, minerals, vitamins, and phytosterols are referred to as functional foods. In addition to serving fundamental nutritional purposes, these foods may also be designed to have physiological benefits and lower the risk of chronic disease. They look like conventional foods and should be included in a regular diet. The phrase functional foods was originally used in Japan in 1980, and it was defined as a food source that contained certain nutrients or non-nutrients that had a particular effect on a person's body functions. Functional food consumption guarantees an adequate supply of nutrients, offering nutritional advantages. Currently, the food industry is concentrating on creating functional meals that lower the glycemic index and cut calories (Vyas, 2022). The creation of functional foods can benefit from the application of nutrigenomics knowledge. By changing specific genes, transgenic organisms or foods that are advantageous for overall health as well as in specific medical situations can be produced economically.

With the development of functional meals that promote particular health benefits, the post-genomic era has begun. In an effort to give humanity a balanced, nutrient-rich, and varied diet, such health claims can profit from the availability of cutting-edge technology, such as DNA chip technology deployed in integrated form on omics platforms. Utilizing cutting-edge technologies such as proteomics, metabolomics, and genomics to boost crop yield and improve functional food sources can also aid in reducing off-putting substances like acrylamide and phytic acid, which will enhance the quality of nutrition even more (Gupta et al., 2020).

7.11 DIETARY SUPPLEMENTS

Dietary supplements are not intended to prevent any diseases; rather, they are intended to enrich the human diet. These come in the form of pills, tablets, and capsules and are intended to fulfill dietary requirements, promote physical fitness, improve overall well-being, and enhance health. These dietary supplements are made up of physiologically active primary or secondary metabolites in either crude or purified form. They fall into several categories, such as supplements for dietary fiber, minerals, weight loss, cold, elderly people, immune system, brain, bone, and heart health, and GIT health, among others.

A study involving almost 40,000 participants between the ages of 40 and 75 revealed that vitamin E can lower the risk of coronary heart disease (CHD). Men who took ≥60 vit E IU/day had a 36% decreased risk of CHD than those who consumed <7.5 IU/day. Another study, which involved about 87,245 female nurses, demonstrated that vitamin E treatment for more than 2 years reduced the subjects' chance of coronary disease damage by 41%. Additionally, arginine consumption provided protection against CVS illnesses. A study comprising 15 patients who were supplemented with arginine hydrochloride at varying dosages (6–12.6 g/d × 6 wk) showed a significant increase in blood flow in the forearm, from 5.1+/−2.8 to 6.6+3.4 mL/min/dL.

It has been demonstrated that secondary metabolites such as pyruvates, conjugated linoleic acid, hydroxy citric acid, and flavonoids are important components of weight reduction supplements that enhance the metabolism of fat and carbohydrates. However, diabetes is also associated with these chemicals. Male C57BL/6 mice were given a high-fat meal supplemented with luteolin (0.002 and 0.01%) for 12 weeks. This helped to improve insulin sensitivity and glucose intolerance in addition to suppressing body weight increase (Xu et al., 2014).

In a pilot study, 13 participants with T1DM demonstrated the benefits of daily omega-3 fatty acid diet supplementation. During 4 weeks, 5.4 g of eicosapentaenoic acid and 2.3 g of docosahexaenoic acid were taken to lower the levels of HDL cholesterol, triglycerides, and blood sugar. Additionally, the study demonstrated the preventive role of cocoa polyphenols in the treatment of inflammatory disorders and CVS. In a meta-analysis, 173 participants with hypertension who received cocoa supplements for 2 weeks saw a drop in blood pressure. In another study, T2DM patients who received chocolate rich in cocoa phenolics had higher levels of HDL cholesterol and lower levels of total and HDL cholesterol ratios. When epigallocatechin gallate (EGCG) supplementation was administered to pathologically afflicted islets, it was demonstrated that T2DM could be avoided and that the number and size of islets increased in db/db mice.

Patients with T2DM were found to benefit from symbiotic cultures of *Lactobacillus* and *Bifidobacterium bifidum*, cultivated at a concentration of 200 ml @ 4 × 208 CFU/100 ml, on their HDL cholesterol, triglyceride levels, and total cholesterol. A randomized double blind controlled experiment was conducted in T2DM patients to investigate the benefits of probiotic yogurt that contained 300g/d × 6 wks of *Lactobacillus acidophilus*, La5 and *Bifidobacterium lactis*, Bb12. HbA1C and fasting glucose levels decreased as a result of the supplementation, whereas erythrocyte SOD, GSH-PX, and antioxidant activity increased (Kaur, 2018).

7.12 ETHICAL ISSUES

The scientific community must address a number of ethical dilemmas and issues raised by research in nutritional genetics in order to further the field's understanding and make it easier for the general public to receive it in an understandable and respectful manner (Ceriani et al., 2023).

Nutrigenomics' involvement in food and public health raises several ethical questions. First and foremost, nutrigenomics education is necessary. Given that every person is unique in their genetic makeup, it is unknown if functional meals, which purport to act at the DNA level to promote or enhance health, are appropriate for everyone.

Second, there should be a fundamental knowledge of which foods directly affect genes, as well as how and why. Since 2001, some businesses, such as Boulder, Colorado-based Sciona Inc., have been providing customized dietary guidance based on an individual's genetic profile. There is still a lot of research to be done, and therefore some scientists are skeptical. Genetics is still too young to guarantee such outcomes at this time. Thus, it makes sense to be concerned about quality control in this field.

Thirdly, professional nutritionists' role in genetic testing and information sharing needs to be carefully considered. When conducting population screening, rules must be followed, because some illnesses may not always be as distinct as PKU. Furthermore, the data obtained from genetic testing can be more appealing to outside parties that have something to gain from it. There is worry that certain people may be unfairly disadvantaged by the use of genetic information by insurance or employers. Thus, the dilemma emerges of who should have access to and where to keep personally relevant information. How would this information be obtained by the nutritionists? Would a sizable population database be accessible, or would people carry smart cards with their genetic profiles on them? There must be rules over who can access large population databases and under what circumstances.

Fourth, it will not be long until each person has access to a customized diet: that is, what a person needs to eat in order to maintain good health, as well as what foods they should stay away from. Can this be considered an infringement on the right to choose what to eat?

Fifth, human patients must be used in clinical trials for the research of nutrient–gene interaction, even when it is carried out in cell cultures and other animal models. Testing on ethnic and culturally varied groups is necessary in a population with a diverse ethnic makeup. The issue of testing on human beings is delicate, since there is a chance that certain institutions and researchers may use people as lab animals or take advantage of the socioeconomically disadvantaged.

Blood is the only source of DNA that is available for nutrition study. Because gene expression varies throughout tissues, it is not appropriate to depend exclusively on the DNA obtained from this source. The only method to obtain DNA from the stomach, kidney, and liver is through biopsies. This approach to sample collection is highly intrusive (Munshi, 2014).

Salloum et al. (2018) looked at US rural and urban citizens' general awareness of genetic testing services, stratified by racial and ethnic groupings. The likelihood that an urban person was aware of direct-to-consumer genetic testing (DTC-GT) was higher than that of a rural resident. Furthermore, a lack of health literacy and language hurdles raise ethical concerns by increasing the possibility that consumers would misinterpret results and by widening the difference in health outcomes.

7.13 FUTURE RESEARCH DIRECTIONS

Nutritional sciences will always be a fascinating and important field of study. Success will depend on determined researchers making use of the quickly advancing technologies to pinpoint the molecular sites of action of bioactive food ingredients and comprehend how these sites contribute to disease prevention. Effective evidence emphasizing wide diversity in reactions to food modifications within a common genetic subgroup has also been demonstrated by research. Thus, it may be argued that working with omic biomarkers to target health advantages for an individual is crucial when it comes to individualized nutrition guidance (Uthpala et al., 2020).

There are still a lot of unanswered research questions concerning nutrition and cancer. How, for example, do interactions between different food ingredients affect the expression of genes inside a cell? Is it possible to confirm in vivo the improved anti-proliferative effects of combining bioactive dietary components discovered in vitro? Furthermore, are responses to bioactive substances similar in different tissues? What effects do gender and age have on the way that food ingredients affect molecular targets? What is the best way to take into account individual differences in food metabolism? How can biomarkers representing the state of nutrients be found and verified? In what ways could the response to dietary intervention initiatives be predicted using exfoliated cells? Does a nutrient's good effect disappear if it interacts with a particular molecular target to block a cancer-related pathway and triggers compensatory activity through other pathways? If there are multiple mechanisms via which nutrients interact with molecular targets relevant to cancer, how might the most significant targets or processes be identified to lower the risk of cancer? Is it possible to find and validate biomarkers that are influenced by nutrition and that function as surrogate endpoint biomarkers for clinical disease? Will the analytical methods and study design now in use in molecular-based nutrition and cancer research be sufficient? (Vyas, 2022).

Since it is doubtful that a single person or institution would have the necessary resources to address every issue, the establishment of successful collaborations between nutrition scientists and other speciality scientists will be crucial to providing solutions to many of these challenges. It is critical to understand that it will require a great deal of patience and time to create and execute this new research paradigm in nutrition and cancer prevention. Even though there will be many obstacles to overcome, there could be huge benefits in terms of reduced cancer-related morbidity and mortality.

Science's previous discoveries have led to a fundamental comprehension of the essential macro and micronutrient requirements for the majority of people (Mullins et al., 2020). Ultimately, in the 21st century, it has led to a one-size-fits-all strategy that is embodied in the majority of recommended dietary regimens, such as "My Plate for the Day", in both developed and developing nations, including India. This approach has had a significant positive impact on the reduction of malnutrition and diseases caused by nutrient deficiencies. The development of nutritional genetics will be a benefit in managing various chronic diseases and eradicating all forms of malnutrition, which will advance any country. Though there has not been enough progress to reach this aim yet, it is hoped that future research will pave the road for customized nutrition to become a reality.

7.14 CONCLUSION

The bioavailability and metabolism of nutrients may be impacted by genetic variability among different individuals. In order to address this variation, the application of genetics to nutritional sciences would result in a revolutionary perspective on food—one that sees it not only as a source of nourishment but also as a medication that can delay the ravages of aging and reverse illness conditions. The nutrigenomics method is similar to pharmacogenomics, which examines the connection between a patient's response to medication and SNPs in the genome to customize treatment. The two are closely related; without nutrigenomics, results from pharmacogenomics cannot be properly interpreted, because food can influence the expression of genes related to drug metabolism.

Because what an individual eats influences a drug's efficacy, pharmaceutical companies should incorporate nutrigenomics into the design of new medications. Most effective dietary suggestions may be paved using the combined knowledge from these two omics. Targeting the genes implicated in the main human disorders, such as cancer, diabetes, heart disease, obesity, and MetS, is a challenge for nutrigenomics research. Currently, a large number of the genes causing these polygenic, chronic illnesses are yet unknown. Foods containing bioactive substances have the potential to activate some genes while inhibiting another group of genes linked to a certain disease.

Significance of biomarkers and completion of biomarker-monitoring clinical trials are prerequisites for the success of this discipline. This technology's wider and more exciting application is the creation of a cell's or organism's metabolic content at a certain moment in time. Combining the fields of nutrition and antimicrobial research can aid in examining the relationship between genetic diversity and disease, which in turn aids in creating long-term objectives for enhancing health and preventing illness. With careful planning and focused actions, this knowledge will need to be applied and used in the future for greater populations.

Global knowledge exchange is also necessary for successful advancement because it is necessary to have experience from a variety of sectors. The increasing amount of nutrigenomics data produced by genome technologies has led to the requirement for databases to safely store trustworthy data. The scientific community as a whole must work together to ensure success in this area. This will aid in the development of a solid database that is validated and supported by solid evidence, enabling our dieticians and physicians to enhance nutritional status. Although the current state of progress is still insufficient to accomplish this goal, we have high hopes that research will pave the road for its realization in the future.

REFERENCES

Aguirreiree F, Brown A, Cho NH, Dahlquist G, Dodd S, Dunning T, Scott, C. *IDF Diabetes Atlas*. 2013. Brussels: International Diabetes Federation. https://diabetesatlas.org/idfawp/resource-files/2010/07/IDF_diabetes_atlas_sixth_edition_en.pdf

Alfaro AC, Young T. Showcasing metabolomic applications in aquaculture: A review. *Rev. Aquacult*. 2018; 10: 135–152.

Barry EL, Rees JR, Peacock JL, Mott LA, Amos CI, Bostick RM, Figueiredo JC, Ahnen DJ, Bresalier RS, Burke CA. Genetic variants in CYP2R1, CYP24A1, and VDR modify the efficacy of vitamin D3 supplementation for increasing serum 25-hydroxyvitamin D levels in a randomized controlled trial. *J. Clin. Endocrinol. Metab.* 2014; 99: E2133–E2137. https://doi.org/10.1210/jc.2014-1389

Barrea L, Annunziata G, Bordoni L, Muscogiuri G, Colao A, Savastano S; Obesity Programs of nutrition, Education, Research and Assessment (OPERA) Group. Nutrigenetics-personalized nutrition in obesity and cardiovascular diseases. *Int. J. Obes. Suppl.* 2020 Jul; 10(1): 1–13. doi: 10.1038/s41367-020-0014-4. Epub 2020 Jul 20. PMID: 32714508; PMCID: PMC7371677.

Benedict M, Zhang X. Non-alcoholic fatty liver disease: An expanded review. *World J. Hepatol.* 2017, 9, 715–732.

Berna G, Oliveras-López MJ, Jurado-Ruíz E, Tejedo J, Bedoya F, Soria B, Martín F. Nutrigenetics and nutrigenomics insights into diabetes etiopathogenesis. *Nutrients.* 2014 Nov 21; 6(11): 5338–5369. doi: 10.3390/nu6115338. PMID: 25421534; PMCID: PMC4245593.

Bertot LC, Adams LA. The natural course of non-alcoholic fatty liver disease. *Int. J. Mol. Sci.* 2016; 17: 774.

Bouchard-Mercier A, Paradis AM, Rudkowska I, Lemieux S, Couture P, Vohl MC. Associations between dietary patterns and gene expression profiles of healthy men and women: A cross-sectional study. *Nutr. J.* 2013; 12: 24.

Braicu C, Mehterov N, Vladimirov B, Sarafian V, Nabavi SM, Atanasov AG, Berindan-Neagoe I. Nutrigenomics in cancer: Revisiting the effects of natural compounds. *Semin. Cancer Biol.* 2017 Oct; 46: 84–106. doi: 10.1016/j.semcancer.2017.06.011. Epub 2017 Jul 1. PMID: 28676460.

Cao, F, Liu, T, Xu, Y, Xu, D, Feng, S. Curcumin inhibits cell proliferation and promotes apoptosis in human osteoclastoma cell through MMP-9, NF-κB and JNK signaling pathways. *Int. J. Clin. Exp. Pathol.* 2015; 8(6): 6037–6045.

Cassidy S, Chau JY, Catt M, Bauman A, Trenell MI. Cross-sectionalstudy of diet, physical activity, television viewing andsleep duration in 233 110 adults from the UK Biobank; the behavioural phenotype of cardiovascular disease and type 2diabetes. *BMJ Open* 2016; 6: e010038. https://doi.org/10.1136/bmjopen-2015-010038

Chadwick AC, Musunuru K. Genome editing for the study of cardiovascular diseases. *Curr. Cardiol. Rep.* 2017; 19: 22.

Chaudhary N, Kumar V, Sangwan P, Pant NC, Saxena A, Joshi S, Yadav AN. Personalized nutrition and -omics. *Compreh. Foodomics.* 2021: 495–507. doi: 10.1016/B978-0-08-100596-5.22880-1. Epub 2020 Nov 12. PMCID: PMC7217104

Chen LZ, Xin YN, Geng N, Jiang M, Zhang DD, Xuan SY. PNPLA3 I148M variant in non-alcoholic fatty liver disease: Demographic and ethnic characteristics and the role of the variant in nonalcoholic fatty liver fibrosis. *World J. Gastroenterol.* 2015; 21: 794–802.

Claussnitzer M, Dankel SN, Kim KH, Quon G, Meuleman W, Haugen C, et al. FTO obesity variant circuitry and adipocyte browning in humans. *N. Engl. J. Med.* 2015; 373: 895–907. https://doi.org/10.1056/NEJMoa1502214.

Coughlin SS. Toward a road map for global-omics: A primer on-omic technologies. *Am. J. Epidemiol.* 2014; 180: 1188–1195.

De Caterina R, El-Sohemy A. Moving toward specific nutrigenetic recommendation algorithms: Caffeine, genetic variation and cardiovascular risk. *Lifestyle Genom.* 2016; 9: 106–115.

Fanning E, O'Shea D. Genetics and the metabolic syndrome. *Clin. Dermatol.* 2018; 36: 9–13.

Farhud D, Zarif Yeganeh M, Zarif Yeganeh M. Nutrigenomics and nutrigenetics. *Iran J. Public Health.* 2010; 39(4): 1–14. Epub 2010 Dec 31. PMID: 23113033; PMCID: PMC3481686.

Ceriani F, Montalvan M, Quintero B, Suárez R, Bautista-Valarezo E, Frias-Toral, E.. Ethics of the clinical practice of nutrigenetics and nutrigenomics. *Clin. Nutri. Open Sci.* 2023; 49: 58–66, ISSN2667- 2685. https://doi.org/10.1016/j.nutos.2023.04.006.

Garg R, Sharma N, Jain SK. Nutrigenomics and nutrigenetics: Concepts and applications in nutrition research and practice. *Acta Med. Int.* 2022; 1(2): 124–130.

Grarup N, Sandholt CH, Hansen T, Pedersen O. Genetic susceptibility to type 2 diabetes and obesity: From genome-wide association studies to rare variants and beyond. *Diabetologia* 2014; 57: 1528–1541.

Gupta E, Sharma H, Devi S, Maurya NK. Nutrigenomics in functional foods and personalized. *Nutrition* 2020; 33(02): 670–686.

Hindorff LA, MacArthur J, Morales J, Junkins HA, Hall PN, Klemm AK, Manolio TA. A catalog of published genome-wide association studies. (accessed on 23 June 2014). Available online: www.genome.gov/gwastudies

Huerta AE, Prieto-Hontoria PL, Sáinz N, Martínez JA, Moreno-Aliaga MJ. Supplementation with α-lipoic acid alone or in combination with eicosapentaenoic acid modulates the inflammatory status of healthy overweight or obese women consuming an energy-restricted diet. *J. Nutr.* 2015; 146(4): 889S–896S.

Irimie AI, Braicu C, Pasca S, Magdo L, Gulei D, Cojocneanu R, Ciocan C, Olariu A, Coza O, Berindan-Neagoe I. Role of key micronutrients from nutrigenetic and nutrigenomic perspectives in cancer prevention. *Medicina (Kaunas).* 2019 Jun 18; 55(6): 283. doi: 10.3390/medicina55060283. PMID: 31216637; PMCID: PMC6630934.

Jiang-Hua Q, De-Chuang J, Zhen-Duo L, Shu-de C, ZhenzhenL. Association of methylenetetrahydrofolate reductase and methioninesynthase polymorphisms with breast cancer risk andinteraction with folate, vitamin B 6, and vitamin B 12 intakes. *Tumour Biol.* 2014; 35: 11895–11901. https://doi.org/10.1007/s13277-014-2456-1

Jyotirmayee B, RajLaxmi S, Sanjukta M, Srikrushna M. Nutrigenetics and nutrigenomics: A brief review with future prospects. *Biomedicine* 2021; 41(4): 714–719.

Karczewski J, Sledzinska E, Baturo A, Jonczyk I, Maleszko A, Samborski P, et al. Obesity and inflammation. *Eur. Cytokine Netw.* 2018; 29: 83–94.

Kaur KK, Allahbadia G, Singh M. Impact of nutrigenomics on various metabolic disorders in relation to life style alteration. *Austin J. Nutri. Food Sci.* 2018; 6(1): 1100.

Kaushik S, Shyam H, Sharma R, Balapure AK. Genistein synergize centchroman action in human breast cancer cells. *Ind. J. Pharmacol.* 2016; 48(6): 637.

Kiani AK, Bonetti G, Donato K, Kaftalli J, Herbst KL, Stuppia L, Fioretti F, Nodari S, Perrone M, Chiurazzi P, Bellinato F, Gisondi P, Bertelli M. Polymorphisms, diet and nutrigenomics. *J. Prev. Med. Hyg.* 2022 Oct 17; 63(2 Suppl 3): E125–E141. doi: 10.15167/2421-4248/jpmh2022.63.2S3.2754. PMID: 36479483; PMCID: PMC9710387.

Larochelle, S. Protein isoforms: More than meets the eye. *Nat. Methods* 2016; 13: 291.

Ludhiadch A, Vasudeva K, Munshi A. Establishing molecular signatures of stroke focusing on omic approaches: A narrative review. *Int. J. Neurosci.* 2020 Dec; 130(12): 1250–1266. doi: 10.1080/00207454.2020.1732964. Epub 2020 Feb 27. PMID: 32075476.

Marcum JA. Nutrigenetics/nutrigenomics, personalized nutrition, and precision healthcare. *Curr. Nutr. Rep.* 2020 Dec; 9(4): 338–345. doi: 10.1007/s13668-020-00327-z. PMID: 32578026.

Mazo DF, Malta FM, Stefano JT, Salles APM, Gomes-Gouvea MS, Nastri ACS, Almeida JR, Pinho JRR, Carrilho FJ, Oliveira CP. Validation of PNPLA3 polymorphisms as risk factor for NAFLD and liver fibrosis in an admixed population. *Ann. Hepatol.* 2019; 18: 466–471.

Meroni M, Longo M, Rustichelli A, Dongiovanni P. Nutrition and genetics in NAFLD: The perfect binomium. *Int. J. Mol. Sci.* 2020; 21: 2986.

Meiliana A, Wijaya AY. Nutrigenetics, nutrigenomics and precision nutrition. Ind. Biomed. J. 2020; 29(2). https://doi.org/10.1177/026010602311672

Mullins VA, Bresette W, Johnstone L, Hallmark B, Chilton FH. Genomics in personalized nutrition: Can you "eat for your genes"? *Nutrients* 2020 Oct 13; 12(10): 3118. doi: 10.3390/nu12103118. PMID: 33065985; PMCID: PMC7599709.

Munshi A, Duvvuri VS. Nutrigenomics: Looking to DNA for nutrition advice. *Ind. J. Biotechnol.* 2008; 7: 32–40.

Munshi A. *Nutrigenomics: Gene Based Personalized Nutrition Advice. Woman and Food Studies from the Indian Sub-Continent.* Lambert Academic Publishing (Chapter 17, pp. 120–135); 2014. ISBN-13: 978-3848430710.

Naureen Z, Miggiano GAD, Aquilanti B, Velluti V, Matera G,Gagliardi L, Zulian A, Romanelli R, Bertelli M. Genetic test for the prescription of diets in support of physical activity. *Acta Biomed.* 2020; 91. https://doi.org/10.23750/abm.v91i13-S.10584.

Nehlig, A. Interindividual differences in caffeine metabolism and factors driving caffeine consumption. *Pharmacol. Rev.* 2018; 70: 384–411.

Puppala J, Bhrugumalla S, Kumar A, Siddapuram SP, Viswa PD, Kondawar M, Akka J, Munshi A. Apolipoprotein C3 gene polymorphisms in Southern Indian patients with nonalcoholic fatty liver disease. *Indian J. Gastroenterol.* 2014 Nov; 33(6): 524–529. doi: 10.1007/s12664-014-0504-9. Epub 2014 Oct 17. PMID: 25319715.

Ramos-Lopez O, Milagro FI, Allayee H, Chmurzynska A, Choi MS, Curi R, De Caterina R, Ferguson LR, Goni L, Kang JX. Guide for current nutrigenetic, nutrigenomic, and nutriepigenetic approaches for precision nutrition involving the prevention and management of chronic diseases associated with obesity. *J. Nutrigenet Nutrigenomics* 2017; 10: 43–62. https://doi. org/10.1159/000477729

Reddy VS, Palika R, Ismail A, Pullakhandam R, Reddy GB. Nutrigenomics: Opportunities & challenges for public health nutrition. *Indian J. Med. Res.* 2018 Nov; 148(5): 632–641. doi: 10.4103/ijmr.IJMR_1738_18. PMID: 30666988; PMCID: PMC6366269.

Salloum RG, George TJ, Silver N, Markham MJ, Hall JM, Guo Y, Bian J, Shenkman EA. Rural-urban and racial-ethnic differences in awareness of direct-to-consumer genetic testing. *BMC Public Health* 2018; 18: 277.

Salzberg SL. Open questions: How many genes do we have? *BMC Biol.* 2018; 16: 94.

Shamim N, Gupta A, Paul V, Vida E. Nutritional genomics: A review. *Pharma Innov.* 2017; 6(4): 17–20.

Simopoulos AP. Genetic variants in the metabolism of omega-6 and omega-3 fatty acids: Their role in the determination of nutritional requirements and chronic disease risk. *Exper. Biol. Med.* 2010; 235: 785–795.

Swati Vyas. Advances in nutrigenomics and applications in public health: A recent update. *Curr. Res. Nutri. Food Sci. J.* 2022; 10(3): 1092–1104.

Takaya J, Iharada A, Okihana H, Kaneko K. A calcium-deficient diet in pregnant, nursing rats induces hypomethylation of specific cytosines in the 11β-hydroxysteroid dehydrogenase-1 promoter in pup liver. *Nutr. Res.* 2013; 33(11): 961–970.

Toro-Martín D, Arsenault BJ, Després J-P, Vohl M-C. Precisionnutrition: A review of personalized nutritional approaches for the prevention and management of metabolic syndrome. *Nutrients* 2017; 9: 913. https://doi.org/10.3945/ajcn.114.099150.

Trepo E, Romeo S, Zucman-Rossi J, Nahon P. PNPLA3 gene in liver diseases. *J. Hepatol.* 2016; 65: 399–412.

Tryndyak VP, Marrone AK, Latendresse JR, Muskhelishvili L, Beland FA, Pogribny IP. MicroRNA changes, activation of progenitor cells and severity of liver injury in mice induced by choline and folate deficiency. *J. Nutr. Biochem.* 2016; 28: 83–90.

Uthpala TG, Marapana RAU, Lakmini KP, Wettimuny DC. Nutritional bioactive compounds and health benefits of fresh and processed cucumber (Cucumis sativus L). *Sumerianz J. Biotechnol.* 2020; 3(9): 75–82. ISSN(e): 2617-3050, ISSN(p): 2617–3123.

Vo TX, Revesz A, Sohi G, Ma N, Hardy DB. Maternal protein restriction leads to enhanced hepatic gluconeogenic gene expression in adult male rat offspring due to impaired expression of the liver X receptor. *J. Endocrinol.* 2013; 218(1): 85–97.

Vorderstrasse AA, Cho A, Voils CI, Orlando LA, Ginsburg GS. Clinical utility of genetic risk testing in primary care: The example of Type 2 diabetes. *Personalized Med.* 2013; 10(6): 549–563.

Voruganti VS. Nutritional genomics of cardiovascular disease. *Curr. Genet. Med. Rep.* 2018 Jun; 6(2): 98–106. doi: 10.1007/s40142-018-0143-z. Epub 2018 Apr 30. PMID: 30581653; PMCID: PMC6300156.

Xu N, Zhang L, Dong J, Zhang X, Chen YJ, Bao B, et al. Low dose supplement of a natural flavanoid, luteolin, ameliorates diet induced obesity and insulin resistance in mice. *Mol. Nutr. Food Res.* 2014; 58: 1258–1312.

8 Assessing the Benefits and Challenges of Promoting Millets for Advancing Food and Nutrition Security

Chhavi Taliwal, Shireesha Mukka, and Maheshwar Mekam

8.1 INTRODUCTION

Millets offer a promising alternative for enhancing food and nutrition security due to their high nutritional content, resilience to climatic changes, and potential health benefits (Chaudhary et al., 2023; Lydia Pramitha et al., 2023; Veerabadhran et al., 2023). These small-grained cereals have been a staple in the Indian subcontinent for centuries, providing essential nutrients for rural populations (Nanje Gowda et al., 2022). Unlike rice and wheat, which often lack key nutrients, millets are rich in vitamins, minerals, and beneficial compounds (Alekhya & Shravanthi, 2019; Ashoka et al., 2020)

However, consumption of millets in India has declined over the years, despite their nutritional and environmental advantages (Ashoka et al., 2020). This decline is due to a combination of historical, cultural, and market factors. The shift towards rice and wheat, perceived as more desirable, has contributed to the reduced popularity of millets (Chera, 2017). Government programs promoting high-yielding varieties of rice and wheat have further decreased millet consumption (Raghunathan et al., 2021). To counter this trend, it is crucial to raise awareness among consumers and farmers about the benefits of millets and provide incentives for their cultivation (Chaudhary et al., 2023). Utilizing millets' nutritional and medicinal properties, along with traditional knowledge and genetic diversity, can enhance food security, dietary diversity, and climate resilience (Bombom et al., 2023; Kaur, 2023).

Efforts to revive millets include government and development organization initiatives, but changing entrenched dietary habits is challenging (Behera, 2017; Chera, 2017). Millet cultivation significantly decreased between 1955 and 2019. Organizations like the Indian Institute of Millets Research (IIMR) and the International Crops Research Institute for the Semi-Arid Tropics (ICRISAT) are working to

DOI: 10.1201/9781003487227-8

improve millet production through new technologies. The Indian government supports millet production and consumption through programs like the All India Coordinated Research Project on Pearl Millet (AICRP-PM), the Initiative for Nutritional Security through Intensive Millets Promotion (INSIMP), and the National Food Security Mission (NFSM), and by including millets in mid-day meals and providing minimum support prices (MSPs) for key millets. Raising awareness about millets' health benefits through campaigns and consumer surveys is essential. Malnutrition may be fought by adding millets to the public food supply and strengthening mid-day meal programs. Additionally, incentives and subsidies for startups in millet-based food production can promote these products (Lokesh, Dudhagara, Mahera et al., 2022).

Despite challenges, promoting millets can significantly enhance India's food and nutrition security. Millets are well-suited to the country's diverse agroclimatic conditions, making them a sustainable crop. Increased millet cultivation and consumption can also benefit small-scale and marginal farmers economically (Ashoka et al., 2020; Behera, 2017).

8.2 THE SIGNIFICANCE OF MILLETS HISTORICALLY IN INDIA

For ages, millets have been a staple food in semi-arid and arid regions of India, where they have been grown for centuries (Director et al., 2023; Maitra et al., 2020). When humans moved from being nomadic to permanent farming communities in the Neolithic era, approximately 10,000 years ago, the millets were among the first cultivated crops. The early cultivation of millets has been established by archaeological evidence from Neolithic sites in India, such as Burzahom in Kashmir and Chirand in Bihar. Results from Harappan sites demonstrate that millets constituted an important part of food production and agriculture throughout the Harappan civilization, which flourished around 2500 BCE. Millets have been identified in several works of ancient Indian literature, such as the Samhita, Purana, and Veda, emphasizing their cultural and nutritional significance. Ayurveda and the Mauryan empire's Kautilya Arthashastra both acknowledge the nutritional and agronomic advantages of millets (Veerabadhran et al., 2023).

Millets have long been an integral part of Indian cuisine; the nation produces about 10% of the world's 30 million tonnes of millets (Mudau et al., 2022). Particularly in the high-altitude regions of the Himalayas and other mountainous areas, these hardy, drought-resistant grains were essential for the food security and nutritional well-being of local communities (Bidinger et al., 2009). However, the declining prevalence of millet cultivation and consumption in these regions has led to a shift towards the consumption of more mainstream grains, such as rice.

Millets have been a cherished and integral part of the Indian culinary landscape for centuries, deeply rooted in the cultural and traditional food systems of the region. These small-grained cereals have long held a significant place in the diets of rural populations, providing a valuable source of nutrition and sustenance. Millet-based dishes and preparations have been passed down through generations, reflecting the historical importance and prominence of these grains in Indian cuisine and food security.

8.3 MILLETS AS TRADITIONAL STAPLES IN MANY PARTS OF INDIA

Historically, millets have been grown and eaten in many parts of India, each with its own variations and cooking customs. Millets have long been a primary food crop in India's high hills and mountains, offering the local inhabitants vital sustenance and nourishment for several generations (Koirala, 2020).

Millets have historically been integral to the agricultural and culinary practices across various regions of India. Numerous millet varieties have been grown and savored throughout the country, with each area highlighting its distinct farming techniques, taste profiles, and traditional cooking methods. Varieties like jowar, ragi, and bajra have served as essential food sources in the high hills and mountainous regions of India for generations, providing vital nutrition and sustenance to local populations. The cultivation of these wholesome grains has not only supported the livelihoods of these communities but has also been instrumental in maintaining local food traditions and culinary heritage. Over centuries of growth and consumption, millets have woven themselves into the very fabric of Indian culture, representing resilience, sustainability, and a profound connection to the land. The diverse practices of millet farming and cooking have crafted a culinary landscape that honors the richness and variety of India's agricultural legacy. As these ancient grains continue to nourish both the body and spirit, they exemplify the lasting relationship between people, their land, and the food they cultivate and share.

8.4 WHY INDIA WILL FACE FOOD SHORTAGES IN COMING YEARS

India is projected to face food shortages for a number of reasons, including a growing population, changing dietary habits, the loss of natural resources, and the effects of climate change. The rapidly increasing population is exerting significant pressure on the country's food production systems, with a marked decline in the per capita availability of pulses, a crucial protein source, from 64 g per day to just 36 g per day, well below the recommended 80 g per day (Pragya et al., 2017).

The focus on primary cereal crops such as wheat and rice has led to a decline in the cultivation and consumption of more nutrient-dense and climate-resilient crops, such as millets. Millets are highly nutritious and can help combat malnutrition and metabolic disorders, yet their production and consumption have declined as polished white rice has become more popular (Nanje Gowda et al., 2022).

The depletion of natural resources due to unsustainable agricultural practices and climate change is another significant threat. The availability of agricultural land is decreasing as more land is used for non-agricultural purposes, further complicating food production (Pragya et al., 2017). Climate change is causing increasing temperatures, erratic rainfall, and extreme weather events, all of which negatively impact crop yields. However, millets, being climate-resilient, offer a viable adaptation strategy (Ajatasatru et al., 2024).

The over-exploitation of natural resources, including water and soil fertility, is leading to declining productivity. The cultivation of water-intensive crops like rice and wheat is unsustainable, while millets, which are more drought-resistant, can help reduce pressure on scarce water resources and maintain soil conditions (Ashoka et al., 2020; Pragya et al., 2017). To address these challenges, the Millets Mission in India aims to revive millet cultivation and consumption, leveraging their nutritional benefits, climate resilience, and potential to enhance food security. This mission focuses on promoting the production, processing, and commercialization of millets to build a more sustainable and resilient agricultural system.

8.5 BENEFITS OF PROMOTING MILLETS FOR ADVANCING SECURITY OF FOOD AND NUTRITION

A varied family of small-seeded cereal grains, millets have long been an essential part of traditional diets across much of the world, but especially in parts of Africa and India. For many communities, millets were a main diet a few generations ago. However, as societies have turned towards more processed and refined grains, like polished white rice, their consumption has drastically decreased over time.

Promoting millets for addressing significant issues related to security of nutrition and food has garnered attention again recently. According to Nanje Gowda et al. (2022), millets are incredibly nutrient-dense, including substantial levels of minerals, vitamins, dietary fiber, and vital amino acids. Since millets are more resistant to environmental stressors like drought and poor soil, compared to main cereal crops, they represent a viable option for providing adequate nourishment in the context of resource scarcity and climate change.

Researchers have shown that millets have the potential to improve malnutrition, notably in India, where a large number of people—especially children—struggle with a variety of nutritional inadequacies. The Indian government, as well as state governments, have implemented a number of initiatives to encourage the production and consumption of millets due to their acknowledged nutritional and environmental advantages (Behera, 2017).

However, transforming food systems and consumer preferences away from millets has been a significant challenge. As Anitha et al. (2021) and Chera (2017) note, the shift away from millets in favor of polished rice was influenced by a complex interplay of historical, cultural, and socioeconomic factors. Overcoming the cultural stigma associated with millets and reintroducing them into the modern diet has required concerted efforts by public health professionals, development agencies, and the commercial sector.

These efforts aim to highlight the nutritional and environmental advantages of millets while addressing the practical challenges of processing, storing, and incorporating them into contemporary food products and culinary traditions. Despite the challenges, promoting millets holds great promise for advancing food and nutrition security, particularly in regions where traditional millet-based farming systems have been neglected or abandoned. By supporting the revival and modernization of millet-based food systems, policymakers, researchers, and development practitioners can contribute to improving the health and well-being of vulnerable populations while also promoting more sustainable and resilient agricultural practices.

Many types of millets have become more well known recently because of their high nutritional content and numerous health advantages (Figure 8.1). The millets

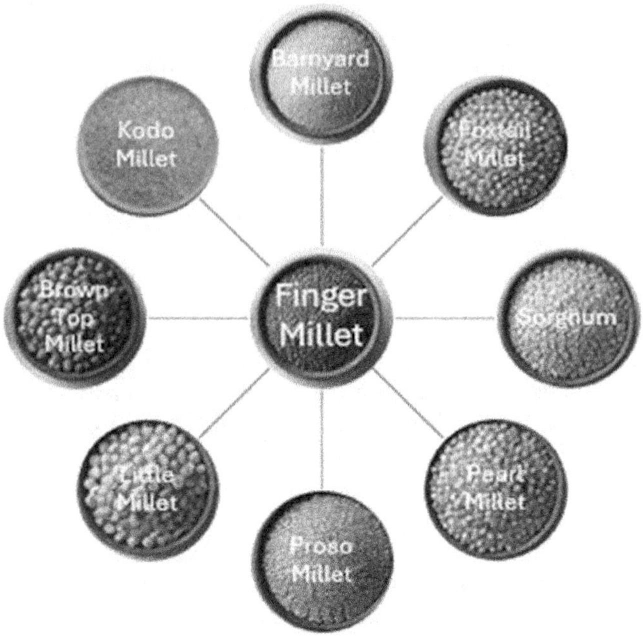

FIGURE 8.1 Different types of millets.

that are regularly consumed now and have historical references (Veerabadhran et al., 2023) are:

nali (pearl millet): *Pennisetum glaucum (L.) R. Br.*
ragi (finger millet): *Eleusine coracana (L.) Gaertn*
chinaka (proso millet): *Panicum miliaceum L.*
shyamaka (barnyard millet): *Echinochloa frumentacea L.*
kangu (foxtail millet): *Setaria italica (L.) P.Beauv.*
little millet: *Panicum sumatrense Roth. ex Roem. & Schult.*

8.6 NUTRITIONAL VALUE AND HEALTH ADVANTAGES OF MILLETS

Packed with dietary fiber, vitamins, and minerals, millets serve as an extremely nutritious food that can help prevent malnutrition and promote general health.

Nutrient profile

In terms of energy and carbohydrates, millets are similar to basic cereals. They are also an excellent source of protein, minerals, and phytochemicals. Millets are composed of 7% to 12% protein, 2% to 5% fat, 65% to 75% carbs, and 15% to 20% dietary fiber.

Millets have unique nutritional qualities (Table 8.1). They are well known for their complex carbohydrates, high dietary fiber content, and special phenolic compounds

TABLE 8.1
Nutritional Comparison of Millets and Other Cereals per 100g at 12% Moisture Content

Grain	Carbo hydrate (g)	Protein (g)	Fat (g)	Energy (kcal)	Dietary fiber (g)	Ca (mg)	P (mg)	Mg (mg)	Zn (mg)	Fe (mg)
				Cereals						
Wheat	64.7	10.6	1.47	321	11.2	39.4	315	125	2.8	3.9
Rice	78.2	7.9	0.52	356	2.8	7.5	96	19	1.2	0.6
				Millets						
Sorghum	67.7	9.9	1.73	334	10.2	27.6	274	133	1.9	3.9
Pearl millet	61.8	10.9	5.43	347	11.5	27.4	289	124	2.7	6.4
Finger millet	66.8	7.2	1.92	320	11.2	364	210	146	2.5	4.6
Kodo millet	66.2	8.9	2.55	331	6.4	15.3	101	122	1.6	2.3
Proso millet	70.4	12.5	1.10	341	—	14.0	206	153	1.4	0.8
Foxtail millet	60.1	12.3	4.30	331	—	31.0	188	81	2.4	2.8
Little millet	65.5	10.1	3.89	341	7.7	16.1	130	91	1.8	1.5
Barnyard millet	65.5	6.2	2.20	307	10.1	20.0	280	82	3.0	5.0

Source: Indian Institute of Millet Research; adapted from Lokesh, Dudhagara, Mahera, Kumar, et al. (2022).

and phytochemicals that have therapeutic uses. They provide a natural supply of vital minerals like calcium, iron, and zinc, all of which are critical in treating India's malnutrition problems (Figure 8.2). Millets are also a good source of calcium, iron, potassium, magnesium, zinc, folic acid, and niacin. Finger millet is the most abundant supplier of calcium, containing 300 mg to 350 mg per 100 g. Other small millets are noteworthy providers of iron and phosphorus. In addition, millets are high in lecithin content, quickly absorbed, and have positive effects on the nervous system (Bhat et al., 2018).

Compared to wheat (11.8%) and rice (6.8%), proso and foxtail millets have greater protein content (12.5% and 12.3%, respectively). Compared to wheat (41 mg/100 g) and rice (10 mg/100 g), finger millets have a substantially greater calcium content (344 mg/100 g), which is even three times more than that of milk. Because finger millets have a high calcium content, mothers in Mumbai, India, as well as in Mali and Indonesia, use them to make baby porridge. Zinc and iron are also abundant in pearl millets. Proso, foxtail, and small millets are among the millets that are rich in sulfur-containing amino acids (methionine and cysteine).

Additionally, millets have higher quantities of micronutrients than rice and wheat, as well as greater concentrations of polyunsaturated and monounsaturated fatty acids (PUFAs and MUFAs) (Hasan et al., 2019). They are a good source of important minerals like iron, magnesium, phosphorus, and zinc, which are needed for energy production, immune system function, bone health, and oxygen transport (Nanje Gowda et al., 2022). Millets also provide essential vitamins, particularly B vitamins

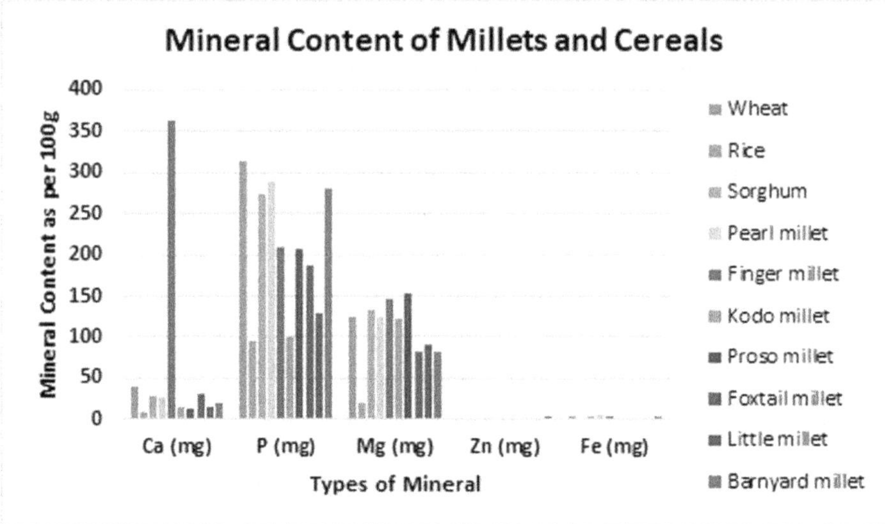

FIGURE 8.2 Mineral contents of millets and cereals per 100 g. (Data from Indian Institute of Millet Research.)

such as riboflavin, thiamin, and niacin, which are essential for energy metabolism and general health (Clemens et al., 2023).

Health benefits and resistance against non-communicable diseases

Scientific research has demonstrated that millets are outstanding, nutrient-dense cereals that are good for human health. Because millets are suitable for these populations, they are especially advised for infants, nursing mothers, elderly people, and those recovering from illness.

Millets are essential for halting the global diabetes pandemic because of their low glycemic index (GI), which implies they release glucose gradually. Individuals who eat millets as a main diet are less likely to develop gastrointestinal problems and diabetes mellitus. Furthermore, millets' high fiber content lowers the incidence of bowel and colon problems and helps avoid constipation (Bhat et al., 2018; Table 8.2).

Hypoglycemic characteristics

The GI for millets is lower than for various cereal crops. Foods are categorized on the GI according to how quickly and how much they increase blood sugar, or glucose levels. Foods are classified as low GI (values 0 to 55), moderate GI (values 56 to 69), and high GI (values above 70).

Millets have a low GI for a variety of reasons, including the hydrolysis of millet starch by the starch, lipids, proteins, polyphenols, and fiber. The spherical and polygonal structure of millet starch contributes to its hypoglycemic qualities. Enzymes that hydrolyze starch can enter more easily thanks to pores in the starch structures of

TABLE 8.2
Dietary Fiber Properties of Millets and Their Health Benefits

Millet Type	Function	Health Benefit
All millets	Water absorption and bulking properties	Provides energy diluents that aid in creating low-calorie diets
Sorghum, finger millet	Enhanced transit time for food in the digestive system	Lowers the risk of inflammatory bowel disease
Pearl millet, sorghum, finger millet	Binding of bile acids and steroids	Promotes hypocholesterolemic activity and decreases the likelihood of cardiovascular issues
Sorghum, pearl millet, finger millet	Slowing carbohydrate absorption and improving glucose tolerance	Aids in the management of certain types of diabetes
Sorghum	Detoxification	Functions as an agent for detoxification

Source: Bhat et al. (2018).

foxtail, proso, and pearl millets. In contrast, the starch granules of finger millets are devoid of holes.

In terms of starch hydrolysis index, millets are ranked as follows (in ascending order): finger, pearl, foxtail, and proso. Reductions in blood glucose, cholesterol, and the risk of type 2 cardiovascular disease and diabetes can all be achieved by lowering the GI of meals. Furthermore, the lack of the protein gluten in millets guards against coeliac disease and its consequences (Hasan et al., 2019; Table 8.3).

Anti-nutrients

Phytic acid, polyphenols, cyanogenic glucosides, tannins, oxalates, and amylase inhibitors are a few examples of the anti-nutrients found in millets (Table 8.4). The body's ability to absorb nutrients from these anti-nutrients can be decreased. However, adopting common home food processing methods like germination, decortication, fermentation, and malting—which enhance nutrient bioavailability—can lower their levels (Hasan et al., 2019; Singh & Sarita, 2016).

Antioxidant properties

Millets possess distinct nutritional benefits. They are recognized for their complex carbohydrates and elevated levels of dietary fiber. In addition, millets contain an abundance of bioactive compounds with antioxidant activity, providing a valuable source of essential nutrients. Antioxidants play a crucial role in promoting human health by mitigating oxidative stress and combating free radicals. The diverse natural phenolic compounds found in millets, such as phenolic acids, flavonoids, and tannins, contribute to their antioxidant properties. Additionally, millets contain insoluble fiber,

TABLE 8.3
Health Benefits of Millets

Health Benefit	Description
Cardiovascular health	Millets are rich in antioxidants, fiber, and phytochemicals that promote heart health and may lower the risk of cardiovascular diseases. Their consumption is linked to better lipid profiles, including lower LDL cholesterol levels.
Diabetes management	Millets have a lower GI than many other grains, helping to regulate blood sugar levels and decrease the risk of type 2 diabetes. Their high fiber content also aids in maintaining stable blood sugar levels.
Digestive health	The fiber in millets supports healthy digestion and may help prevent constipation. Additionally, millets have prebiotic properties that encourage the growth of beneficial gut bacteria, enhancing overall gut health.
Weight management	The high fiber content in millets promotes a sense of fullness, aiding in weight management and appetite control. They are a nutritious choice for weight-loss diets due to their low caloric content and high nutrient density.
Gluten-free option	Millets are naturally free of gluten, making them suitable for those with celiac disease or gluten sensitivity. Incorporating millet into gluten-free diets can enhance nutrient intake and variety.
Antioxidant benefits	Millets are abundant in antioxidants, such as phenolic compounds and flavonoids, which help combat free radicals and mitigate oxidative stress. These antioxidants play a role in overall health and may lower the risk of chronic diseases.
Nutrient-rich food source	Millets provide a wealth of essential nutrients, including proteins, vitamins, and minerals. Adding millets to the diet can help fulfill nutritional needs and promote better health and well-being.
Sustainable agriculture	Millets are hardy crops that can thrive in challenging environmental conditions, requiring less water and resulting in a smaller carbon footprint than major cereals. Growing millets supports sustainable agricultural practices and contributes to food security.

Source: Tripathi et al. (2023).

xylo-oligosaccharides (XOs), and peptides, further enhancing their nutritional profile. Similarly, lipophilic antioxidants like carotenoids and vitamin E are widely present in various millet varieties, offering a well-rounded antioxidant support system.

With such a rich array of nutrients and antioxidants, millets have the potential to be utilized as a nutraceutical food resource. As a plentiful source of these beneficial compounds, millets help to protect cells from the damage caused by the action of free radicals, unstable molecules that contribute to oxidative stress. Incorporating millets into our diet can effectively neutralize harmful free radicals, thereby reducing the risk of various diseases linked to oxidative stress, such as cardiovascular problems, cancers, and age-related conditions. By incorporating millets into the diet, individuals can benefit from their protective effects against diseases and their overall contribution to maintaining optimal health and well-being. Embracing millets as part of a

TABLE 8.4
Processing Techniques to Mitigate the Impact of Anti-nutrients in Millet-Based Meals

No.	Processing Technique	Function
1	Soaking	Reduces levels of phytic acid and polyphenolic compounds Enhances protein digestibility
2	Germination	Lowers tannin content (from 1.6% to 0.83%) Improves the bioavailability of key minerals, such as calcium, iron, and zinc
3	Fermentation	Facilitates the production of various food products with improved flavors and textures Decreases anti-nutrient content and increases protein availability and digestibility
4	Popping or puffing	Uses a high-temperature short-time (HTST) method for starch gelatinization, causing the endosperm to expand and burst Enhances flavor and aroma, making millet products more palatable

Source: Singh & Sarita (2016); Hasan et al. (2019).

balanced diet can help reduce the risk of illnesses and support overall health through their diverse array of bioactive compounds and antioxidant content (Liang & Liang, 2019; Harish et al., 2024).

Sustainable reservoirs of bioactive compounds

Millets are recognized as an essential source of bioactive compounds. These nutrient-rich grains are becoming more popular due to their sustainable characteristics, acting as a treasure trove of antioxidants, vitamins, and minerals vital for our overall health. Their distinctive makeup enables millets to contribute significantly to sustainable agricultural practices and bolster global food security. With their ability to thrive in various climates and with minimal resources, millets are viewed as an ecofriendly crop option that can help tackle challenges like climate change and soil degradation. Moreover, the bioactive compounds present in millets, including phenolic compounds and flavonoids, provide a range of health advantages, such as antioxidant and anti-inflammatory effects that can help fight various diseases and promote longevity. As a sustainable source of bioactive compounds, millets emerge as a versatile and nutritious food choice that meets the increasing demand for environmentally friendly and health-oriented options in contemporary food systems. Adopting millets as a fundamental part of our diet can pave the way for a healthier and more sustainable future for both individuals and the planet (Priya et al., 2023).

Nutraceutical properties

Millets play a significant nutrigenomic role and positively impact human health through their various properties, including hypoglycemic, anti-tumorigenic, anti-atherosclerogenic, antioxidant, anti-hypertensive, anti-inflammatory, and antimicrobial effects. As millets are rich in various essential nutrients, they provide both preventive and therapeutic benefits from chronic diseases. They are highly nutritious, promote optimal bodily functions, and rival the top cereals in terms of health benefits (Saleem et al., 2023).

8.7 BENEFITS OF MILLETS FOR CLIMATE RESILIENCE AND FARMER ECONOMICS

Climate resilience

Millets support climate-resilient agriculture by thriving in challenging environments with minimal inputs, ensuring food security in vulnerable regions (Behera, 2017; Millets for Climate Resilience and Food Security in India, n.d.).

- *Drought tolerance:* Millets are perfect for water-scarce places since they grow well in arid and semi-arid climates and use a lot less water than staple crops like rice and wheat (Millets: Recipe for Environmental Resilience, n.d.).
- *Short growing season:* Their short growing cycle allows millets to mature quickly, even with erratic rainfall patterns, making them adaptable to unpredictable weather (Serba & Yadav, 2016).
- *Heat and cold tolerance:* Millets can withstand extreme temperatures, both hot and cold, enabling cultivation in regions with wider temperature fluctuations (Bidinger et al., 2009).
- *Nutrient use efficiency:* Efficient in using soil nutrients, millets reduce the need for synthetic fertilizers, which have environmental drawbacks.

Economic benefits for farmers

- *Lower input costs:* Millets require fewer inputs, such as water and fertilizers, making them cost-effective to cultivate, especially for resource-limited farmers (Behera, 2017; Kumar et al., 2018).
- *Market demand and premium prices:* Growing awareness of millets' nutritional benefits has increased market demand, allowing farmers to sell millets at premium prices, boosting their income (Chaudhary et al., 2023; Millets for Climate Resilience and Food Security in India, n.d.).
- *Government support and initiatives:* Governments are promoting millet cultivation through policies and programs that include subsidies, MSPs, and research support, providing economic incentives for farmers (NITI Aayog Hails Millet Revival in Odisha – The Hindu, n.d.).
- *Value-added products:* Farmers can enhance their income by producing and selling millet-based products like flour, flakes, snacks, and ready-to-eat meals.
- *Climate resilience and yield stability:* Millets' resilience to climate change and adaptability to harsh environments provide yield stability, mitigating risks associated with climate change and ensuring reliable income for farmers (Kumar et al., 2018).

Benefits for sustainability and soil health

Cultivating millets supports a sustainable and equitable food system while enhancing farmers' economic well-being. Millets offer significant advantages for both biodiversity and soil health.

- *Promoting crop diversity:* Millets, with their various species and varieties suited to different agro-ecological zones, contribute to on-farm biodiversity, which is vital for resilience against pests, diseases, and climate change (Six Reasons to Bring Millets to the Market!, n.d.).
- *Supporting pollinators:* Many millet species attract beneficial insects, including pollinators like bees and butterflies, thus supporting a healthier ecosystem and the pollination of nearby crops (Mother of Grains: What Millet Teaches Us about Biodiversity – CGIAR, n.d.).
- *Reducing pesticide use:* Millets' natural resilience to pests and diseases allows for reduced reliance on synthetic pesticides, preserving beneficial insects and maintaining ecosystem balance.
- *Improving soil structure:* Millets' deep root systems enhance soil structure, aeration, and water infiltration, which is particularly beneficial in arid and semi-arid regions facing soil degradation (Sajjan et al., 2019).
- *Enhancing nutrient cycling:* Millets efficiently utilize soil nutrients and contribute to nutrient cycling, reducing the need for synthetic fertilizers that can harm soil health (Sajjan et al., 2019).
- *Preventing soil erosion:* The extensive root systems of millets help bind soil and prevent erosion by wind and water, maintaining topsoil fertility and preventing land degradation (Sajjan et al., 2019).

Promoting millet cultivation fosters sustainable agricultural practices, supports biodiversity, improves soil health, and contributes to a resilient and equitable food system.

8.8 CHALLENGES IN PROMOTING MILLETS FOR FOOD AND NUTRITION SECURITY

The promotion of millets to advance food and nutrition security faces several challenges (Figure 8.3).

Consumer perception and dietary habits

Historically, in many cultures, millets were staples when more expensive grains were scarce. This has led to a lingering perception of them as "inferior" or less desirable, especially as people's incomes rise (What Will It Take to Revive India's Almost Forgotten Grain?, n.d.). In many regions, millets are perceived as "poor man's food" or "birdseed" and lack the culinary appeal of more commonly consumed grains like rice and wheat. Changing ingrained dietary habits and promoting millets as tasty and versatile ingredients is crucial for increasing consumer demand (Chera, 2017)

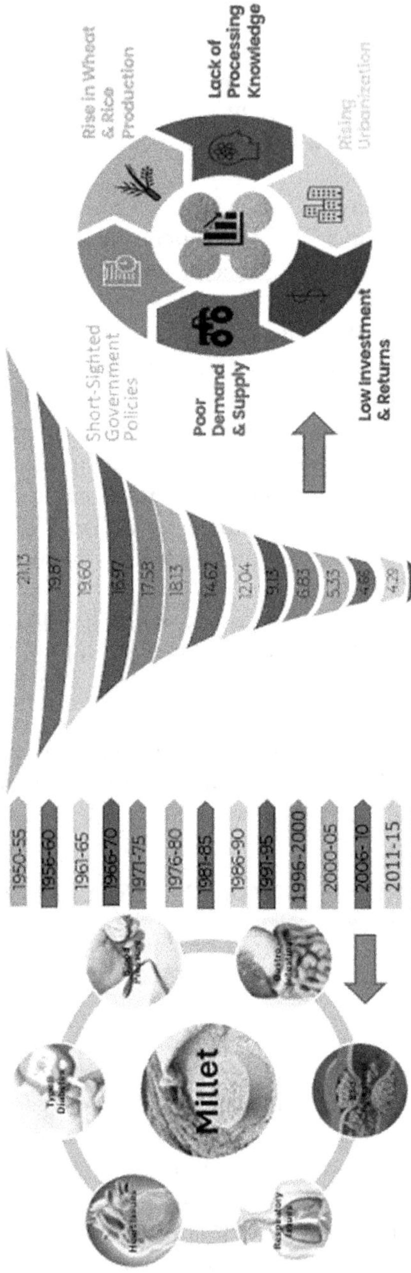

FIGURE 8.3 Millets: health benefits, production, and challenges in India. (Data from various issues of DES-GOI (2021); adapted from Priya et al., 2023.)

Entrepreneurs have highlighted that the perception of millets as "inferior" food is a significant barrier to their demand. Research shows that political, agricultural, and economic changes, such as the Green Revolution and MSPs, led most Indians to substitute millets with wheat and rice, which are seen as more desirable. Millets are often viewed as a poor man's food, while rice is associated with upper-caste status, wealth, and ritual celebration. One entrepreneur noted the rural bias that millets are considered cattle feed and not suitable for high-class people.

Lack of awareness

The biggest challenge in the current Indian market for millets is creating customer demand, given the lack of awareness about their nutritional, environmental, and economic benefits. Many customers are unfamiliar with millets and often do not recognize them even when using regional names. This confusion extends to dieticians and nutritionists, who recommend limited millet recipes, thus discouraging their consumption. Entrepreneurs have noted regional differences in millet awareness; northern Indians are more familiar with major millets, while southern Indians are more aware of minor millets.

Cooking with millets presents another challenge, as they are gluten-free and require specific preparation methods, such as soaking overnight, to avoid issues like hard texture and digestive discomfort. Entrepreneurs address this by organizing cooking workshops, maintaining blogs, introducing recipe books, and using social media to spread awareness. Clear cooking instructions are also printed on packaging to help customers use millets correctly and enjoyably (Shah et al., 2023).

Stigma and perception

The view of millets as "poor man's food" or "birdseed" undermines their appeal compared to staples like rice and wheat (Chera, 2017). Entrepreneurs in the Indian millet market face significant challenges due to customer reluctance to try their products, stemming from a lack of familiarity. This reluctance is rooted in consumer inertia, as habits formed post-Green Revolution shifted dietary preferences from millets to more accessible and affordable wheat and rice. Younger generations are unfamiliar with millets, while older generations have become accustomed to wheat and rice.

Despite efforts to market millets as a superfood and highlight their benefits, customers resist incorporating them into their regular diets. Behavioral research indicates that eating habits are influenced more by habit and external factors than by a rational assessment of benefits. To counter this, entrepreneurs have organized tasting sessions and provided free samples to introduce customers to the taste of millets, hoping to foster a preference for these products (Shah et al., 2023).

Taste and texture

Entrepreneurs have reported that taste and texture are major barriers to millet demand. Millets are naturally bitter and have a coarse texture compared to wheat and rice, making them less appealing to consumers despite their health benefits. To improve taste, entrepreneurs add flavors like coconut, chocolate, and orange. Regional differences have been noted, with southern Indians being more familiar with millets and more flexible in accepting their taste compared to northern Indians.

Entrepreneurs have also highlighted the challenge of making millet-based foods palatable. Innovations and experimentation with spice blends and flavors were necessary to improve the taste of millet snacks. Additionally, many entrepreneurs export millet products to Africa, the Middle East, and Asia, where meeting international sensory preferences is crucial (Shah et al., 2023).

Limited recipe knowledge

Another significant barrier identified is the lack of convenience in cooking with millets. Millets require cleaning, grinding, and soaking overnight before cooking, which takes longer than preparing wheat and rice. This inconvenience discourages customers who prefer easy-to-prepare food products. Additionally, millets have a "sad" and "boring" image due to their association with limited recipes, such as porridge. The lack of gluten in millets makes them difficult to use for chapatis, a staple in northern India, further discouraging their use.

To address these challenges, entrepreneurs have used social media to build millet communities for sharing recipes and motivating others to try millets. They offer ready-to-eat and ready-to-cook millet products for convenience and use packaging to increase recipe awareness. South Indians find it easier to replace rice with millets in their diets, while North Indians struggle to replace wheat dishes with millets. Entrepreneurs have identified that regular customers consume millets only once or twice a week, and increasing this frequency to make millets a staple remains a challenge. To combat the misconception that only limited recipes can be made with millets, entrepreneurs have introduced a wider range of ready-to-eat and ready-to-cook millet offerings (Shah et al., 2023). Nevertheless, there is a lack of widespread knowledge about how to prepare millets in appealing ways, making it harder to integrate them into modern diets.

High cost of millets

Millets are highly nutritious grains rich in essential vitamins and minerals, yet they often come with a higher price tag than traditional cereals. This price disparity poses challenges for individuals with limited financial means, making it difficult for them to afford these healthy grains. The increased cost of millets, when compared to more commonly available staples, can hinder low-income consumers from accessing nutritious food. As a result, marginalized people and economically disadvantaged individuals may struggle to include these valuable grains in their diets, which could restrict their intake of the diverse nutrients that millets provide. Additionally, external influences like market demand, transportation costs, and the broader agricultural environment can also affect millet prices. It is crucial for consumers to recognize these price variations and influencing factors when planning their budgets for millets or evaluating their nutritional benefits. However, people can make choices about including these types of healthy grains in to their diets while managing the costs of the millets (Harish et al., 2024).

Insufficient production

The inadequate productivity of millets represents a considerable barrier to achieving global food security. Despite their significant nutritional benefits, millets are frequently neglected and encounter various challenges related to cultivation efficiency and yield. This restricted productivity complicates efforts to ensure a consistent and sustainable food supply for an expanding global population. To tackle this challenge, it is essential for agricultural researchers and policymakers to prioritize the development of innovative strategies and technologies that aim to improve millet yields. Enhancing millet productivity not only strengthens food security but also encourages the cultivation of diverse and resilient crops, which are vital for sustaining a healthy and balanced diet. Given the rising global food demand, addressing the low productivity of millets is imperative for guaranteeing that communities have access to a sufficient and varied food supply. Ultimately, devising solutions to boost millet productivity is fundamental to overcoming food security issues and fostering sustainable agricultural practices in the future (Harish et al., 2024; Kheya et al., 2023).

Challenges in agriculture

The cultivation of millet is frequently associated with low yields and limited profitability, presenting considerable challenges for farmers and often deterring them from pursuing this agricultural endeavor. The inadequate production levels and financial limitations tied to millet farming create significant hurdles that farmers must navigate, resulting in a hesitance to allocate time and resources toward these crops. Given the widespread belief that millet is a less profitable choice compared to alternative crops, farmers tend to deprioritize its cultivation, thereby overlooking potential advantages that could arise from this traditional agricultural practice. Additionally, the restricted market demand and corresponding lack of profitability further dissuade farmers from engaging in millet cultivation, intensifying the existing barriers to entry in this field. In light of these difficulties, it is clear that addressing the fundamental issues surrounding millet cultivation—such as enhancing yield efficiency and increasing market value—is essential for encouraging farmers to reconsider and possibly reassess their commitment to millet farming practices over the long term (Harish et al., 2024).

Value chain and market access

- *Infrastructure problems:* Inadequate processing, storage, and transportation infrastructure might result in post-harvest losses and deterioration of quality (Kumar et al., 2018).
- *Fragmented value chains:* The millet value chain is frequently fragmented, resulting in inefficiencies and variable quality (Developing Inclusive Food Systems in Kenya and the United Republic of Tanzania, n.d.).
- *Processing capacity:* The creation of millet products with added value is hampered by the lack of specialized equipment (Kumar et al., 2018). The creation of millet-based products that provide a superior value proposition faces considerable obstacles due to the lack of specialized machinery and tools

essential for effective processing, formulation, and packaging. This shortfall not only disrupts the efficiency of production processes but also limits the variety of products that could appeal to a broader market. Without the appropriate equipment designed for millet processing, manufacturers struggle to enhance the nutritional content, flavor, texture, and presentation of their offerings, which restricts their capacity to satisfy consumer preferences and market needs. Investing in cutting-edge machinery and technology specifically for millet processing can pave the way for innovative opportunities to develop a wide array of value-added millet products that align with the changing demands of health-conscious consumers looking for alternatives to conventional staple foods. Adopting modern processing equipment tailored for millet production not only improves operational efficiency and product quality but also strengthens the overall competitiveness of the millet sector by promoting innovation, sustainability, and product differentiation. Ultimately, acquiring and integrating specialized equipment is a crucial step toward overcoming current challenges and realizing the full potential of millets as a versatile and nutritious ingredient in food processing and manufacturing.

- *Rivalry with major crops:* Subsidized staple crops such as wheat and rice provide millets with fierce competition (Developing Inclusive Food Systems in Kenya and the United Republic of Tanzania, n.d.). The presence of subsidized staple crops, particularly wheat and rice, presents a formidable challenge to millets due to their lower prices and widespread availability, which intensifies market competition. The affordability and accessibility of these staples render them more appealing to consumers, resulting in a decline in the demand for nutrient-dense millets. As a result, millet farmers find it increasingly difficult to secure a competitive position in the market against these dominant crops. The substantial government support and subsidies allocated to wheat and rice production further complicate the situation for millet producers, hindering their ability to compete effectively. Consequently, the promotion and consumption of millets encounter significant barriers stemming from these heavily subsidized staples, which obstruct the growth and sustainability of the millet sector. To mitigate this challenge, it is essential to enhance awareness regarding the nutritional advantages and intrinsic value of millets, alongside the implementation of policies that create a more equitable market environment for millet farmers. By cultivating a deeper understanding of the necessity for diversifying staple crop options and bolstering millet cultivation, a more balanced agricultural ecosystem can be fostered, ensuring the ongoing availability and consumption of this nutritious grain (Harish et al., 2024).

Research and development

There has been less research on millets compared to major staples, affecting improvements in yield and processing (Ashoka et al., 2020). Research on millets has been significantly less comprehensive than research on major staple crops. This lack of emphasis on millets has adversely affected the agricultural sector, particularly by limiting advancements in yield improvement and processing optimization. While major staples attract more attention and resources, millet cultivation practices have not received equivalent examination and innovation. This imbalance in research funding is reflected in the difficulties encountered in boosting the efficiency and sustainability of millet farming systems. By reallocating more scientific research and financial support towards millets, there is substantial potential for major improvements in cultivation methods and processing technologies, ultimately benefiting both farmers and consumers. Given this disparity, it is crucial to prioritize and expand research initiatives focused on millets to realize their full potential and encourage their integration into food systems, fostering a more diverse and resilient agricultural environment (Kheya et al., 2023).

Policy and subsidy structures

- *Subsidy disparities:* Government subsidies often favor major staples, making millets less competitive in terms of price (Fuglie et al., 2020).
- *Procurement policies:* Government procurement programs prioritize major staples, creating a market bias against millets (Sebayang et al., 2019).
- *Research focus:* Historical R&D investments have predominantly supported major staples, neglecting millet research (Chodavarapu et al., 2016).
- *Trade policies:* Trade policies may favor major staples with lower tariffs, making it harder for millets to compete (Sebayang et al., 2019).
- *Marketing and promotion:* Government marketing often overlooks millets, limiting consumer awareness and demand (Kaitibie et al., 2010).

Addressing these challenges requires a coordinated approach involving consumers, farmers, researchers, policymakers, and industry players to fully leverage millets' potential to provide a wholesome and sustainable food system.

8.9 OBJECTIVES AND CURRENT TRENDS OF THE MILLETS MISSION IN INDIA

The goal of the Millets Mission in India is to promote the dietary advantages and climate resilience of millets while revitalizing their production, consumption, and commercialization. Once a staple in many Indian diets, millets had been overshadowed by major cereals like rice and wheat. However, recent initiatives seek to re-popularize these "neglected and underutilized species" by addressing various challenges. The mission focuses on boosting millet production and productivity through the development of specialized technologies and infrastructure, such as advanced post-harvest processing equipment. Additionally, it seeks to increase consumption and awareness of millets, particularly in urban areas where their popularity has waned. This includes promotional campaigns and integrating millets into diverse food products to underscore their health benefits.

Current trends show a resurgence in interest, driven by heightened awareness of millets' nutritional and environmental advantages. Government initiatives, including incorporating millets into public distribution systems and launching the National Mission on Millets, have been crucial in promoting these grains. Efforts by various stakeholders are challenging previous negative perceptions of millets and fostering a shift toward more sustainable food systems. To further promote millets, several recommendations are proposed. Policymakers should re-evaluate subsidy structures to favor millets, diversify procurement programs, and invest in research and development. Additionally, increasing consumer awareness through public campaigns and collaborating with chefs to develop appealing recipes can drive demand. Supporting farmers through training and infrastructure development, as well as investing in processing technologies, will also be vital. Successful examples include Karnataka's millet programs, which enhance market development and public distribution, and Odisha's Millet Mission, which focuses on increasing production and improving infrastructure. Together, these efforts aim to leverage millets' potential to advance food security, improve nutrition, and support sustainable agriculture.

8.10 CONCLUSION

Promoting millets offers significant benefits for advancing food and nutrition security, particularly in regions vulnerable to climate change and food scarcity. However, addressing the challenges requires a comprehensive approach that encompasses consumer education, market expansion, farmer training, and supportive policies. By leveraging the benefits of millets and addressing their limitations, it is possible to foster sustainable agricultural practices, improve agricultural sustainability, and promote better nutrition.

Promoting millet consumption requires a multipronged approach that addresses production, awareness, and accessibility. As this chapter has shown, millets possess significant nutritional and environmental advantages over major staples, offering a path towards greater food security and sustainability. Successful initiatives, like those implemented in Karnataka and Odisha, demonstrate the effectiveness of farmer training programs, market development strategies, and the integration of millets into public distribution systems. However, overcoming challenges such as consumer perception and limited market access will require continued investment in research, infrastructure development, and engaging public awareness campaigns.

By learning from these case studies and implementing the policy recommendations outlined, governments, communities, and individuals can collectively contribute to a future where millets reclaim their rightful place as dietary staples. Embracing millets is not simply a dietary shift; it is an investment in a healthier, more sustainable, and equitable food system for all. Let us rediscover the potential of these ancient grains and cultivate a future where millets nourish both people and the planet.

REFERENCES

Ajatasatru, A., Prabhu, V., Pal, B. D., & Mukhopadhyay, K. (2024). Economy-wide impact of climate smart agriculture in India: A SAM framework. *Journal of Economic Structures*, *13*(1), 4. https://doi.org/10.1186/s40008-023-00320-z

Alekhya, P., & Shravanthi, A. R. (2019). Buying behaviour of consumers towards millet based food products in Hyderabad district of Telangana, India. *International Journal of Current Microbiology and Applied Sciences*, *8*(10), 223–236. https://doi.org/10.20546/ijcmas.2019.810.023

Anitha, S., Kane-Potaka, J., Tsusaka, T. W., Botha, R., Rajendran, A., Givens, D. I., Parasannanavar, D. J., Subramaniam, K., Prasad, K. D. V., Vetriventhan, M., & Bhandari, R. K. (2021). A systematic review and meta-analysis of the potential of millets for managing and reducing the risk of developing diabetes mellitus. *Frontiers in Nutrition*, *8*(July), 1–18. https://doi.org/10.3389/fnut.2021.687428

Ashoka, P., Gangaiah, B., & Sunitha, N. H. (2020). Millets- foods of 21 century. *International Journal of Current Microbiology and Applied Sciences*, *9*(12), 2404–2410. https://doi.org/10.20546/IJCMAS.2020.912.285

Behera, M. K. (2017). Assessment of the state of millets farming in India. *MOJ Ecology & Environmental Sciences*, *2*(1). https://doi.org/10.15406/MOJES.2017.02.00013

Bhat, B. V., Rao, B. D., & Tonapi, V. A. (2018). *The Story of Millets*. Karnataka State Department of Agriculture, Bengaluru, India WithICAR-Indian Institute of Millets Research, Hyderabad, India. https://ruralindiaonline.org/en/library/resource/the-story-of-millets/

Bidinger, F. R., Yadav, O. P., & Weltzien Rattunde, E. (2009). Genetic improvement of pearl millet for the arid zone of northwestern India: Lessons from two decades of collaborative ICRISAT-ICAR research. *Experimental Agriculture*, *45*(1), 107–115. https://doi.org/10.1017/S0014479708007059

Bombom, A., Kaweesi, T., Walugembe, F., Bhebhe, S., Maphosa, M., Bombom, A., Kaweesi, T., Walugembe, F., Bhebhe, S., & Maphosa, M. (2023). Millets: Traditional "poor man's" crop or future smart nutri-cereals? *Millets – Rediscover Ancient Grains*. https://doi.org/10.5772/INTECHOPEN.110534

Chaudhary, J., Shelar, R., Thakur, K., Singh, R., & Rimpika. (2023). Millets in India: Production, consumption and impact on food security. *Asian Journal of Agricultural Extension, Economics & Sociology*, *41*(8), 151–162. https://doi.org/10.9734/ajaees/2023/v41i81991

Chera, M. (2017). Transforming millets: Strategies and struggles in changing taste in Madurai. *Food, Culture & Society*, *20*(2), 303–324. https://doi.org/10.1080/15528014.2017.1305830

Chodavarapu, S., Giertz, A., & Jaeger, P. (2016). *Agribusiness in South Asia*. https://doi.org/10.1596/25116

Clemens, R., Rao, P. G., Elouafi, I., Oniang'o, R., Chandrasekara, A., Pressman, P., & Yadav, J. (2023). A commentary on millets for enhancing agri-economy, nutrition, environmental, and sustainable development goals. *Journal of Food Bioactives*, *22*, 1–4. https://doi.org/10.31665/jfb.2023.18342

Developing Inclusive Food Systems in Kenya and the United Republic of Tanzania. Lessons Learned from the Agribusiness Support for Smallholders Project in Kenya and the Southern Highlands Food Systems Programme in Tanzania |Policy Support and Governance| Food and Agriculture Organization of the United Nations. (n.d.). Retrieved August 7, 2024, from www.fao.org/policy-support/tools-and-publications/resources-details/en/c/1401158/

Director, E., El-Hashash, E. F., Al-Habeeb, A., Bakri, H., & Yassin Majjami, A. (2023). A comprehensive review of pearl and small millets: Taxonomy, production, breeding and future prospects in Saudi Arabia. *Asian Journal of Research in Crop Science*, *8*(4), 151–166. https://doi.org/10.9734/AJRCS/2023/V8I4196

Fuglie, K., Gautam, M., Goyal, A., & Maloney, W. F. (2020). Harvesting prosperity: Technology and productivity growth in agriculture. *Harvesting Prosperity: Technology and Productivity Growth in Agriculture*. https://doi.org/10.1596/978-1-4648-1393-1

Harish, M. S., Bhuker, A., & Chauhan, B. S. (2024). Millet production, challenges, and opportunities in the Asia-pacific region: A comprehensive review. *Frontiers in Sustainable Food Systems*, *8*(March), 1–16. https://doi.org/10.3389/fsufs.2024.1386469

Hasan, M., Maheshwari, C., Garg, N., & Kumar, M. (2019). Millets: Nutri-cereals. *Biotexh Express*, *6*(69 April). www.researchgate.net/publication/332495842

Kaitibie, S., Omore, A., Rich, K., & Kristjanson, P. (2010). Kenyan dairy policy Change: Influence pathways and economic impacts. *World Development*, *38*(10), 1494–1505. https://doi.org/10.1016/J.WORLDDEV.2010.06.008

Kaur, C. (2023). Millet: A therapeutic grain. *The Pharma Innovation*, *12*(5), 2289–2293. https://doi.org/10.22271/tpi.2023.v12.i5ab.20202

Kheya, S. A., Talukder, S. K., Datta, P., Yeasmin, S., Rashid, M. H., Hasan, A. K., Anwar, M. P., Islam, A. K. M. A., & Islam, A. K. M. M. (2023). Millets: The future crops for the tropics – Status, challenges and future prospects. *Heliyon*, *9*(11), e22123. https://doi.org/https://doi.org/10.1016/j.heliyon.2023.e22123

Koirala, U. (2020). Health and nutritional aspect of underutilized high-value food grain of high hills and mountains of Nepal. *Nutritional and Health Aspects of Food in South Asian Countries*, 195–209. https://doi.org/10.1016/B978-0-12-820011-7.00023-X

Kumar, A., Tomer, V., Kaur, A., Kumar, V., & Gupta, K. (2018). Millets: A solution to agrarian and nutritional challenges. *Agriculture and Food Security*, *7*(1), 1–15. https://doi.org/10.1186/S40066-018-0183-3/FIGURES/2

Liang, S., & Liang, K. (2019). Millet grain as a candidate antioxidant food resource: A review. *International Journal of Food Properties*, *22*(1), 1652–1661. https://doi.org/10.1080/10942912.2019.1668406

Lokesh, K., Dudhagara, C. R., Mahera, A. B., Kumar, S., & Patel, H. D. (2022). Millets: The future smart food. *The Pharma Innovation Journal*, *4*, 75–84. www.thepharmajournal.com

Lokesh, K., Dudhagara, C. R., Mahera, A. B., Kumar, S., & Patel, H. (2022). Millets: The future smart food. *The Pharma Innovation Journal*, *11*(4S), 75–84. www.thepharmajournal.com/special-issue?year=2022&vol=11&issue=4S&ArticleId=11762

Lydia Pramitha, J., Ganesan, J., Francis, N., Rajasekharan, R., & Thinakaran, J. (2023). Revitalization of small millets for nutritional and food security by advanced genetics and genomics approaches. *Frontiers in Genetics*, *13*(January), 1–21. https://doi.org/10.3389/fgene.2022.1007552

Maitra, S., Pine, S., Shankar, T., Pal, A., & Pramanick, B. (2020). Agronomic management of Foxtail millet (Setaria italica L.) in India for production sustainability: A review. *International Journal of Bioresource Science Citation: IJBS*, *7*(1), 11–16. https://doi.org/10.30954/2347-9655.01.2020.3

Millets: Recipe for Environmental Resilience. (n.d.). Retrieved August 7, 2024, from https://organiser.org/2023/03/23/165904/bharat/millets-recipe-for-environmental-resilience/

Millets for Climate Resilience and Food Security in India. (n.d.). Retrieved August 7, 2024, from www.orfonline.org/expert-speak/millets-for-climate-resilience-and-food-security-in-india

Mother of Grains: What Millet Teaches Us About Biodiversity – CGIAR. (n.d.). Retrieved August 7, 2024, from www.cgiar.org/news-events/news/mother-of-grains-what-millet-teaches-us-about-biodiversity

Mudau, M., Mashau, M. E., & Ramashia, S. E. (2022). Nutritional quality, antioxidant, micro-structural and sensory properties of spontaneously fermented gluten-free finger millet biscuits. *Foods*, *11*(9), 1265. https://doi.org/10.3390/FOODS11091265/S1

Nanje Gowda, N. A., Siliveru, K., Vara Prasad, P. V., Bhatt, Y., Netravati, B. P., & Gurikar, C. (2022). Modern processing of Indian millets: A perspective on changes in nutritional properties. *Foods*, *11*(4), 499. https://doi.org/10.3390/FOODS11040499

NITI Aayog Hails Millet Revival in Odisha – The Hindu. (n.d.). Retrieved August 7, 2024, from www.thehindu.com/news/national/other-states/niti-aayog-hails-millet-revival-in-odisha/article33505460.ece

Pragya, U. D., E, P. V, & K, S. T. (2017). Available online. In *Advances in Food Science and Technology* (Vol. 5, Issue 8). www.internationalscholarsjournals.org

Priya, V. R. K., Lakhawat, S., Yadav, V. K., Gacem, A., Abbas, M., Yadav, K. K., Park, H. K., Jeon, B. H., & Mishra, S. (2023). Millets: Sustainable treasure house of bioactive components. *International Journal of Food Properties*, *26*(1), 1822–1840. https://doi.org/10.1080/10942912.2023.2236317

Raghunathan, K., Headey, D., & Herforth, A. (2021). Affordability of nutritious diets in rural India. *Food Policy*, *99*, 101982. https://doi.org/10.1016/J.FOODPOL.2020.101982

Sajjan, A. S., Esh, L., Patil, S. B., & Patil, M. B. (2019). Enhancement of plant stand establishment through seed priming and seed treatment on growth, seed yield and quality in Foxtail millet [Setaria italica (L.) Beauv.]. *International Journal of Current Microbiology and Applied Sciences*, *8*(9), 2674–2687. https://doi.org/10.20546/IJCMAS.2019.809.309

Saleem, S., Mushtaq, N. U., Shah, W. H., Rasool, A., Hakeem, K. R., Seth, C. S., Tahir, I., & Rehman, R. U. (2023). Millets as smart future food with essential phytonutrients for promoting health. *Journal of Food Composition and Analysis*, *124*, 105669. https://doi.org/10.1016/j.jfca.2023.105669

Sebayang, V. B., Sinaga, B. M., Harianto, H., & Kariyasa, I. K. (2019). The impact of domestic policy on farmers' welfare and maize processing industry in Indonesia. *International Journal of Economics and Financial Issues*, *9*(3), 225–232. https://doi.org/10.32479/IJEFI.7910

Serba, D. D., & Yadav, R. S. (2016). Genomic tools in pearl millet breeding for drought tolerance: Status and prospects. *Frontiers in Plant Science*, *7*(November2016), 220903. https://doi.org/10.3389/FPLS.2016.01724/BIBTEX

Shah, P., Dhir, A., Joshi, R., & Tripathy, N. (2023). Opportunities and challenges in food entrepreneurship: In-depth qualitative investigation of millet entrepreneurs. *Journal of Business Research*, *155*(PB), 113372. https://doi.org/10.1016/j.jbusres.2022.113372

Singh, E., & Sarita. (2016). Potential of millets: Nutrients composition and health benefits. *Journal of Scientific and Innovative Research*, *5*(2), 46–50. www.jsirjournal.com

Six Reasons to Bring Millets to the Market! (n.d.). Retrieved August 7, 2024, from www.fao.org/newsroom/story/Six-reasons-to-bring-millets-to-the-market!/en

Tripathi, G., Jitendrakumar, P. H., Borah, A., Nath, D., Das, H., Bansal, S., Singh, N., & Singh, B. V. (2023). A review on nutritional and health benefits of millets. *International Journal of Plant & Soil Science*, *35*(19), 1736–1743. https://doi.org/10.9734/ijpss/2023/v35i193722

Tripathi, T., & Vyas, S. (2023). From ancient grains to modern solutions: A history of millets and their significance in agriculture and food security. *International Journal of Home Science*, *9*(2), 72–78.

Veerabadhran, V., Palakuru, H. R., Pratap, G. P., Rajeshwari, B., Prasad, G. P., Srikanth, N., & Acharya, R. (2023). A critical review of the history and practices of millets in India. *Journal of Drug Research in Ayurvedic Sciences*, *8*(Suppl 1), S18–S25. https://doi.org/10.4103/jdras.jdras_113_23

What Will it Take to Revive India's Almost Forgotten Grain? (n.d.). Retrieved August 7, 2024, from www.ndtvprofit.com/opinion/what-will-it-take-to-revive-indias-almost-forgotten-grain

9 Assessing Low Carbon Footprint Diets

Pathways to Sustainable Food Choices

Naga Jyothi Ala, Jharna Puppala, and Maheshwar Mekam

9.1 INTRODUCTION

The term *carbon footprint* has gained significant traction in public discourse and has gained widespread acceptance in recent years. It is now a catchphrase used by the government, corporate sector, and media (Chen et al., 2021; Matuštík & Kočí, 2021). The concept of carbon footprint can be traced to the idea of *ecological footprint* proposed by Wackernagel and Rees in 1996 (Syrovátka, 2020; Pandey et al., 2010). Ecological footprint can be said to represent "the area continuously required to generate a quantity of photosynthetic biomass energy and material equivalent to the amount used and dissipated by the population's consumption" (Kitzes et al., 2009: 1991). It is a measure of how dependent humans are on natural resources. According to this notion, carbon footprint refers to the land area needed to incorporate the entire amount of carbon dioxide produced by mankind during its lifetime (Pandey et al., 2010). It can also be described as a measurement of the total quantity of greenhouse gas emissions, including carbon dioxide emissions, that are accumulated throughout the course of a product's life and are generated by actions, both directly and indirectly (Chen et al., 2021; Hertwich, 2021).

Rising carbon emissions are the main factor causing global climate change, endangering ecosystems and human security. Studies have been conducted to quantify carbon emissions by establishing CO_2 equivalents, known as global warming potential (GWG) (Amicarelli et al., 2021; Lannelongue et al., 2021; Scuderi et al., 2023). The usual perception of the public is that the widespread use of coal and steel as well as the improvement of industrial technology are important factors contributing to the accelerations in greenhouse gas emissions, which in turn increase the carbon footprint. Coal became a crucial power asset following the industrial revolution. Natural gas, coal, and oil reserves around the world are depleting fast, while emissions of carbon monoxide, carbon dioxide, and methane are rising quickly. Due to the simultaneous rise of industrialization through trade and capital investment, the global economy has grown, which in turn has caused highly polluting and highly energy-intensive industries to shift from developed to developing countries. In comparison to

DOI: 10.1201/9781003487227-9

sectors like the metal, paper, and chemical production industries, the food business is less energy-intensive and produces less pollution. However, the food business has a big influence on a country's economy, people's quality of life, economic growth, and boosting domestic demand (Lin & Lei, 2015).

9.2 THE FOOD INDUSTRY

Food is a major requirement for mankind's existence, and so the food industry has its own unique importance. The majority of the food consumed by people worldwide is supplied by the food industry, which is a complicated and varied field of labor (Tadini & Gut, 2022). With manufacturing ranging from enormous investments and highly mechanized processes to small, traditional, family-owned businesses that are heavily labor-intensive, the food industry has become extremely diverse. The majority of the food industry depends on regional farming, fisheries, produce, and/or livestock farms. Because of the application of scientific discoveries and technological breakthroughs in the field, the modern food business has experienced rapid growth (Lin & Lei, 2015). Our eating habits have a considerable environmental cost associated with farming, production, packaging, freezing, cooking, and waste disposal, in addition to industrial operations. Reviewing various options on the path to a healthy and sustainable diet should take into account pertinent data on both the nutritional value and carbon footprint of each diet pattern, given the growing public awareness of a variety of dietary choices.

9.3 FOOD SUSTAINABILITY

India is witnessing a rapidly challenging food landscape in the context of lifestyle changes, food habits, and scientific findings. New estimates show that 56.4% of the total disease burden in the country is due to unhealthy diets. Food systems are responsible for one third of the greenhouse gas emissions (ICMR – National Institute of Nutrition, n.d.). In this regard, sustainable eating helps address the problems with the country's food systems. Food sustainability simply means producing food in a way that protects the environment. It involves balancing environmental, social, and economic factors to ensure that food systems are biologically responsible, socially impartial, and economically feasible (Vågsholm et al., 2020). Some key aspects of food sustainability include the following.

Environment

Sustainable food systems aim to minimize environmental degradation and conserve natural resources such as water, soil, and biodiversity. This includes practices such as organic farming, agroecology, conservation tillage, and crop rotation to reduce chemical inputs, soil erosion, and habitat destruction.

Climate change mitigation

Agriculture is a significant contributor to greenhouse gas emissions through activities like deforestation, livestock farming, and fertilizer use. Once all direct and indirect

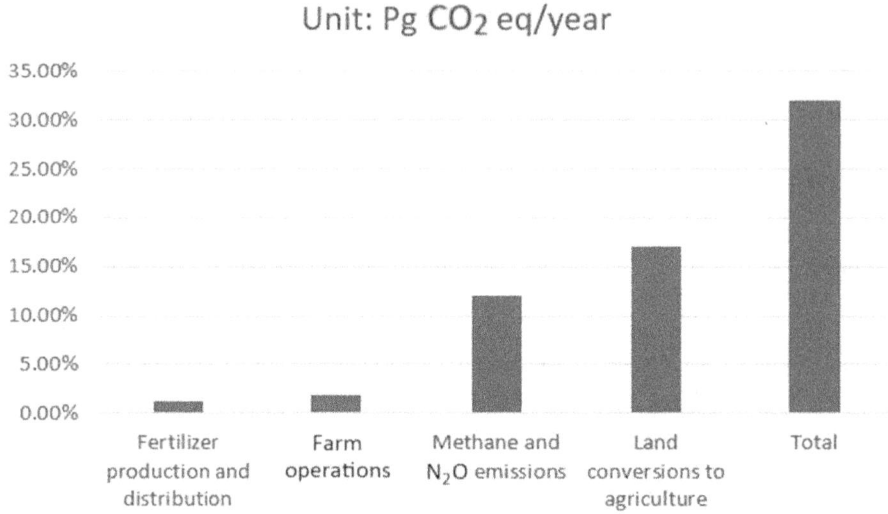

FIGURE 9.1 Agriculture's contribution to global gas emissions. (Data from Garnett, 2013.)

impacts are summed, agriculture's contribution to the global emissions total has been estimated to account for as much as 30% (Figure 9.1). Sustainable food systems focus on reducing emissions, sequestering carbon in soils, and adapting to climate change through practices such as agroforestry, renewable energy use, and carbon farming techniques (Garnett, 2013).

Biodiversity conservation

Protecting biodiversity is essential for resilient and sustainable food systems. Preserving genetic diversity in crops and livestock helps maintain resilience to pests, diseases, and environmental stresses. Sustainable agriculture practices promote habitat preservation, wildlife corridors, and the preservation of indigenous and heirloom

Resource efficiency

Sustainable food production seeks to optimize resource use and minimize waste. This includes reducing water consumption, improving energy efficiency, minimizing food loss and waste throughout the supply chain, and promoting circular economy principles such as composting and recycling.

Social equity and food justice

Food sustainability encompasses social dimensions such as equity, access to nutritious food, fair labor practices, and community empowerment. It involves supporting small-scale farmers, indigenous food systems, fair trade practices, and ensuring food access for vulnerable populations.

Health and nutrition

Sustainable food systems prioritize human health and nutrition by promoting diverse, nutrient-rich diets based on whole foods (Grosso et al., 2020). This includes reducing the consumption of processed foods, excessive meat, and dairy products, and promoting plant-based diets rich in fruits, vegetables, whole grains, legumes, and nuts.

Economic feasibility

Sustainable food systems need to be economically viable for farmers, producers, and workers throughout the supply chain. This involves fair pricing, transparent supply chains, investment in rural infrastructure, access to markets, and support for small-scale and family farmers.

9.4 IMPACT OF CARBON FOOTPRINT ON FOOD

All phases of food intake result in the production of a carbon footprint, from the initial extraction of the raw material until its disposal (Figure 9.2). The carbon footprint contribution differs at each stage. Cultivating crops and rearing animals for food is part of the process of extraction of raw resources, which is the first stage in the life cycle of food production. When fossil fuels are used in agricultural tools, fertilizers, and other activities, this stage can add to greenhouse gas emissions. After the stage of agricultural production, the food is packaged and processed in preparation for consumption and distribution. This phase will also result in carbon emissions due to increased energy-intensive processes including heating, cooling, and transportation (Nabipour Afrouzi et al., 2023).

Food is then transported to retailers, dealers, and other local distributors from the processing and packaging plants. A significant amount of greenhouse gas emissions can be seen at this stage because of transportation, due to its utilization and dissipation of fuels, especially when food is transported over longer distances. Food preparation and consumption by the population is involved in the fourth step, which is acquisition and consumption. Energy utilization while cooking, holding, and storing the food also contributes to the carbon footprint of food production. Finally, food waste disposal is a crucial step in the cycle of food production in which methane, which is a potent greenhouse gas, will be produced when waste food is dumped in landfills, adding to climate change (McAuliffe et al., 2019). Let us now consider all the parameters in detail.

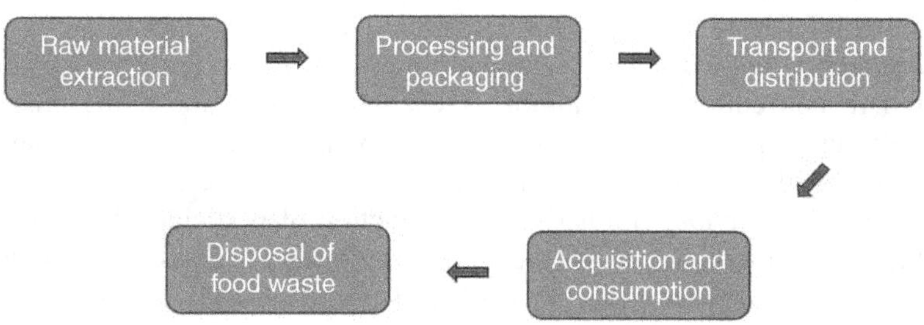

FIGURE 9.2 Food consumption life cycle. (Data from Nabipour Afrouzi et al., 2023.)

TABLE 9.1
Greenhouse Gas Emissions from the Production of Different Foods

	Greenhouse Gas Emissions (g kg-1)			
Animal/Crop	**CH_4**	**N_2O**	**CO_2**	**GWP (CO_2 eq.)**
Apple	0.0	1.0	41.7	331.4
Banana	0.0	0.2	10.0	71.6
Brinjal	0.0	0.1	12.5	31.1
Cauliflower	0.0	0.1	13.3	28.2
Egg	0.0	2.0	1.0	588.4
Fish	25.0	0.3	18.8	718.3
Milk	29.2	0.0	0.0	729.2
Mutton	482.5	0.0	0.0	12,062.7
Oilseed	0.0	1.3	50.0	422.5
Potato	0.0	0.1	10.0	24.9
Poultry meat	0.0	2.7	50.0	846.5
Pulse	0.0	0.8	83.3	306.8
Rice	43.0	0.2	75.0	1221.3
Rice, basmati	53.7	0.3	82.5	1515.4
Spice	0.0	2.5	100.0	845.0
Wheat	0.0	0.3	45.0	119.5

Note: CH_4 = methane, N_2O = nitrous oxide, CO_2 = carbon dioxide, GWP = global warming potential.

Raw material extraction

The increase in food consumption brought about by the growing human population has increased the amount of agricultural production. The extraction of raw materials in food production refers to the initial stages of agriculture, including planting, growing, and harvesting crops, as well as raising livestock and cultivating fish (Nabipour Afrouzi et al., 2023). While these activities are essential for food production, they can also contribute to the carbon footprint through various processes (Table 9.1).

- *Land use change:* Converting natural ecosystems such as forests, grasslands, or wetlands into agricultural land releases stored carbon into the atmosphere. This occurs through deforestation, drainage of wetlands, or conversion of other natural habitats to make way for agricultural activities.
- *Fertilizer production:* The manufacturing of synthetic fertilizers, commonly used in conventional agriculture, is energy-intensive and emits greenhouse gases during production. Furthermore, applying fertilizers to soils may cause the powerful greenhouse gas nitrous oxide (N_2O) to be released.
- *Pesticide production:* Similarly, the production of pesticides, herbicides, and other agricultural chemicals involves energy-intensive processes and can contribute to the carbon footprint. Chemical pesticides may also release greenhouse gases during application and degradation.

- *Mechanized farming:* The use of heavy machinery such as tractors, combines, and irrigation systems in agriculture relies on fossil fuels, contributing to greenhouse gas emissions. Energy use for irrigation, including pumping water from underground sources or surface water bodies, also adds to emissions.
- *Livestock emissions:* Ruminant animals like cattle and sheep produce methane during digestion, a greenhouse gas that has a role in climate change. Manure management practices, such as storage and treatment, can also release methane and nitrous oxide.
- *Aquaculture:* Fish farming, or aquaculture, requires energy for water management, aeration, feed production, and waste management. Energy use in aquaculture facilities, as well as emissions from feed production and waste treatment, contribute to the carbon footprint of fish production (Jiang et al., 2022).

At the farm level, animal food production, otherwise known as prime production, is where most of the resource use and emissions take place. One of the main components of primary goods is the work involved in producing poultry and cattle. The manufacture of animal feed, animals, direct energy usage on farms, and enteric fermentation caused by handling and storing manure are sources of greenhouse gas emissions. Researchers have contended that the direct emissions of carbon dioxide that animals and poultry breathe in should also be taken into account when determining their carbon footprint. In 2008, the United Nations Environment Programme (Zervas & Tsiplakou, 2012) published data on the emissions associated with producing 100 kcal of food, highlighting the foods that have the biggest carbon dioxide emissions (Figure 9.3).

Reducing the carbon footprint of raw material extraction in food production requires adopting sustainable farming practices that minimize environmental impacts. Organic farming, agroecology, precision agriculture, integrated pest control, rotational grazing, and sustainable aquaculture techniques are a few examples of these

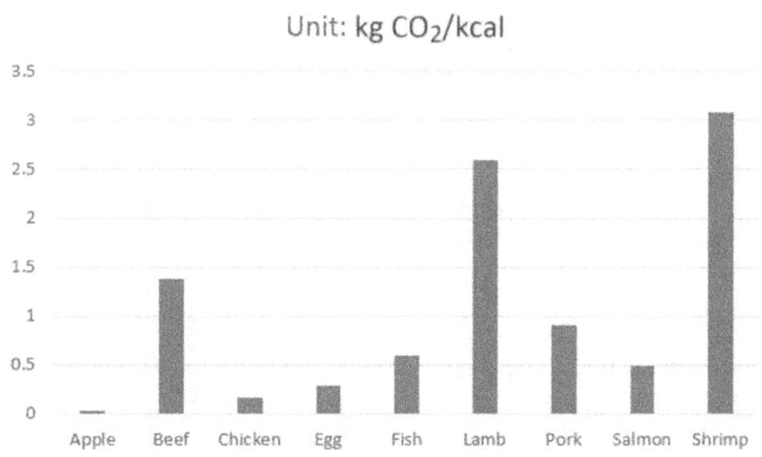

FIGURE 9.3 Carbon emissions of different foods. (Data from Nabipour Afrouzi et al., 2023.)

practices. Additionally, increasing efficiency in resource use, reducing reliance on fossil fuels, and promoting soil conservation and carbon sequestration can help mitigate emissions associated with food production.

Processing and packaging

This is an essential phase in the food production process because it helps to lessen the problems that the food contains. Raw foods are susceptible to spoilage due to the presence of bacteria or mold, which can present a health risk to consumers. Food must be processed and packaged in order for it to be ready for delivery to retail establishments. The processing stage here accounts for a significant amount of carbon emissions through involvement in energy use, as food processing often requires significant energy inputs in the form of cooking, drying, freezing, or canning. The type of energy used (either fossil fuels or renewable energy) greatly affects the carbon footprint (Parashar et al., 2020). Transportation, another inbuilt aspect in food processing, contributes to emissions through the movement of raw ingredients to processing facilities and finished products to distribution centers or markets, particularly if transportation involves long distances or inefficient modes like usage of trucks instead of trains or ships. Food processing can generate waste, such as trimmings or byproducts, which may emit methane if not properly managed (Shabir et al., 2023).

The packaging stage describes the method used to package food in order to maintain its quality. The manufacture of packaging materials like plastic, glass, metal, and paper requires energy and resources, emitting carbon dioxide and other greenhouse gases. Packaging materials need to be transported to the processing facilities, adding to emissions. Improper disposal of packaging, particularly non-biodegradable materials like plastics, can result in long-lasting emissions as they degrade or are incinerated (Castillo-Benancio et al., 2022).

There are several strategies involved in lowering the carbon footprint of food manufacturing and packaging.

- *Energy effectiveness:* Processing-related emissions can be decreased by utilizing energy-efficient technologies and renewable energy sources.
- *Sustainable packaging:* Opting for ecofriendly packaging materials that are recyclable, biodegradable, or made from renewable resources can help mitigate the environmental impact.
- *Local sourcing:* Reducing transportation distances by sourcing ingredients locally can cut down on emissions related to transportation.
- *Waste reduction:* Minimizing waste through better production processes and recycling can lower emissions associated with waste disposal.

Transport and distribution

Food can be transported using ground vehicles, sea vessels, or even aircraft, and different modes of transportation have varying levels of efficiency and emissions. Food often travels long distances from farms or processing facilities to distribution centers, retailers, and ultimately consumers. The further the distance, the more fuel is consumed, contributing to higher carbon emissions. The type of fuel used also affects emissions. Generally, transportation contributes less greenhouse gas emissions (Figure 9.4); however, diesel-powered trucks emit more carbon dioxide than vehicles running on alternative fuels like natural gas or electricity.

Food distribution involves various activities such as warehousing, sorting, and repackaging, all of which consume energy and contribute to emissions. Perishable foods often require refrigeration during transportation and storage to maintain freshness. Refrigeration units on trucks or in warehouses consume energy, predominantly from fossil fuels, leading to emissions. Packaging materials used for transportation and distribution, such as cardboard boxes, plastic wraps, and pallets, contribute to the carbon footprint due to their production and disposal. Hence, the global community may be quite concerned about the carbon footprint that comes from the distribution and transportation of food.

Reducing the carbon footprint of transportation and distribution in food production involves several strategies:

- *Optimizing transportation routes:* Efficient route planning and consolidation of shipments can reduce the distance traveled and overall emissions.
- *Modal shift:* Utilizing more sustainable modes of transportation where possible, such as trains or ships instead of trucks, can lower emissions.
- *Improving vehicle efficiency:* Investing in fuel-efficient vehicles, using alternative fuels, or transitioning to electric or hybrid vehicles can reduce emissions per unit of transported goods.
- *Cold chain efficiency:* Implementing technologies to improve the energy efficiency of refrigeration systems and reducing food waste in the cold chain can lower emissions.

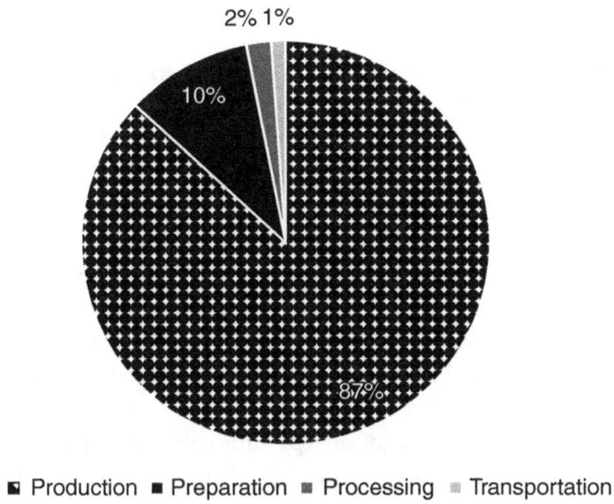

FIGURE 9.4 Stages of the food life cycle and their contributions to global warming. (Data from Pathak et al., 2010.)

- *Packaging optimization:* Using lightweight, recyclable, and reusable packaging materials can reduce emissions associated with packaging during transportation and distribution.

Acquisition and consumption

Food acquisition and consumption also contribute to the carbon footprint. The methods used in agriculture, such as conventional vs. organic farming, livestock vs. plant-based production, and the use of fertilizers and pesticides, all influence the carbon footprint. For example, conventional agriculture often relies heavily on fossil fuel-based inputs, leading to higher emissions. Deforestation or conversion of natural habitats for agriculture releases carbon stored in trees and soil, contributing to the carbon footprint. Irrigation practices, particularly in water-stressed regions, can lead to emissions due to energy consumption for pumping and treating water.

Food consumption takes place both in households and in food service establishments. It was observed that dining out has a significantly higher carbon footprint than consuming food at home (Nabipour Afrouzi et al., 2023). The other factors which affect greenhouse gas emissions during food consumption include the following.

- *Food choices:* Different foods have vastly different carbon footprints. Animal-based products generally have higher emissions than plant-based foods due to the resource-intensive nature of livestock farming, including feed production, methane emissions, and manure management.
- *Food waste:* Wasting food results in emissions associated with its production, transportation, and disposal. Food waste decomposes anaerobically in landfills, releasing the powerful greenhouse gas methane.
- *Cooking methods:* The energy source and efficiency of cooking appliances influence the carbon footprint of food preparation. For example, using a gas stove emits carbon dioxide, while electricity emissions depend on a mix of energies.

Reducing the carbon footprint during acquisition and consumption involves various strategies such as the following.

- *Sustainable agriculture:* Encouraging applications like forest farming, conservation tillage, and ecological farming can bring down emissions from agricultural production.
- *Dietary shifts:* Promoting plant-based diets or reducing the consumption of high-carbon foods like red meat can significantly lower carbon footprints.
- *Reducing food waste:* Implementing measures to prevent food waste at the consumer level, such as meal planning, proper storage, and composting, can reduce emissions.
- *Energy-efficient cooking:* Use of energy-efficient appliances, cooking methods (e.g., boiling vs. baking), and renewable energy sources can lower emissions during food preparation.

Disposal of food waste

Food waste is a necessary component of the food supply chain at every point, including the extraction, production, distribution, and trash generated from food in homes or markets (Nabipour Afrouzi et al., 2023). The carbon footprint associated with food disposal primarily stems from the decomposition of organic matter in landfills, leading to the release of methane, a potent greenhouse gas. Agricultural production generates byproducts and waste, such as crop residues, damaged or unsold produce, and inedible parts of plants or animals. When these materials are not properly managed, they can decompose and release methane in landfills or during on-farm disposal. Food processing facilities produce waste in the form of trimmings, peelings, and other byproducts. If not repurposed or recycled, this waste can contribute to emissions through landfill decomposition or incineration. Packaging materials used during food production, such as cardboard, plastic, and metal, contribute to the carbon footprint when disposed of. Incineration of packaging waste releases carbon dioxide, while landfill disposal leads to methane emissions. Unsold or expired food products at retail establishments contribute to food waste. When consumers discard food at home, whether due to spoilage or excess, it adds to the overall carbon footprint of food disposal.

Food waste decomposes anaerobically in landfills because there is little oxygen present. During this process, methane is created, a greenhouse gas with a significantly bigger potential for global warming than carbon dioxide. Methane emissions from landfills contribute to climate change by trapping heat in the atmosphere, thereby exacerbating global warming. Transporting food waste to landfills requires fuel, usually from fossil sources, which emits carbon dioxide. The emissions from transportation depend on the distance traveled and the efficiency of the vehicles used.

Reducing the carbon footprint of food disposal involves various strategies.

- *Food waste prevention:* Minimizing food waste in the first place reduces the amount of organic matter sent to landfills. This can be achieved through better meal planning, proper storage, portion control, and reducing over-purchasing.
- *Composting:* Instead of sending food waste to landfills, composting it can significantly reduce emissions. Aerobic decomposition in compost piles produces carbon dioxide instead of methane, which has a lower impact on climate change. Additionally, compost can be used to enrich soil and reduce the need for synthetic fertilizers.
- *Anaerobic digestion:* In order to break down organic waste in a controlled environment and produce biogas for energy production, some facilities use anaerobic digestion. This process helps mitigate methane discharge while generating renewable energy.
- *Landfill gas capture:* In some cases, landfills are equipped with gas capture systems to collect methane emissions and prevent their release into the atmosphere. Captured methane can be used for energy generation, reducing reliance on fossil fuels.

- *Waste reduction:* Practices for minimizing waste generation at each stage of the food production process include better inventory management, optimization of production processes to reduce byproducts, and improvements in packaging efficiency.
- *Recycling and repurposing:* Finding alternative uses for food waste, such as composting agricultural and processing byproducts or recycling packaging materials, can divert waste from landfills and reduce emissions.
- *Energy recovery:* Utilizing waste-to-energy technologies such as anaerobic digestion or incineration with energy recovery can convert organic waste into biogas or electricity, cutting back on fossil fuel use and lowering emissions.
- *Consumer education:* Educating consumers about the environmental impact of food waste and providing guidance on proper storage, portion control, and meal preparation can contribute to a decrease in household waste.

9.5 CARBON FOOTPRINTS OF DIETS IN INDIA

Dietary patterns in India

Food holds great importance in Indian culture and symbolizes unity, love, and celebration. Indian food traditions and customs are deeply rooted in the country's history, religion, and regional diversity. Different types of cuisines across India reflect its diverse cultural heritage (Vecchio et al., 2014). But the evolving food landscape influenced by factors like globalization and urbanization has led to a shift in the consumption patterns away from the typical traditional Indian diet and towards many other Westernized diets (Tak et al., 2019). Dietary patterns include the following.

- *Plant-based diets:* Consuming mostly plant-based foods, such as fruits, vegetables, grains, nuts, seeds, and legumes, and minimizing or abstaining from animal products, such as dairy, eggs, and meat, is known as a plant-based diet (Rabès et al., 2020). People choose plant-based diets for various reasons, including health benefits, environmental concerns, and ethical considerations regarding animal welfare. Plant-based diets are often associated with numerous health benefits, including lower risk of heart disease, type 2 diabetes, certain cancers, and obesity. They typically provide ample fiber, vitamins, minerals, and antioxidants while being lower in saturated fats and cholesterol compared to diets heavy in animal products.
- *Vegetarian diets:* Vegetarian diets exclude meat, poultry, and seafood but typically include other animal-derived products like dairy and eggs. However, there are different types of vegetarian diets, each with its own variations regarding which animal products are excluded (Hargreaves et al., 2021).
    - *Lacto-ovo-vegetarian diets:* This is the most popular kind of vegetarian diet, which omits meat, poultry, fish, and shellfish but allows dairy products and eggs.
    - *Lacto-vegetarian diets:* This diet includes dairy products but excludes eggs, meat, poultry, fish, and seafood.
    - *Ovo-vegetarian diets:* Eggs are allowed on this diet, but dairy, meat, poultry, fish, and shellfish are not.

- *Vegan diets:* A plant-based diet known as a vegan diet avoids all products made from animals, such as meat, chicken, seafood, dairy, eggs, honey, and any other ingredients derived from animals. Veganism extends beyond dietary choices and often encompasses a lifestyle that seeks to minimize harm to animals in all aspects of life, including clothing, cosmetics, and other consumer goods. Similar to vegetarian diets, vegan diets offer numerous health benefits, including reduced risk of heart disease, type 2 diabetes, certain cancers, and obesity. They are typically high in fiber, vitamins, minerals, and antioxidants while being lower in saturated fats and cholesterol compared to diets heavy in animal products (Dawczynski et al., 2022). Ethical and environmental considerations are often driving factors for adopting a vegan lifestyle.
- *Flexitarian diets:* A flexitarian diet is primarily plant-based eating with the flexibility to include small amounts of meat and other animal products. The term *flexitarian* is a combination of *flexible* and *vegetarian*. Flexitarians primarily focus on eating fruits, vegetables, whole grains, nuts, seeds, and legumes, but they occasionally incorporate meat, poultry, fish, eggs, and dairy into their meals. The emphasis is on consuming plant-based foods for their health benefits and environmental sustainability while still allowing for some animal products if desired. Flexitarians may choose to eat meatless meals several times a week or only include meat on occasion, such as on special occasions or when dining out. This approach offers the benefits of a predominantly plant-based diet, such as increased intake of fiber, vitamins, and minerals, while also providing the flexibility to meet individual preferences and nutritional needs (Bruns et al., 2023). Flexitarianism is becoming increasingly popular as people seek ways to improve their health and reduce their environmental impact without committing to a strict vegetarian or vegan diet.
- *Carnivore diets:* Carnivore diets, also known as all-meat diets or zero-carb diets, involve consuming only animal products, predominantly meat, and sometimes including other animal-derived foods like eggs and dairy. They are essentially an extreme form of the low carbohydrate high fat (LCHF), or ketogenic diet, with the exclusion of plant-based foods (Dawczynski et al., 2022). Advocates of carnivore diets claim various health benefits, including weight loss, improved mental clarity, reduced inflammation, and relief from autoimmune conditions (Lennerz et al., 2021). However, scientific evidence supporting these claims is limited, and the long-term health effects of following a carnivore diet are not well understood.
- *Omnivorous diets:* Omnivorous diets include a variety of foods from both plant and animal sources. Humans are natural omnivores, meaning we are biologically adapted to consume and derive nutrients from both plant-based and animal-based foods. An omnivorous diet typically includes plant- and animal-based foods. With the flexibility and variety this diet offers in terms of food options, people can satisfy their nutritional requirements while also savoring a broad variety of flavors and textures (Dawczynski et al., 2022). Numerous health advantages of a well-planned omnivorous diet include increased nutritional intake, decreased risk of nutrient deficiencies, and support for general health and well-being.

Assessing low carbon footprint diets

Religion and tradition are the main factors influencing Indian food. Being a nation of Hindus, the majority of Indians abstain from eating beef and pork, which makes them vegetarians. Even though the contribution of greenhouse gas emissions from Indian diets are low compared to countries like the USA and Germany (Table 9.2), a shift in diet pattern by many Indians towards a mixed diet, such as combining vegetables and meat, can change the emissions impact (Kovacs et al., 2021).

Analyzing diets based on both consumption patterns and their associated carbon footprints is an important aspect of sustainable food systems (Willits-Smith et al., 2020). Here is a breakdown of how different diets can impact carbon footprint based on consumption.

- *Plant-based diets:* These diets generally have lower carbon footprints compared to diets rich in animal products (Rabès et al., 2020). Plants require fewer resources such as water and land and produce fewer greenhouse gas emissions during production. Additionally, plant-based foods often require less processing and transportation, further reducing their carbon footprint.
- *Vegetarian diets:* Vegetarian diets typically have lower carbon footprints compared to diets that include meat. While dairy and egg production contribute to carbon emissions, they generally have lower environmental impacts than meat production, particularly red meat and processed meats (O'Malley et al., 2023).
- *Vegan diets:* Vegan diets tend to have the lowest carbon footprints among all diets. By excluding animal products entirely, vegan diets greatly reduce greenhouse gas emissions associated with livestock farming, land use change, and feed production (Rabès et al., 2020).
- *Flexitarian diets:* Flexitarian diets are primarily plant-based but occasionally include small amounts of meat, seafood, dairy, or eggs. Flexitarian diets can vary in their carbon footprint depending on the frequency and quantity of animal products consumed. Generally, they have lower carbon footprints than

TABLE 9.2
Greenhouse Gas Emissions of Daily Food Group Recommendations for 2000 kcal Diet Patterns in Different Countries (kg of CO_2-Eq. Per Day)

Country	Protein	Diary	Grains	Fruits	Vegetables	Oils/Fats	Total
Germany	0.98	0.81	0.05	0.12	0.20	0.09	2.25
India	0.03	0.41	0.11	0.05	0.17	0.08	0.86
Netherlands	1.12	0.89	0.08	0.08	0.12	0.15	2.86
Oman	1.24	0.17	0.20	0.39	0.27	0.26	2.53
Thailand	0.63	0.33	0.31	0.47	0.09	N/A	1.83
Uruguay	1.50	0.65	0.03	0.18	0.18	0.04	2.42
USA	1.84	1.10	0.02	0.16	0.16	0.03	3.83

Source: Kovacs et al. (2021).

diets that include meat in every meal but may have higher footprints than strict vegetarian or vegan diets (Dixon et al., 2023).

- *Meat-heavy diets:* A meat-heavy diet is one that includes large quantities of meat, especially red meat and processed meats. Meat-heavy diets typically have higher carbon footprints than plant-based diets. Methane emissions are a significant source of carbon emissions from livestock production, especially the raising of ruminant animals such as cattle (Karandikar et al., 2022). Additionally, meat production requires significant amounts of land, water, and feed, contributing to environmental degradation and carbon emissions.
- *Omnivorous diets:* Omnivorous diets, which include a combination of plant-based foods and animal products, can have varying carbon footprints depending on factors such as the types and quantities of foods consumed, as well as agricultural and production practices. In general, the carbon footprint of an omnivorous diet tends to be higher than that of a vegetarian or vegan diet, primarily due to the inclusion of animal products (Rabès et al., 2020). However, the carbon footprint can be influenced by individual food choices within the omnivorous diet, with options like poultry, pork, and sustainably sourced seafood generally having lower environmental impacts than beef and lamb. Additionally, adopting sustainable agricultural practices, reducing food waste, and choosing locally sourced and minimally processed foods can help lower the carbon footprint of an omnivorous diet (Gaillac & Marbach, 2021).

9.6 BALANCED DIET APPROACH

A balanced diet is a wholesome and nutritionally adequate diet that helps in performing a wide range of functions in the body by providing ample amounts of calories, proteins, vitamins, minerals and fiber (ICMR – National Institute of Nutrition, n.d.). Calculating the precise carbon footprint of a balanced diet requires detailed information about specific food choices, production methods, and transportation routes. Nevertheless, adopting a balanced diet approach can significantly decrease carbon footprint by choosing sustainable food options, such as shifting from red meat to lean meat sources, focusing on plant products, choosing seasonal foods, selecting eco-friendly packaging material, and reducing waste.

A study revealed the global warming potential of different meal patterns followed in India (Figure 9.5). Considering the foods that are frequently components of meals in India, according to this study an adult male consumes 1165 g of food per day and emits 723.7 g of CO_2 equivalent of greenhouse gases per day. Emissions 20% lower were observed from adult female vegetarians. However, a 40% hike was seen in the greenhouse gas emissions for a non-vegetarian diet. In a common lacto-vegetarian diet, rice accounted for the largest proportion of the carbon footprint at 49%, followed by milk at 22%. At 35%, mutton made up the major contribution of a non-vegetarian diet towards greenhouse gas emission, closely followed by rice at 34% (Table 9.3).

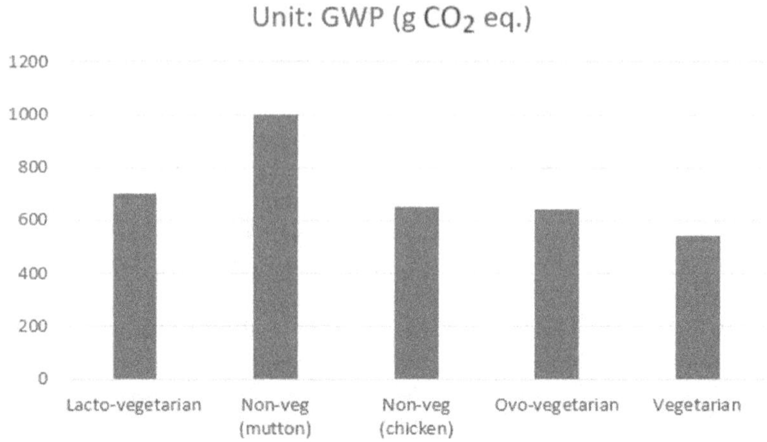

FIGURE 9.5 Global warming potential (GWP) of vegetarian and non-vegetarian diets in India. (Pathak et al., 2010.)

TABLE 9.3
Greenhouse Gas Emissions (GHG) for Different Food Items in Balanced Vegetarian and Non-Vegetarian Diets

Food Item	GHG Emissions in Balanced Vegetarian Diet (%)	GHG Emissions in Balanced Non-Vegetarian Diet (%)
Egg	—	2
Fruits	1	1
Milk	22	8
Mutton	—	35
Oil	2	2
Pulses	3	2
Rice	49	34
Sugar	5	3
Vegetables	7	5
Wheat	11	8

Source: Pathak et al. (2010).

9.7 PATHWAYS TO SUSTAINABLE FOOD CHOICES

Choosing sustainable food options is an impactful way to contribute to environmental conservation and promote healthier living. Several pathways are available that would help in reducing the carbon footprint for a better ecosystem.

Shifting to plant-based diets

Plant-based diets, such as vegetarian and vegan diets, typically have lower carbon footprints than diets rich in animal products. This is because the production of plant-based foods generally requires fewer resources, such as land, water, and energy, and emits fewer greenhouse gases compared to animal agriculture (Macdiarmid, 2021). Shifting towards a plant-based diet can significantly reduce the ecological footprint and is widely recognized as one of the most sustainable food choices for the following reasons.

- *Reduced carbon footprint:* Plant-based diets generally have a lower carbon footprint than diets high in animal products. The production of meat and dairy involves significant greenhouse gas emissions, primarily from methane released by livestock and carbon dioxide produced by grazing and feed crop deforestation.
- *Conservation of resources:* When compared to animal goods, plant-based foods usually require fewer natural resources to produce, such as land, water, and energy. We can protect land and water resources, which are frequently overused in modern animal agriculture, by switching to plant-based diets.
- *Mitigation of deforestation:* Animal agriculture is a leading driver of deforestation, particularly in regions like the Amazon rainforest where land is cleared for cattle ranching and feed crops. Choosing plant-based foods reduces the demand for land conversion, helping to preserve critical ecosystems and biodiversity.
- *Water conservation:* Plant-based diets require significantly less water compared to animal-based diets. Producing one kilogram of beef, for example, can require thousands of gallons of water, primarily for growing feed crops and providing drinking water for livestock. Most plant foods have a much lower water footprint per calorie or gram of protein.
- *Reduced pollution:* Plant-based agriculture tends to produce fewer pollutants such as nitrogen and phosphorus runoff, which can lead to water pollution and ecosystem degradation. Animal waste from concentrated animal feeding operations (CAFOs) can contaminate waterways with harmful pathogens and nutrients, presenting dangers to aquatic ecosystems and human health.
- *Biodiversity conservation:* Industrial animal agriculture often involves the destruction of natural habitats and ecosystems to create space for livestock production and feed crops. By transitioning to plant-based diets, we can help mitigate habitat loss and support biodiversity conservation efforts.
- *Health benefits:* Plant-based diets are associated with numerous health benefits, including reduced risk of chronic diseases such as heart disease, diabetes, and certain cancers. By promoting healthier eating patterns, plant-based diets can alleviate pressure on healthcare systems and improve overall well-being.
- *Ethical considerations:* Many people adopt plant-based diets for ethical reasons, including worries regarding animal welfare in industrial agriculture. Choosing plant-based foods supports more compassionate and humane treatment of animals.

Reducing meat consumption

Reducing the consumption of high-impact meats, such as beef and lamb, can significantly lower the carbon footprint. These meats have higher GHG emissions per calorie or gram of protein compared to other animal products like poultry, pork, or seafood. Transitioning to poultry, pork, or plant-based protein sources can help reduce the carbon footprint associated with food (Lucas et al., 2023).

Choosing locally sourced foods

Choosing locally sourced and seasonal produce can lessen the carbon footprint associated with the transportation of food. Locally grown foods often require less energy for transportation compared to foods that are transported over long distances (Stein & Santini, 2021). Additionally, seasonal produce is more likely to be grown outdoors, reducing the energy required for climate control in greenhouses. Locally produced food is a sustainable choice with several benefits, such as the following.

- *Reduced carbon emissions:* Locally sourced foods typically travel shorter distances from farm to plate compared to imported or long-distance foods. This reduces transportation-related carbon emissions, including those from fuel consumption in trucks, ships, and airplanes. By supporting local producers, consumers help mitigate the effects of long-distance food transportation on the environment.
- *Support for local economies:* Purchasing locally sourced foods supports local farmers, ranchers, and food producers, contributing to the vitality of rural and regional economies. This helps create jobs, sustain livelihoods, and strengthen community resilience. Additionally, money spent on local products tends to circulate within the community, benefiting local businesses and services. Good places to find fresh, locally grown produce are farm-to-table dining establishments, farmers' markets, and community-supported agriculture (CSA) programs.
- *Preservation of farmland and green spaces:* Supporting local agriculture helps preserve farmland and green spaces in the region. When farmers have a viable market for their products, they are more likely to continue farming rather than selling their land for development. Preserving farmland supports biodiversity, soil health, and ecosystem services such as water filtration and carbon sequestration.
- *Promotion of food diversity:* Local food systems often offer a greater variety of seasonal produce and artisanal products that reflect the cultural and agricultural heritage of the region. By supporting local peasant markets, CSA programs, and restaurants that serve food from farms to tables, consumers can relish a good range of fresh, flavorful foods while fostering culinary traditions and food sovereignty (Egli et al., 2023).
- *Enhanced food traceability and transparency:* Customers can get to know their food origin locality and how it gets produced by purchasing directly from regional producers or through open supply chains. This promotes food traceability, quality assurance, and accountability in food production practices.

Consumers can make informed choices based on factors such as farming methods, sustainability certifications, and ethical standards.

- *Seasonal eating and food security:* Local foods have better flavor, higher nutritional content, and are more enjoyable to eat since they are frequently harvested when they are at their ripest and freshest. By embracing seasonal eating, consumers can reconnect with the natural rhythms of the local food system and reduce reliance on imported or out-of-season produce. Encouraging local food production also improves food security since it diversifies food supplies and lessens reliance on unstable global supply lines.
- *Community engagement and education:* Initiatives centered around local food, such as farmers' markets, community gardens, and farm tours, offer opportunities for social interaction, education, and community involvement. These platforms foster connections between producers and consumers, promote agricultural literacy, and raise awareness about sustainable food systems, environmental stewardship, and food justice issues.

Selecting organic foods

Supporting organic farming practices can contribute to lower carbon footprints by decreasing reliance on industrial fertilizers and pesticides, which are energy-intensive to produce and can contribute to greenhouse gas emissions (Das et al., 2020). Sustainable farming methods such as agroforestry, crop rotation, and zero-till farming can also help to sequester carbon in the soil, further mitigating the carbon footprint of food production. Natural pest control methods, biodiversity, and soil health are given top priority in organic farming practices, minimizing the application of artificial fertilizers and insecticides that can harm ecosystems and human health. Choosing organic foods can offer several other benefits, such as the following.

- *Reduction of chemical inputs:* Natural inputs and methods are prioritized in organic farming operations in order to reduce the usage of artificial pesticides, herbicides, and fertilizers. Because organic agriculture does not use hazardous chemicals, it reduces pollution and environmental degradation and helps maintain the quality of the land, water, and air.
- *Soil health:* The goal of organic farming techniques is to improve and preserve soil health by using techniques like crop rotation, cover crops, and composting. Healthy soils are more resilient to erosion, nutrient depletion, and drought, promoting long-term agricultural sustainability. Organic farming also enhances soil biodiversity and microbial activity, contributing to ecosystem functioning and carbon sequestration.
- *Biodiversity conservation:* Organic farms tend to support higher levels of biodiversity compared to conventional monoculture systems. Beneficial insects, birds, and other wildlife find homes in organic agriculture since it does not use artificial pesticides and promotes a variety of habitats. Protecting biodiversity is essential for pollination, pest control, and ecosystem resilience.
- *Water conservation:* Drip irrigation, mulching, and soil conservation are examples of organic farming techniques that help save water and minimize the

need for irrigation. By improving soil structure and water retention, organic agriculture mitigates the impacts of drought and water scarcity. Organic farms also reduce the threat of water pollution associated with chemical fertilizers and pesticides.

- *Climate change mitigation:* By storing carbon in soils and cutting greenhouse gas emissions, organic farming may help mitigate the effects of climate change. Reduced tillage, agroforestry, and cover crops are examples of practices that improve soil carbon storage and encourage carbon sequestration, which helps lessen the effects of climate change (Rancilio et al., 2022).
- *Health benefits:* Organic foods are produced without synthetic pesticides, genetically modified organisms (GMOs), or artificial additives, making them a healthier choice for consumers. Organic farming prioritizes natural methods of pest and disease management, reducing exposure to potentially harmful chemicals in food and the environment. By choosing organic foods, consumers can support their own health and well-being.
- *Support for sustainable farming communities:* Choosing organic foods supports farmers who adhere to environmentally sustainable and socially responsible practices. Organic farming often involves smaller-scale, family-owned operations that prioritize soil stewardship, animal welfare, and community engagement. Customers can help to maintain the health of local economies and rural communities by purchasing products from organic farmers.
- *Certification and transparency:* Organic certification provides consumers with an assurance that foods have been produced according to strict organic standards, verified by independent certifying bodies. Organic labels help consumers make informed choices about the foods they buy, promoting transparency and accountability in the food system.

Seasonal eating

Seasonal eating is a sustainable food choice that aligns consumption with the natural rhythms of local food production. Eating seasonally means consuming foods that are grown and harvested locally. As a result, there is less demand for long-distance driving, which requires more fuel for cars, ships, and airplanes, and this can reduce greenhouse gas emissions. By choosing seasonal, locally grown food, consumers may lessen their carbon impact and encourage more sustainable agricultural systems (Puigdueta et al., 2021).

Support for local farmers

Seasonal eating supports local farmers and producers by creating demand for their seasonal crops. This provides economic stability for farmers and strengthens local food systems. By purchasing directly from farmers' markets, consumers can invest in their local agricultural communities and foster connections with the people who grow their food (Karwacka et al., 2020).

- *Promotion of biodiversity:* Eating seasonally encourages diversity in diets and supports a wide variety of crops grown in different seasons. This promotes biodiversity in agricultural landscapes, as farmers cultivate a range of fruits, vegetables, grains, and legumes adapted to local growing conditions. Biodiversity is essential for ecosystem resilience, soil health, and pollinator habitat conservation.

- *Optimal flavor and nutrition:* Seasonal foods are harvested at peak freshness and ripeness, offering superior flavor, texture, and nutritional value compared to out-of-season produce that may be picked prematurely or transported long distances. By consuming foods in season, consumers can enjoy the full spectrum of flavors and nutrients that nature has to offer, enhancing culinary enjoyment and nutritional diversity.
- *Connection to nature:* Seasonal eating fosters a deeper connection to the natural world and the changing seasons. By tuning into the seasonal availability of foods, consumers can appreciate the cyclical rhythms of nature and gain a greater understanding of the agricultural processes that sustain life. This connection to nature promotes mindfulness, gratitude, and environmental stewardship.
- *Reduction of food waste:* Eating seasonally can help reduce food waste by aligning consumption with production cycles. When foods are abundant in season, there is less likelihood of excess inventory being wasted or discarded. By embracing seasonal eating and preserving surplus produce through techniques such as canning, freezing, or fermenting, consumers can minimize food waste and make the most of seasonal abundance.
- *Educational opportunities:* Seasonal eating provides opportunities for learning about local food traditions, culinary techniques, and agricultural practices. Farmers' markets, cooking classes, and community events centered around seasonal foods offer educational experiences for consumers of all ages. Learning about seasonal eating can inspire creativity in the kitchen, promote food literacy, and empower consumers to make informed food choices.

Reducing food waste

Approximately one third of the food produced worldwide is lost or discarded, which adds to resource depletion and greenhouse gas emissions. Wasted food is a significant contributor to carbon emissions, as it represents a waste of the resources and energy used in production, transportation, and disposal. By minimizing food waste through better meal planning, storage, and composting, individuals can reduce the carbon footprint associated with their diets (Reisch et al., 2021). Reducing food waste is a critical aspect of promoting sustainability in the food system, and the growing population can make a difference through the following channels.

- *Conservation of resources:* Significant resources like land, water, energy, and labor are needed for food production. These resources are consumed needlessly when food is wasted. People can contribute to the preservation of natural resources and lessen the environmental effect of food production by cutting down on food waste.

- *Mitigation of greenhouse gas emissions:* Greenhouse gas emissions are exacerbated by food waste, which is a contributing factor throughout the food supply chain. Methane is a strong greenhouse gas that is produced during the decomposition of organic waste in landfills and contributes to climate change. People can help offset these emissions and fight global warming by cutting food waste.
- *Preservation of biodiversity:* Food production often involves the conversion of natural habitats into agricultural land, leading to habitat loss and biodiversity decline. By wasting less food, individuals can reduce the demand for agricultural expansion and help protect ecosystems and wildlife habitats.
- *Support for food security:* Food waste exacerbates issues of food insecurity and hunger by diverting edible food away from those in need. By decreasing food waste, people help to ensure that more food reaches those who are food-insecure and to promote food security and equitable access to nutrient-dense food.
- *Economic savings:* The financial losses incurred by people, households, corporations, and governments due to food waste are substantial. By wasting less food, individuals can save money on grocery bills, reduce disposal costs, and increase economic efficiency throughout the food supply chain.
- *Promotion of sustainable consumption:* Reducing food waste encourages more mindful and sustainable consumption patterns. By planning meals, shopping strategically, and using leftovers creatively, individuals can minimize excess food purchases and consumption, leading to more sustainable lifestyles.
- *Innovation and technology:* Innovation and technical developments in food processing, storage, and delivery are fueled by efforts to minimize food waste. Through the implementation of strategies like enhanced packaging, refrigeration technology, and supply chain optimization, individuals can help to tackle the underlying causes of food waste and construct a more robust and efficient food system.
- *Educational opportunities:* Educating people about the negative effects of food waste and disseminating waste reduction techniques can inspire them to take action in their daily lives. Campaigns, community programs, and educational initiatives can offer helpful advice, materials, and encouragement for cutting down on food waste at home, in schools, and in the workplace.

Home gardening

Home gardening is a sustainable food choice that offers numerous benefits for individuals, families, and communities, for the following reasons.

- *Local food production:* Home gardening allows individuals to produce their own fruits, vegetables, and herbs where they live, reducing reliance on store-bought produce that may have traveled long distances. By growing food locally, gardeners can minimize transportation emissions and support more sustainable food systems (Wiedenhofer et al., 2018).

- *Reduction of food miles:* Food grown in home gardens travels zero miles from garden to plate, further reducing carbon emissions associated with transportation. By lowering reliance on fossil fuels for food distribution, this helps mitigate climate change and leaves a reduced carbon imprint.
- *Promotion of biodiversity:* By offering a home for pollinators, birds, and beneficial insects, home gardens can promote biodiversity. By cultivating diverse plant species, gardeners create ecosystems that are more resilient to pests, diseases, and environmental stresses, reducing the need for chemical pesticides and fertilizers.
- *Conservation of resources:* Home gardening promotes resource conservation by utilizing organic gardening practices such as composting, mulching, and water-efficient irrigation techniques. By recycling organic waste into compost and using rainwater harvesting systems, gardeners can minimize waste and conserve water, soil, and nutrients.
- *Healthy eating:* Home-grown fruits and vegetables are often fresher, tastier, and more nutritious than store-bought produce, as they will be picked when fully matured and can be consumed immediately. By incorporating home-grown produce into their diets, individuals can enjoy the health benefits of fresh, nutrient-rich foods and support their overall well-being.
- *Food security:* Home gardening enhances food security by providing a reliable source of fresh produce, especially during times of economic uncertainty or food shortages. By growing their own food, individuals can supplement their diets with home-grown produce and reduce dependence on commercial food systems.
- *Educational opportunities:* Home gardening provides valuable scholastic opportunities for individuals of all ages to learn about plant biology, gardening techniques, and environmental stewardship. By involving children in gardening activities, families can inculcate a sense of duty, self-sufficiency, and connection to nature.
- *Community building:* Home gardening can foster community connections by offering a chance for neighbors to share resources, knowledge, and produce. Community gardens, neighborhood seed swaps, and gardening clubs offer social spaces where individuals can come together to cultivate friendships, exchange ideas, and support each other's gardening endeavors.
- *Resilience and self-sufficiency:* Home gardening promotes resilience and self-sufficiency by empowering individuals to take control of their food supply and reduce dependence on external food sources. By growing a wide variety of crops and saving seeds for future plantings, gardeners can adapt to changing environmental conditions and ensure long-term food security.

Choosing low-impact food processing methods

Food processing can significantly increase the carbon footprint of food products, especially when energy-intensive methods such as deep frying or freezing are involved (Piscitelli et al., 2023). Choosing minimally processed or lightly processed foods can help in bringing down the carbon footprint associated with food consumption.

Educating yourself and others
Educating consumers about the environmental effects of food options and providing information on low carbon footprint diets can empower individuals to make sustainable food choices (Hudha et al., 2020). Additionally, policies that incentivize sustainable farming practices, support local food systems, and reduce food waste can further promote low carbon footprint diets at the societal level. Individuals can keep up with food sustainability-related concerns and impart knowledge to friends, family, and neighbors. They can also advocate for policies and initiatives that support sustainable agriculture, food access, and environmental conservation.

Supporting sustainable brands
Consumers can choose products from companies and brands that prioritize sustainability throughout their supply chains, from sourcing ingredients to packaging and distribution (Rondoni & Grasso, 2021; Lemken et al., 2021).

9.8 CONCLUSION

Carbon footprint is definitely a highly destructive element that is a major threat to the environment, and food patterns and diet systems contribute a significant amount to greenhouse gas emissions (González-García et al., 2018). Choosing food products that have fewer negative effects on the environment is one strategy that can be used to cut greenhouse gas emissions. Strategies to lower food consumption's carbon footprint include eating more locally grown food, consuming less meat, and substituting alternative vegetable proteins for meat and milk. However, when it comes to replacing food products, nutritional benefits like vitamins, proteins, and minerals are just as crucial as calorific value and greenhouse gas emissions. To effectively implement climate-wise diets, more information is needed about the life cycle impact of individual products, relationships between diets, and the effects of different diets on the food chain. Indian food products have a global warming potential that is typical for the Indian context; other countries cannot directly utilize these to design choices to cut emissions to a given level.

Not only food, but the entire life cycle of food consumption contributes to an increase in global warming potential. The adoption of sustainable farming practices, efficient use of resources, optimization of transportation routes, energy-efficient cooking, and proper waste disposal can all help in decreasing carbon emissions. Individual responsibilities also matter, in the form of education and promotion of biodiversity, encouragement of locally grown foods, home gardening, support for sustainable brands, and economic savings. By considering these pathways and making informed choices about food consumption, individuals can contribute to mitigating climate change and promoting sustainability through low carbon footprint diets. Thus, each person has a responsibility to contribute to resolving this global problem in order to give future generations a sustainable future via improved ecosystems.

REFERENCES

Amicarelli, V., Lagioia, G., & Bux, C. (2021). Global warming potential of food waste through the life cycle assessment: An analytical review. *Environmental Impact Assessment Review*, *91*, 106677. https://doi.org/10.1016/j.eiar.2021.106677

Bruns, A., Nebl, J., Jonas, W., Hahn, A., & Schuchardt, J. P. (2023). Nutritional status of flexitarians compared to vegans and omnivores – A cross-sectional pilot study. *BMC Nutrition*, *9*(1). https://doi.org/10.1186/s40795-023-00799-6

Castillo-Benancio, S., Alvarez-Risco, A., Esquerre-Botton, S., Leclercq-Machado, L., Calle-Nole, M., Morales-Ríos, F., De Las Mercedes Anderson-Seminario, M., & Del-Aguila-Arcentales, S. (2022). Circular economy for packaging and carbon footprint. In A. Alvarez-Risco, S.S. Muthu, S. Del-Aguila-Arcentales (eds.), *Circular Economy Circular: Impact on Carbon and Water Footprint* (pp. 115–138). London: Springer Nature. https://doi.org/10.1007/978-981-19-0549-0_6

Chen, R., Zhang, R., & Han, H. (2021). Where has carbon footprint research gone? *Ecological Indicators*, *120*, 106882. https://doi.org/10.1016/j.ecolind.2020.106882

Das, S., Chatterjee, A., & Pal, T. K. (2020). Organic farming in India: A vision towards a healthy nation. *Food Quality and Safety*, *4*(2), 69–76. https://doi.org/10.1093/fqsafe/fyaa018

Dawczynski, C., Weidauer, T., Richert, C., Schlattmann, P., Dawczynski, K., & Kiehntopf, M. (2022). Nutrient intake and nutrition status in vegetarians and vegans in comparison to omnivores – The Nutritional Evaluation (NuEva) study. *Frontiers in Nutrition*, *9*. https://doi.org/10.3389/fnut.2022.819106

Dixon, K. A., Michelsen, M. K., & Carpenter, C. L. (2023). Modern diets and the health of our planet: An investigation into the environmental impacts of food choices. *Nutrients*, *15*(3), 692. https://doi.org/10.3390/nu15030692

Egli, L., Rüschhoff, J., & Priess, J. (2023). A systematic review of the ecological, social and economic sustainability effects of community-supported agriculture. *Frontiers in Sustainable Food Systems*, *7*. https://doi.org/10.3389/fsufs.2023.1136866

Gaillac, R., & Marbach, S. (2021). The carbon footprint of meat and dairy proteins: A practical perspective to guide low carbon footprint dietary choices. *Journal of Cleaner Production*, *321*, 128766. https://doi.org/10.1016/j.jclepro.2021.128766

Garnett, T. (2013). Food sustainability: Problems, perspectives and solutions. *Proceedings of the Nutrition Society*, *72*(1), 29–39. https://doi.org/10.1017/s0029665112002947

González-García, S., Esteve-Llorens, X., Moreira, M. T., & Feijoo, G. (2018). Carbon footprint and nutritional quality of different human dietary choices. *Science of the Total Environment*, *644*, 77–94. https://doi.org/10.1016/j.scitotenv.2018.06.339

Grosso, G., Mateo, A., Rangelov, N., Buzeti, T., & Birt, C. (2020). Nutrition in the context of the Sustainable Development Goals. *European Journal of Public Health*, *30*(Supplement_1), i19–i23. https://doi.org/10.1093/eurpub/ckaa034

Hargreaves, S. M., Raposo, A., Saraiva, A., & Zandonadi, R. P. (2021). Vegetarian diet: An overview through the perspective of quality of life domains. *International Journal of Environmental Research and Public Health*, *18*(8), 4067. https://doi.org/10.3390/ijerph18084067

Hertwich, E. G. (2021). Increased carbon footprint of materials production driven by rise in investments. *Nature Geoscience*, *14*(3), 151–155. https://doi.org/10.1038/s41561-021-00690-8

Hudha, M. N., Hamidah, I., Permanasari, A., Abdullah, A. G., Rachman, I., & Matsumoto, T. (2020). Low carbon education: A review and bibliometric analysis. *European Journal of Educational Research*, *9*(1), 319–329. https://doi.org/10.12973/eu-jer.9.1.319

ICMR – National Institute of Nutrition. (n.d.). www.nin.res.in/dietaryguidelines/index.html

Jiang, Q., Bhattarai, N., Pahlow, M., & Xu, Z. (2022). Environmental sustainability and footprints of global aquaculture. *Resources, Conservation and Recycling*, *180*, 106183. https://doi.org/10.1016/j.resconrec.2022.106183

Karandikar, H., Serota, M. W., Sherman, W. C., Green, J. R., Verta, G., Kremen, C., & Middleton, A. D. (2022). Dietary patterns of a versatile large carnivore, the puma (Puma concolor). *Ecology and Evolution*, *12*(6). https://doi.org/10.1002/ece3.9002

Karwacka, M., Ciurzyńska, A., Lenart, A., & Janowicz, M. (2020). Sustainable development in the agri-food sector in terms of the carbon footprint: A review. *Sustainability*, *12*(16), 6463. https://doi.org/10.3390/su12166463

Kitzes, J., Galli, A., Bagliani, M., Barrett, J., Dige, G., Ede, S., Erb, K., Giljum, S., Haberl, H., Hails, C., Jolia-Ferrier, L., Jungwirth, S., Lenzen, M., Lewis, K., Loh, J., Marchettini, N., Messinger, H., Milne, K., Moles, R., . . . Wiedmann, T. (2009, May 1). A research agenda for improving national Ecological Footprint accounts. *Ecological Economics*, 68(7), 1991–2007. https://doi.org/10.1016/j.ecolecon.2008.06.022

Kovacs, B., Miller, L., Heller, M. C., & Rose, D. (2021). The carbon footprint of dietary guidelines around the world: A seven country modeling study. *Nutrition Journal*, *20*(1). https://doi.org/10.1186/s12937-021-00669-6

Lannelongue, L., Grealey, J., & Inouye, M. (2021). Green algorithms: Quantifying the carbon footprint of computation. *Advanced Science*, *8*(12). https://doi.org/10.1002/advs.202100707

Lemken, D., Zühlsdorf, A., & Spiller, A. (2021). Improving consumers' understanding and use of carbon footprint labels on food: Proposal for a climate score label. *EuroChoices*, *20*(2), 23–29. https://doi.org/10.1111/1746-692x.12321

Lennerz, B. S., Mey, J. T., Henn, O. H., & Ludwig, D. S. (2021). Behavioral characteristics and self-reported health status among 2029 adults consuming a "carnivore diet." *Current Developments in Nutrition*, *5*(12), nzab133. https://doi.org/10.1093/cdn/nzab133

Lin, B., & Lei, X. (2015). Carbon emissions reduction in China's food industry. *Energy Policy*, *86*, 483–492. https://doi.org/10.1016/j.enpol.2015.07.030

Lucas, E., Guo, M., & Guillén-Gosálbez, G. (2023). Low-carbon diets can reduce global ecological and health costs. *Nature Food*, *4*(5), 394–406. https://doi.org/10.1038/s43016-023-00749-2

Macdiarmid, J. I. (2021). The food system and climate change: Are plant-based diets becoming unhealthy and less environmentally sustainable? *Proceedings of the Nutrition Society*, *81*(2), 162–167. https://doi.org/10.1017/s0029665121003712

Matuštík, J., & Kočí, V. (2021). What is a footprint? A conceptual analysis of environmental footprint indicators. *Journal of Cleaner Production*, *285*, 124833. https://doi.org/10.1016/j.jclepro.2020.124833

McAuliffe, G. A., Takahashi, T., & Lee, M. R. F. (2019). Applications of nutritional functional units in commodity-level life cycle assessment (LCA) of agri-food systems. *The International Journal of Life Cycle Assessment*, *25*(2), 208–221. https://doi.org/10.1007/s11367-019-01679-7

Nabipour Afrouzi, H., Ahmed, J., Mobin Siddique, B., Khairuddin, N., & Hassan, A. (2023). A comprehensive review on carbon footprint of regular diet and ways to improving lowered emissions. *Results in Engineering*, *18*, 101054. https://doi.org/10.1016/j.rineng.2023.101054

O'Malley, K., Willits-Smith, A., & Rose, D. (2023). Popular diets as selected by adults in the United States show wide variation in carbon footprints and diet quality. *The American Journal of Clinical Nutrition*, *117*(4), 701–708. https://doi.org/10.1016/j.ajcnut.2023.01.009

Pandey, D., Agrawal, M., & Pandey, J. S. (2010). Carbon footprint: Current methods of estimation. *Environmental Monitoring and Assessment, 178*(1–4), 135–160. https://doi.org/10.1007/s10661-010-1678-y

Parashar, S., Sood, G., & Agrawal, N. (2020). Modelling the enablers of food supply chain for reduction in carbon footprint. *Journal of Cleaner Production, 275*, 122932. https://doi.org/10.1016/j.jclepro.2020.122932

Pathak, H., Jain, N., Bhatia, A., Patel, J., & Aggarwal, P. (2010). Carbon footprints of Indian food items. *Agriculture, Ecosystems & Environment, 139*(1–2), 66–73. https://doi.org/10.1016/j.agee.2010.07.002

Piscitelli, L., De Boni, A., Roma, R., & Ottomano Palmisano, G. (2023). Carbon farming: How to support farmers in choosing the best management strategies for low-impact food production. *Land, 13*(1), 5. https://doi.org/10.3390/land13010005

Puigdueta, I., Aguilera, E., Cruz, J. L., Iglesias, A., & Sanz-Cobena, A. (2021). Urban agriculture may change food consumption towards low carbon diets. *Global Food Security, 28*, 100507. https://doi.org/10.1016/j.gfs.2021.100507

Rabès, A., Seconda, L., Langevin, B., Allès, B., Touvier, M., Hercberg, S., Lairon, D., Baudry, J., Pointereau, P., & Kesse-Guyot, E. (2020). Greenhouse gas emissions, energy demand and land use associated with omnivorous, pesco-vegetarian, vegetarian, and vegan diets accounting for farming practices. *Sustainable Production and Consumption, 22*, 138–146. https://doi.org/10.1016/j.spc.2020.02.010

Rancilio, G., Gibin, D., Blaco, A., & Casagrandi, R. (2022). Low-GHG culturally acceptable diets to reduce individual carbon footprint by 20%. *Journal of Cleaner Production, 338*, 130623. https://doi.org/10.1016/j.jclepro.2022.130623

Reisch, L. A., Sunstein, C. R., Andor, M. A., Doebbe, F. C., Meier, J., & Haddaway, N. R. (2021). Mitigating climate change via food consumption and food waste: A systematic map of behavioral interventions. *Journal of Cleaner Production, 279*, 123717. https://doi.org/10.1016/j.jclepro.2020.123717

Rondoni, A., & Grasso, S. (2021). Consumers behaviour towards carbon footprint labels on food: A review of the literature and discussion of industry implications. *Journal of Cleaner Production, 301*, 127031. https://doi.org/10.1016/j.jclepro.2021.127031

Scuderi, A., Timpanaro, G., & Cammarata, M. (2023). Analysis of global warming potential: Organic vs. conventional tomatoes. *Agricultural Economics (Zemědělská Ekonomika), 69*(7), 267–275. https://doi.org/10.17221/104/2023-agricecon

Shabir, I., Dash, K. K., Dar, A. H., Pandey, V. K., Fayaz, U., Srivastava, S., & Nisha, R. (2023). Carbon footprints evaluation for sustainable food processing system development: A comprehensive review. *Future Foods, 7*, 100215. https://doi.org/10.1016/j.fufo.2023.100215

Stein, A. J., & Santini, F. (2021). The sustainability of "local" food: A review for policymakers. *Review of Agricultural, Food and Environmental Studies, 103*(1), 77–89. https://doi.org/10.1007/s41130-021-00148-w

Syrovátka, M. (2020). On sustainability interpretations of the ecological footprint. *Ecological Economics, 169*, 106543. https://doi.org/10.1016/j.ecolecon.2019.106543

Tadini, C. C., & Gut, J. A. W. (2022). The importance of heating unit operations in the food industry to obtain safe and high-quality products. *Frontiers in Nutrition, 9*. https://doi.org/10.3389/fnut.2022.853638

Tak, M., Shankar, B., & Kadiyala, S. (2019). Dietary transition in India: Temporal and regional trends, 1993 to 2012. *Food and Nutrition Bulletin, 40*(2), 254–270. https://doi.org/10.1177/0379572119833856

Vågsholm, I., Arzoomand, N. S., & Boqvist, S. (2020). Food security, safety, and sustainability—Getting the trade-offs right. *Frontiers in Sustainable Food Systems, 4*. https://doi.org/10.3389/fsufs.2020.00016

Vecchio, M. G., Paramesh, E. C., Paramesh, H., Loganes, C., Ballali, S., Gafare, C. E., Verduci, E., & Gulati, A. (2014). Types of food and nutrient intake in India: A literature review. *The Indian Journal of Pediatrics*, *81*(S1), 17–22. https://doi.org/10.1007/s12098-014-1465-9

Wiedenhofer, D., Smetschka, B., Akenji, L., Jalas, M., & Haberl, H. (2018). Household time use, carbon footprints, and urban form: A review of the potential contributions of everyday living to the 1.5 °C climate target. *Current Opinion in Environmental Sustainability*, *30*, 7–17. https://doi.org/10.1016/j.cosust.2018.02.007

Willits-Smith, A., Aranda, R., Heller, M. C., & Rose, D. (2020). Addressing the carbon footprint, healthfulness, and costs of self-selected diets in the USA: A population-based cross-sectional study. *The Lancet Planetary Health*, *4*(3), e98–e106. https://doi.org/10.1016/s2542-5196(20)30055-3

Zervas, G., & Tsiplakou, E. (2012). An assessment of GHG emissions from small ruminants in comparison with GHG emissions from large ruminants and monogastric livestock. *Atmospheric Environment*, *49*, 13–23. https://doi.org/10.1016/j.atmosenv.2011.11.039

10 Revolutionizing Food Security

Harnessing Artificial Intelligence for Enhanced Nutritional Outcomes

Aparna Chaudhary and Shikha Saxena

10.1 INTRODUCTION

Since 2015, the percentage of people suffering from hunger and food insecurity has continued to rise. In 2022, about 735 million people globally faced chronic hunger, while 2.4 billion people were found to be moderately or severely food-insecure (The Sustainable Development Goals Report, 2023). Regardless of efforts made globally, food insecurity remains an urgent concern in numerous countries (FAO et al., 2019, as cited in Bilali et al., 2020). A joint report from the FAO, IFAD, UNICEF, WFP, and WHO suggests that rapidly growing population, overuse and exhaustion of natural resources, and climate change will likely exacerbate global food insecurity (The State of Food Security, 2022, as cited in Sarku et al., 2023).

Sustainable Development Goal (SDG) 2 aims to eradicate hunger by improving food security and nutrition while advocating for sustainable agricultural practices (The Sustainable Development Goals Report, 2023). Meeting the objective of eradicating global hunger, per SDG 2, often involves supplying food to those in need (Jorgensen et al., 2016, as cited in Chamara et al., 2020). It has been estimated that by 2050, there will be a need for availability of 70% more food to be consumed by humans than current consumption levels, to feed approximately 9.7 billion people (Cole et al., 2018).

Moreover, because of increased food demand and diminished crop yields, higher food costs coupled with income disparities could detrimentally impact the accessibility and availability of food for poor households. The agricultural sector is critical in enhancing food availability and attaining food security (Pawlak & Kołodziejczak, 2020). Novel automated techniques are being introduced to fulfill food demands, as traditional farming methods prove inadequate for meeting these needs (Javaid et al., 2023). The utilization of AI in agriculture has gained importance since 2015 (Lakshmi & Corbett, 2020, as cited in Chamara et al., 2020). Conventional farms rely on laborers for seeding, irrigating, harvesting, weeding, and other necessary activities. AI assists in resolving these challenges by offering automation solutions (Javaid et al., 2023). AI encompasses analytical tools like data analytics, machine

DOI: 10.1201/9781003487227-10

learning, and optimization models, enabling the utilization of historical data and real-time information for making informed decisions (Soori et al., 2023 as cited in Sarku et al., 2023).

10.2 FOOD SECURITY

According to the 1996 World Food Summit, food security exists when all people always have physical, social, and economic access to sufficient, safe, and nutritious food that fits their dietary needs and food preferences for an active and healthy life (Policy Brief, 2006). Food security is compromised when challenges are faced periodically while accessing food, adversely affecting nutritional status. Factors such as unfavorable weather, political instability, or economic issues like lack of employment and rising food costs can affect the ability to maintain food security (FAO, 2008, as cited in Mohamed, 2017).

Food insecurity is a situation that exists when one, some, or all of the dimensions of food security are disturbed (FSIN and Global Network Against Food Crises, 2024). When a household's food intake drops below 80% of the daily recommended calories needed for an individual to stay active and healthy, it is classified as food-insecure (Devereux, 2000, as cited in Mohamed, 2017). Acute food insecurity signifies a scenario wherein populations experience food scarcity that jeopardizes lives or means of survival, irrespective of the underlying causes, circumstances, or duration. Chronic food insecurity is characterized by the ongoing or repetitive inability to access sufficient nutrition for a healthy and active lifestyle, primarily stemming from structural issues such as poverty, marginalization, and limited access to essential services (FSIN and Global Network Against Food Crises, 2024).

10.3 DIMENSIONS OF FOOD SECURITY

The four dimensions of food security are availability, accessibility, utilization, and stability (Policy Brief, 2006).

- *Food availability* refers to having enough food of suitable quality accessible either through local production or imports, which may include food aid (Policy Brief, 2006). Three elements that contribute to food availability are production, distribution, and exchange (Ericksen, 2008, as cited in Capone et al., 2014).
- *Food accessibility* can be described as individuals having sufficient income or resources to obtain suitable food domestically, either through home production, purchasing from local markets, exchanging goods, receiving gifts, borrowing, or accessing food aid (Gunaratne et al., 2021). Access to food relies on the household's income, how that income is distributed within the household, and food prices in the market, as well as factors such as an individual's access to the markets and their social and institutional rights (Kuwornu et al., 2011, as cited in Mohamed, 2017). In rural households where food is self-produced, access depends on land availability and the capacity to cultivate sufficient food for sustenance. Conversely, urban households rely on economic means to access food supplies through retail distribution systems (Erickson & Fausti, 2021). Food

accessibility can be characterized by three components: affordability, distribution, and preference (Ericksen, 2008, as cited in Capone et al., 2014).

- Providing a balanced diet, clean water, sanitation, and healthcare ensures *food utilization* and nutritional well-being, meeting all physiological needs (Policy Brief, 2006). Food utilization can also be described as correct biological food utilization, necessitating a diet that provides adequate energy and essential nutrients, alongside knowledge of food storage, processing, fundamental nutrition, childcare, and managing illnesses (Mohamed, 2017). The three components of food utilization are nutritional value, social value, and food safety (Ericksen, 2008, as cited in Capone et al., 2014).
- *Food stability* is present when there is consistent access to adequate food, without the threat of losing access due to sudden shocks like economic or climatic crises, or events like seasonal food insecurity. Therefore, the notion of stability encompasses both food availability and accessibility (Policy Brief, 2006).

10.4 FOOD SYSTEMS

A food system functions within and is affected by social, political, economic, and environmental circumstances. It affects not just what people consume and the methods of production and acquisition but also who has access to food and the nutritional quality of their diet (Capone et al., 2014). The food system encompasses the production, processing, distribution, storage, procurement, consumption, and wastage of food (Ahmed et al., 2022, as cited in Namkhah et al., 2023).

Sustainability has emerged as a central principle and primary objective for human development (IPCC, 2012, as cited in Allen & Prosperi, 2016). A sustainable food system can be described as a system that provides nutritious food to meet present needs while safeguarding healthy ecosystems for future generations, with minimal adverse effects on the environment. It promotes local production and distribution networks, ensures the availability, accessibility, and affordability of nutritious food for all, and upholds principles of fairness and justice, safeguarding the welfare of everyone, including the people working on farms and the people consuming food (Story et al., 2009, as cited in Allen & Prosperi, 2016).

The agricultural supply chain encompasses various stages, starting with farming activities in the fields and progressing through intermediate storage, transportation to processing plants, and finally reaching clients and consumers. At each stage, data collection is crucial, necessitating numerous decision-making processes. The collected data extend from the field to the eventual use of the product by processors or consumers, with storage typically occurring in cloud-based systems (De Baerdemaeker, 2023).

10.5 ARTIFICIAL INTELLIGENCE

Artificial intelligence (AI) encompasses emulating human intelligence in machines (Russell & Norvig, 2016, as cited in Chamara et al., 2020). These machines are programed to replicate human thought processes and behaviors across a spectrum of tasks, ranging from simple to intricate. They possess the capability of learning from experience, modifying their responses based on new inputs, and thereby executing tasks like humans. Through extensive training, AI systems can process vast amounts of data, identifying patterns within them. Ultimately, AI functions as a data processing system or computational framework, transforming inputs into user-friendly outputs (De Baerdemaeker, 2023).

10.6 AI TECHNOLOGIES IN THE AGRICULTURE SUPPLY CHAIN

Ensuring food and nutrition security persists as a pivotal policy concern worldwide, with the ongoing global malnutrition crisis posing an immediate challenge for both developed and developing nations (Allen & Prosperi, 2016). One out of every three individuals globally grapples with moderate to severe food insecurity. It is projected that over 600 million people worldwide will encounter hunger by 2030. Achieving zero hunger by 2030 demands prompt, collaborative actions and policy measures to address enduring inequalities, transform food systems, and advocate for sustainable agricultural practices (The Sustainable Development Goals Report, 2023).

Given the growing population and finite resources, sustainable agricultural production plays a vital role in ensuring food security (Liu et al., 2023). Ensuring food security for the entire human population may require a substantial increase in agricultural production (estimated to be around 70% to 100%) by 2050 to accommodate the projected population growth (Bradshaw & Brook, 2014, as cited in Ehrlich & Harte, 2015).

Precision agriculture is a management approach that involves collecting, processing, and analyzing temporal, spatial, and individual data. These data are then integrated with other information to guide management decisions, taking into account the estimated variability within production systems. This integration enhances resource utilization, leading to enhanced productivity, production efficiency, quality, profitability, and sustainability in agriculture (ISPA, 2021, as cited in Erickson & Fausti, 2021). Precision agriculture additionally promotes sustainability and environmental conservation (Javaid et al., 2023).

In farms using innovative technology, field management differs depending on the operational cycle depicted in Figure 10.1. The management system begins with the specific crop to be managed, leveraging its inherent variability both spatially and temporally. The platform encompasses the use of sensors to obtain objective data. These data comprise information collected from parameters that are measured within the crop, soil, or environment. The data from the sensors can be obtained through various methods, such as inserting a pen drive into a USB port to access files or obtaining data from software applications that are synchronized with the Internet. Data filtering methods and AI algorithms help growers make informed decisions by extracting only relevant data. After this, equipment that can receive orders from a computerized control unit executes the decision system's commands. The cycle begins and ends at the crop level. Specialized sensors monitor the crop's response, and the loop continues until harvesting, ending the crop's life cycle (Saiz-Rubio & Rovira-Más, 2020).

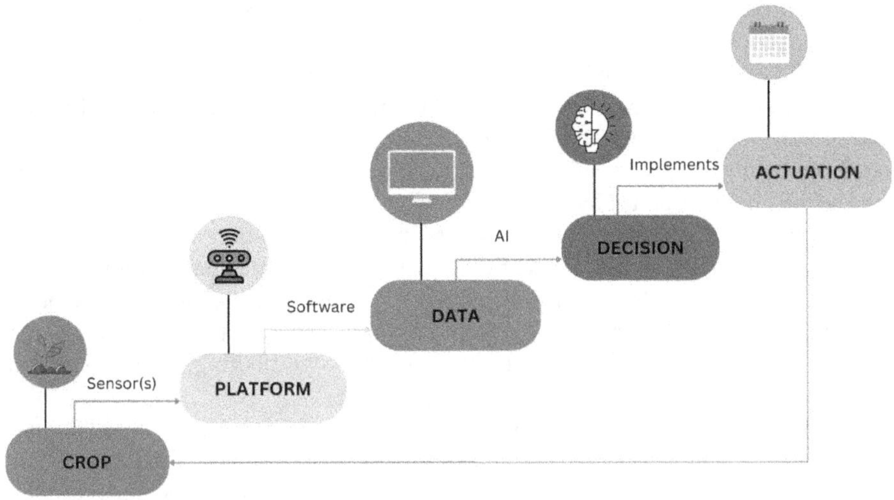

FIGURE 10.1 Cycle of field management. (Adapted from Saiz-Rubio & Rovira-Más, 2020.)

Precision agriculture primarily influences the production aspect of the supply chain by enhancing the efficiency of crop production inputs, as well as increasing production scale effects, yields, and yield stability. Integrating precision agriculture information systems with blockchain technology will broaden the diversity within food supply systems and is expected to bolster food security. Connecting farm production data with supply chain logistics holds promise for reducing food costs and enhancing efficiency in food delivery systems (Erickson & Fausti, 2021). Blockchain technology can ensure end-to-end trackability and integrity of each transaction along the agri-food supply chain (AFSC), provided that all parties involved in agri-food production are transparent along all the processes. Transportation operators can monitor crucial parameters such as time, temperature, and humidity inside the containers using appropriate sensors. Any deviation beyond the established safety limits triggers an immediate alarm. Furthermore, predictive analysis of transportation data enables anticipation of delays in product delivery, allowing for proactive measures like active cooling or selecting faster routes. Retailers can utilize transportation data reports to make informed decisions about accepting or rejecting goods, particularly critical for handling sensitive and refrigerated products (De Baerdemaeker, 2023).

Precision agriculture harnesses the power of AI, which can spearhead an agricultural revolution at a critical juncture where the global demand for food necessitates producing more with fewer resources. AI is viewed as a promising technology capable of providing innovative solutions for agriculture. By integrating image classification techniques along with remote and local sensing data, AI can significantly enhance the efficiency of farm machinery, particularly in tasks such as weed eradication, early disease detection, crop harvesting, and grading. Furthermore, AI can analyze data collected to assess the environmental impact of different dosages and kinds of fertilizers, identifying optimal doses that minimize harm while maximizing production.

AI tools have the potential to aid farmers in reducing waste, improving product quality, and expediting access to markets. Automated tractors are employed to prepare the farm for planting and harvesting. Drones collect data, oversee the health of crops from far away, and transmit the gathered data. AI identifies the key plants on the farm and aids in pest control by determining the pesticides to be used and their appropriate quantities. Predictive analytics can estimate precipitation and evapotranspiration. By combining soil samples and other data obtained, machine learning models can be trained to provide useful information regarding soil moisture, temperature, and overall condition. By leveraging this information, farmers can irrigate crops more effectively, thereby enhancing their profitability and contributing to environmental sustainability (Javaid et al., 2023).

As a scientific field, AI encompasses various methodologies and techniques. These include machine learning, machine reasoning, and robotics. Machine learning is exemplified by deep learning and reinforcement learning, while machine reasoning encompasses planning, scheduling, knowledge representation and reasoning, search, and optimization. Robotics involves control, perception, sensors, actuators, and the incorporation of other techniques into cyber-physical systems (De Baerdemaeker, 2023). Figure 10.2 illustrates different AI techniques described in Table 10.1.

AI utilizes machine and deep learning algorithms to gain insights from data and replicate human intelligence. Predictions are generated by these networks by

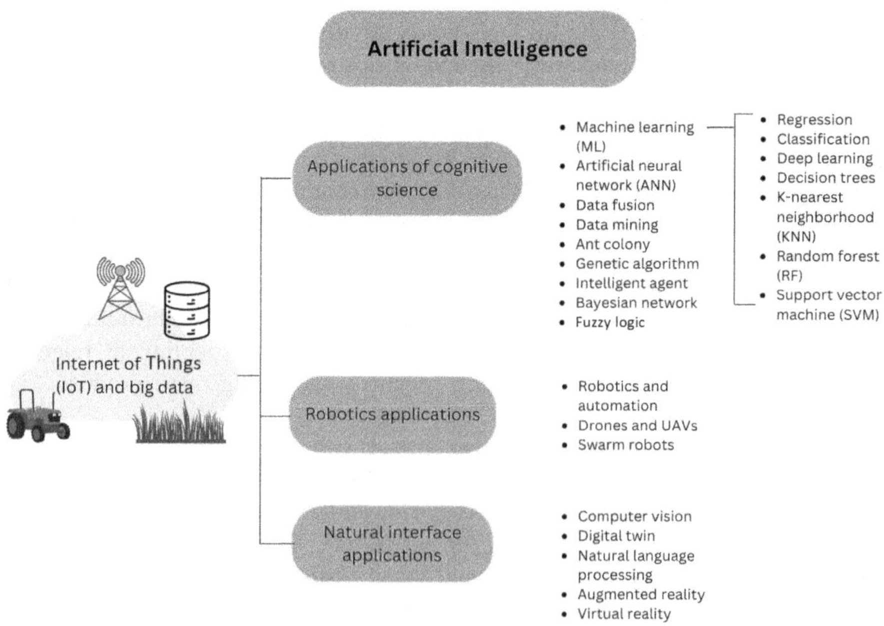

FIGURE 10.2 Various techniques of artificial intelligence. (Adapted from Oliveira & Silva, 2023.)

TABLE 10.1
Techniques of Artificial Intelligence

Technique	Description
Robotics and automation	Machines, computer applications, and other technologies used to execute tasks to reduce human labor
Drones and unmanned aerial vehicles (UAVs)	Unmanned aircraft that can be controlled remotely, without a pilot on board
Machine learning (ML)	A system capable of independently adjusting its behavior through its own experiences, utilizing various algorithms to enhance its accuracy
Artificial neural networks (ANNs)	Machine learning programs modeled after human cognition, capable of learning and adapting to novel and dynamic environments
Deep learning: convolutional neural network (CNN)	Relies on a collection of machine learning algorithms to detect patterns within images for object, class, and category recognition
Genetic algorithm (GA)	ML algorithms employed based on biological evolution processes to address problems and produce top-notch solutions
Computer vision	Encompasses tasks like object detection, motion tracking, and action recognition, employing techniques to automatically acquire, analyze, and comprehend extracted images
Digital twins	A virtual model aimed at maximizing productivity and efficiency
Internet of things (IoT)	Facilitates crop management by linking various intelligent equipment
Cloud computing	Provides immediate accessibility of resources like data storage and computational capacity as needed
Big data	Gathers, handles, and evaluates data

Source: Oliveira & Silva (2023).

connecting input and output variables dynamically, offering solutions to both simple and intricate scenarios (Javaid et al., 2023).

Machine learning

Machine learning (ML) uses statistics, probability theory, and convex optimization to solve problems faced in computer vision, sound detection, natural language processing, robotics management, and other fields (Jordan & Mitchell, 2015, as cited in Liu et al., 2023).

ML finds utility in various domains: food availability and security, weed control, soil management, crop monitoring, and weather forecasting, among others. ML algorithms are deployed to optimize crop yields and reduce input costs by discerning intricate patterns, trends, and interrelations within the multifaceted, diverse agricultural data. These algorithms facilitate precise predictions and furnish a robust framework for enhancing agricultural decision-making and operational management (De

Baerdemaeker, 2023). Support vector machines (SVM), K-nearest neighbors (KNN), and random forest (RF) are some of the ML techniques that have been employed for predicting agricultural production and facilitating precision fertilization (Liu et al., 2023).

Furthermore, ML methods can forecast market prices, making AI-based techniques increasingly favored by producer organizations and cooperatives. These techniques efficiently enhance supply chain performance, boost productivity and profitability, optimize inventory and resource management, minimize expenditure and waste, and elevate customer satisfaction (De Baerdemaeker, 2023).

Deep learning

When contrasted with alternative ML methods, deep learning (DL) demonstrates exceptional proficiency in tasks such as recognition of images and speech, prediction of molecules, analysis of data obtained from particle accelerators, reconstruction of circuits of the brain, and more (LeCun et al., 2015, as cited in Liu et al., 2023). DL methods empower machines to attain performance levels that are competitive with, or even surpass, those of humans (Zhou et al., 2019, as cited in Liu et al., 2023).

DL architectures offer essential resources for predicting crop diseases and automating farm monitoring in agriculture. Despite the absence of information or prior knowledge, artificial neural network (ANN) models can still discern non-linear relationships and forecast dependent responses. As a result, they have been employed in tasks such as food image analysis, food safety evaluation, yield prediction, crop distribution, and diverse thermal and non-thermal food processing operations.

Combining convolutional neural network (CNN)-based image processing with techniques like gene technology, cloud computing, remote sensing, and the Internet of Things (IoT) has enhanced the efficacy of the entire food supply chain. Numerous instances demonstrate the utilization of CNN models for monitoring and forecasting leaf diseases. Conversely, recurrent neural network (RNN), biological neural network (BNN), and various ML models like SVM, support vector regression (SVR), radio frequency (RF), and adaptive neuro-fuzzy inference system (ANFIS) have been utilized to predict yields. Moreover, the adoption of model predictive control methods in greenhouses, field management, agricultural infrastructure, and product processing is cultivating the shift from traditional to precision agriculture (Liu et al., 2023).

Decision support systems

A decision support system (DSS) is a software tool designed to assist end-users in efficiently and swiftly utilizing intricate data to enhance decision-making. Consequently, the raw data and the results obtained after analysis can be transformed into actionable insights and presented via a user-friendly interface. A DSS aids in making more informed decisions, particularly while dealing with complex and ambiguous data.

Internet of Things and wireless sensor networks

Utilizing IoT-based systems with wireless sensor networks (WSNs) enables the provision of continuous, automated, and real-time information regarding the storage of crop products. This empowers managers to make informed decisions about prioritizing the handling or removal of specific products to prevent losses or deterioration (De Baerdemaeker, 2023).

10.7 NEED FOR AI IN AGRICULTURE SUPPLY CHAINS

Agriculture is witnessing an increasing demand for automation due to the rising population and the corresponding need for more agricultural production. AI plays a significant role in assisting farmers across various components, technologies, and applications, as shown in Figure 10.3. Predictive analytics and enhanced farm management systems ensure the quality and production of crops. Enterprises can leverage big data and AI technologies to forecast costing and yield, and to recognize insect infestations. Furthermore, these enterprises can guide farmers regarding levels of demand, optimal varieties of crops for profitability, pesticide usage, and future pricing trends (Javaid et al., 2023).

By optimizing resource allocation more efficiently, AI can assist farmers in increasing outputs while minimizing inputs. It can aid in reducing spoilage and wastage of food by forecasting yields and demand with greater accuracy. Additionally, AI facilitates managing environmental factors pertinent to food safety, thus reassuring consumers regarding the safety and origin of their food. This is achieved by tracking all food items or batches across the agriculture supply chain including production, handling, packaging, and transportation using blockchain technology.

The agricultural sector is poised to gain considerable advantages from the enhanced predictive capabilities of various forecasts relevant to its operations. These forecasts

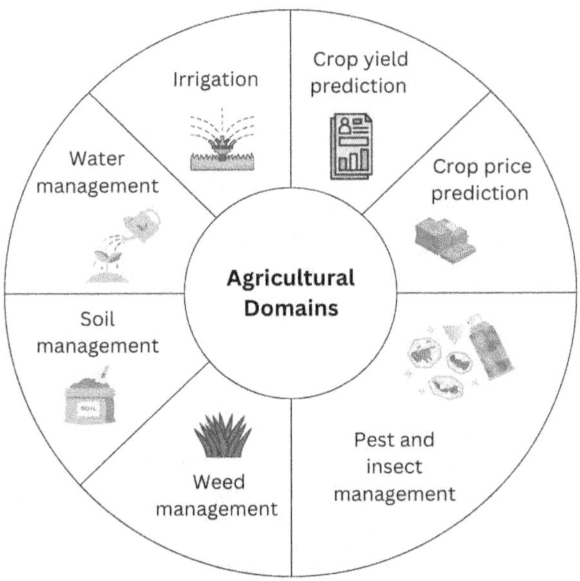

FIGURE 10.3 Agricultural domains monitored by artificial intelligence. (Adapted from Oliveira & Silva, 2023.)

encompass climate models and long-term weather predictions, assessments of the probability of pest and disease outbreaks, as well as forecasts regarding their spread, and broader economic modeling.

Expanding the range of tasks executed by robots could help the agricultural sector surmount productivity constraints stemming from labor shortages. Advances in machine vision, facilitated by ML, may enable farmers to employ robots for weed eradication without relying on herbicides. If AI systems effectively reduce the quantities of pesticides, fertilizers, and water necessary for food production, this would offer environmental benefits in addition to aiding farmers (Sparrow et al., 2021).

10.8 APPLICATIONS OF AI IN THE AGRICULTURE SUPPLY CHAIN

The quest for a sustainable food system has led to the adoption of AI technologies in agriculture to bolster food security (Sarker, 2021, as cited in Sarku et al., 2023). A key contrast between traditional and modern farming, beyond the level of mechanization, lies in the collection of data directly from crops. In traditional farming, decisions are often based on visual assessments, making them relative and subjective. In contrast, modern farming emphasizes quantitative data for making objective decisions (De Baerdemaeker, 2023).

10.9 AI IN FOOD PRODUCTION

Food production involves yield, soil attributes, and irrigation requirements (Ben Ayed & Hanana, 2021, as cited in Namkhah et al., 2023).

Crop yield prediction

Certain pivotal elements like the temperature of the soil, amount of moisture, crop stress, diseases, and pests could influence crop yields. IBM's Watson Decision Platform for Agriculture integrates AI and cloud-based solutions to produce research-backed insights into the previously mentioned influential factors (Torero, 2021).

Precise forecasting of crop yields serves as a potent tool for enhancing food production. AI technology is poised to assume a crucial role in future yield predictions. Beyond direct yield forecasts, ANN models possess the capacity to encompass other influential variables in agricultural production. In one study, researchers crafted an ANN model proficient in predicting energy consumption and greenhouse gas (GHG) emissions within systems used for cultivating watermelons (Nabavi-Pelesaraei et al., 2016, as cited in Chamara et al., 2020).

Insect, pest, and disease management

Effectively managing insects, pests, and diseases in crops is crucial for bolstering yields and, consequently, overall production. Estimates suggest that crop yield losses attributable to diverse pests and diseases are 20% to 40% and 40%, respectively, for the most critical food crops annually (AGRIVI, 2020, as cited in Chamara et al., 2020).

AI holds the potential for phenotyping, enabling the analysis of plant biomass and traits. AI technology can detect the precise causes of diseases by pinpointing analogous trends among infected crops and scrutinizing variations in the biomass of plants alongside environmental conditions (Javaid et al., 2023). Insect, pest, and disease control predominantly rely on diverse pesticide applications, which can have adverse impacts on both the environment and human health. Consequently, there has been a push to explore ecofriendly alternatives.

Bestelmeyer et al. (2020) have developed tools based on AI to manage scientific and big data specific to the site to advance research in agriculture. Their goal is to aid farmers and managers in making site-specific decisions. These techniques detect pest and disease outbreaks early and simplify sustainable farmland management.

Peixoto et al. (2015) devised a method employing fuzzy systems to comprehend the population dynamics and management of soybean aphids (*Aphis glycines*). They applied a methodology based on fuzzy sets theory to depict how the soybean aphid interacts with its predator *Orius insidiosus*. The model, which encompasses various environmental factors, biotic and abiotic, suggests chemical treatments for managing the soybean aphid population. Moreover, it has been proven valuable in forecasting the optimal timing and deployment of predators for controlling soybean aphids biologically.

Chandra Karmokar et al. (2015) have utilized ANN technology to devise a system to recognize disease in tea leaves. The method involves capturing an image of the leaf and employing a combined neural network to recognize patterns on the leaf, thereby identifying any disease present (Chamara et al., 2020). Pham et al. (2020) and Anandhakrishnan and Jaisakthi (2022) have individually utilized ANN and deep convolutional neural networks (DCNN) to identify early diseases characterized by small spots on plant leaves (Liu et al., 2023). Additionally, technologies like GIS and satellite remote sensing have been utilized for predicting yields of potatoes and identifying instances of blight disease and infestations of whiteflies (Torero, 2021).

Weed management

Weeds have a great impact on both the quantity and quality of crop yield. Chemical control remains the predominant method for managing weeds in numerous agricultural settings. However, prolonged and excessive herbicide use can pose risks to human health and the environment. Identifying weeds directly in the field is crucial for effective weed management. Nevertheless, AI techniques offer a promising avenue for reducing herbicide application in agricultural fields through selective targeting. Numerous AI-assisted systems for weed identification and classification have been developed, with many of these systems leveraging ANN technology (Eddy et al., 2008; Barrero et al., 2016, as cited in Chamara et al., 2020).

Weeds can be eradicated through intelligent spraying methods that target herbicides only where weeds are detected, thus avoiding any application onto the soil or cultivated plants. AI tools, including ML techniques, particularly DL, have greatly expanded the capabilities of computer vision, enhancing the accuracy of weed detection in crops. Blue River Technology, a US company, pioneered the "see & spray" technology, utilizing machine vision to eliminate weeds in lettuce production (De Baerdemaeker, 2023). Perez-Oritz et al. (2016) have introduced an innovative approach to weed management by integrating UAVs, image processing, and ML. These UAVs offer ultra-high spatial resolution (Chamara et al., 2020).

Plant breeding

Advancements in food crop breeding will play a fundamental role in addressing future food insecurity by developing cultivars with high yields and protecting the harvest. Genetically breeding the crops has yielded cultivars endowed with favorable characteristics like high yield, stability of yield under fluctuating climate, enhanced endurance to environmental stressors, improved nutrient utilization efficiency, resistance to disease, and superior quality. Leveraging computer science techniques, breeders can swiftly assess the performance of plants in specific climates, identify genes conducive to plant adaptation, and optimize gene combinations through crossbreeding to enhance yield and mitigate the impacts of climate change.

Ampatzidis and Partel (2019) have devised a methodology utilizing small UAVs, CNN, and multispectral imaging to gather data and process images for evaluating phenotypic traits in citrus crops. Employing image analysis with close-range sensors can expedite the process of selection in plant breeding, thereby enhancing breeding efficacy. However, the precision of procured phenotypic characteristics is significantly influenced by the size of pixels in images. Breeders often target rapid estimation of ground coverage (GC) when developing new varieties, which presents a challenge. Hua et al. (2019) employed an ML model-based classification to categorize pixels in original images, frequently captured using visual-spectrum cameras across various platforms. This classification of images into vegetation or background classes aids in computing their GC (Chamara et al., 2020).

Crop harvesting

The automated harvester developed by Harvest CROO Robotics emulates human pickers while maintaining existing crop cultivation methods. Each robot harvester requires 8 seconds to harvest a strawberry plant and 1.5 seconds to transition to the next plant. With the capacity to cover 8 acres per day, a single robot harvester's efficiency is comparable to that of 30 human laborers (Torero, 2021).

Robots can incorporate hardware components such as an autonomous vehicle, a manipulator, and an end-effector. Robots equipped with AI technologies like computer vision systems have been created for cucumber harvesting and can accurately detect cucumbers' ripeness (Van Henten et al., 2002, as cited in Namkhah et al., 2023).

Crop price forecasting

The FAO's Agricultural Market Information System (FAO-AMIS) utilizes ML to conduct sentiment-based market and crop forecasting for wheat, maize, rice, and soybeans. Drawing from supply-and-demand data, along with satellite information calibrated and tested on the ground, the system forecasts prices, taking into account probable short-term developments and outliers (Torero, 2021).

Soil quality

AI solutions have the potential to detect nutrient deficiencies and soil issues by analyzing data obtained from sensors embedded in the soil, collected by drones during soil studies, or images captured by phone cameras (Javaid et al., 2023). Traditionally, farmers have relied on chemical analysis to assess soil quality, a method that is both complex and time-consuming. For instance, AgroPad, a phone application by IBM, analyzes soil and provides the necessary information to small-scale farmers. This application utilizes AI algorithms and sensors, enabling farmers to comprehend the chemical composition of the soil, and to observe soil and water health (Torero, 2021).

An ANN model can forecast the texture of the soil by leveraging hydrographic data extracted from a digital elevation model (DEM), which encompasses parameters such as sediment delivery ratio, terrain factor, and slope position (Zhao et al., 2009, as cited in Namkhah et al., 2023).

Soil water monitoring

Climate variability has heightened weather unpredictability, posing challenges to forecasting. Fluctuating between stormy, high-rainfall periods and dry spells, the climate shift exacerbates crop stress from elevated temperatures, excessive rain, or floods. While heat-resistant crop varieties offer one solution, implementing strategic, long-term sustainable water management practices is imperative.

In agricultural contexts, soil water monitoring via in situ sensors encompasses various techniques such as tensiometers, time domain reflectometry (TDR), capacitance measurements, or electrical conductivity analysis. In many cases, temperature measurement within the same sensor is conducted to enable temperature correction. Among these methods, sensors based on electrical conductivity offer the most economical option and are straightforward to oversee. Typically, these sensors incorporate an outer porous material coating around internal electrodes, allowing the water content within the material to reach equilibrium with the soil moisture. The electrical conductivity measured between the electrodes correlates closely with soil water content, provided that soil salinity levels are not excessively high.

Tensiometers yield particularly valuable data, as they measure water potential, directly reflecting the ease of water extraction by plant roots. Nonetheless, they require consistent monitoring and maintenance. Advancements now enable digital real-time monitoring of tensiometers, facilitating swift identification of malfunctions.

TDR and frequency domain reflectometry (FDR) sensors, while offering precise measurements, are typically considered too costly for economical agricultural applications and generally do not necessitate calibration. FDR sensors have the advantage of integrating electronics within the sensor itself. In contrast, TDR operates at a higher frequency, enabling measurement of water content in soil and electrical conductivity simultaneously. However, TDR measurements often require complex multiplexing connections to a specific monitor, rendering them less practical for extensive fields and the most expensive option. It is worth noting that remote sensing techniques such as radar or microwave methods predominantly capture data from the shallow topsoil layer, typically up to about 1 cm deep. Most of these methods rely on modeling to infer characteristics of deeper soil layers (De Baerdemaeker, 2023).

Athani et al. (2017) developed a soil moisture monitoring system tailored for pasture growers in North Karnataka, India, leveraging IoT technology integrated with Arduino sensors. The study harnesses data from input sensors, managed through neural network algorithms and correction factors for monitoring purposes. By employing readily available components, the technology substantially reduces manufacturing and maintenance expenses, enhancing affordability for small-scale farmers in rural regions (Chamara et al., 2020).

Irrigation

To achieve optimal yield, crops require timely watering. The integration of intelligent irrigation systems has emerged as a solution. These systems typically comprise two main elements: a machine-learning model to determine soil moisture levels, and the utilization of IoT devices for hardware implementation. Embracing such advanced agricultural technologies contributes significantly to the pursuit of sustainability objectives in agriculture (Javaid et al., 2023).

Typically, irrigation scheduling relies on estimates of crop evapotranspiration (ET), rainfall data, and soil water management, ideally supplemented by soil moisture sensing and weather predictions for accurate updates (De Baerdemaeker, 2023). The cutting-edge ML applications currently focus on estimating daily, weekly, or monthly evapotranspiration, facilitating optimized irrigation system utilization. Additionally, there are advancements in predicting daily dew point temperature, aiding in anticipating weather patterns and estimating evapotranspiration and evaporation rates (Javaid et al., 2023).

Sensors deployed within the plants enable each plant or plant monitoring unit to convey its requirements promptly. Each plant is considered as the most appropriate entity in communicating the need for water in real time. The sensors facilitate in determining the optimal timing and quantity of watering, as well as assessing the plant's tolerance for thirst before potentially affecting the anticipated yield (Owino & Söffker, 2022, as cited in De Baerdemaeker, 2023). Figure 10.4 depicts the future of precision irrigation control using AI.

In pursuit of maximum productivity, farming practices often involve supplying crops with more water than their total requirement. Plant roots absorb water for growth, necessitating consideration of the entire root zone rather than just the surface layers. Additionally, accounting for the growth stage is crucial; for instance, pear cultivation in Belgium demands meticulous irrigation tailored to specific growth stages.

The recent development of remote sensing for monitoring above-ground crop status has introduced thermal imaging and multispectral or hyperspectral imaging for stress detection. While these methods are valuable for remote sensing and research

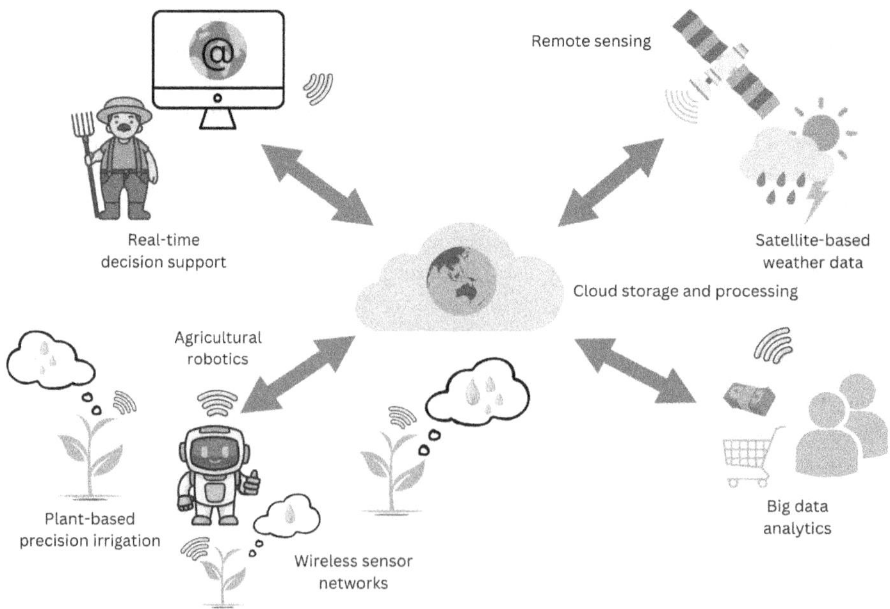

FIGURE 10.4 Future of precision irrigation control. (Adapted from Owino & Söffker, 2022.)

purposes, they often detect water stress too late for effective irrigation scheduling. Utilizing drones or satellites for remote sensing, with regular passing intervals, proves beneficial. Despite limitations such as susceptibility to cloud cover, normalized difference vegetation index (NDVI) methods remain instrumental in tracking biomass growth and identifying variations in growth across fields.

Optimal irrigation scheduling, coupled with comprehensive soil water management across the entire root zone, gains significant advantages from real-time, onsite measurements. AI plays a crucial role in assimilating these live data streams to refine the root–soil water balance and enhance scheduling precision. This necessitates a blend of cost-effective sensors, spatial 3D root zone monitoring, and vegetation surveillance. Achieving more efficient and strategic water usage for crop development involves a synergistic approach encompassing modeling, soil water sensing within the root zone, remote monitoring of crop biomass, and weather forecasting. Effective irrigation scheduling hinges on closely monitoring water levels within the crop's root zone (De Baerdemaeker, 2023).

Evaluating water level in plants is crucial for devising irrigation schedules. Valdes-Vela et al. (2015) introduced a computing technique and constructed a model to estimate stem water potential in plants by leveraging water content in the soil and meteorological data. Employing fuzzy rules, this model offers enhanced approximation capabilities in its outputs (Chamara et al., 2020).

Water supply monitoring

Real-time monitoring of flow data in irrigation pipes or canals is achievable through IoT-enabled sensors powered by solar panels and connected to the Internet. This enables wireless tracking of water quantity at any point within the irrigation system. Particularly in pressurized irrigation systems, continuous leak detection is possible, allowing for swift responses. This enhances the precision of water administration to crops and helps prevent accidental losses. Additionally, hydraulic structures are recommended for canal installations, with water levels monitored using pressure transducers or ultrasonic sensors.

Reduction of water use

The technique of employing a moving rain gun necessitates high pressure and is prone to significant wind-drift losses. In contrast, using a spray boom enables considerable water conservation, particularly in windy conditions. Moreover, the substantially lower pressure required for a spray boom results in significant energy savings. The uniform irrigation achieved by the spray boom facilitates monitoring of pressures and discharges within the system, thereby enabling more precise and differential irrigation across the field.

Drip irrigation supplies water precisely to the root zone, mitigating losses from wind drift and soil evaporation. While it requires permanent installation, it lacks the flexibility of other systems. Nevertheless, drip irrigation systems can be remotely controlled, with pressures monitored internally. This allows for highly precise and timely fertilizer application, minimizing nutrient losses to the underlying aquifer. Implementing an AI system for either the spray boom or drip irrigation, which integrates water supply measurement with soil water monitoring, enhances efficiency and reduces overwatering (De Baerdemaeker, 2023).

Table 10.2 summarizes the various applications of AI in food production as discussed before in detail.

TABLE 10.2
AI in Food Production

Study	Domain	Technique	Application
Nabavi-Pelesaraei et al. (2016)	Crop yield prediction	ANN	Predicted energy usage and GHG emissions from watermelon production systems
Peixoto et al. (2015)	Pest management	Fuzzy systems	Forecasted the optimal timing of deployment of predators for controlling soybean aphids biologically
Chandra Karmokar (2015)	Disease management	ANN	Identified tea leaf disease
Pham et al. (2020) Anandhakrishnan & Jaisakthi (2022)	Disease management	ANN and DCNN	Identified early diseases characterized by small spots on plant leaves
Torero (2021)	Crop yield prediction and disease management	Satellite remote sensing and GIS techniques	Predicted potato yields and detected blight disease and whiteflies
Eddy et al. (2008); Barrero et al. (2016)	Weed management	ANN	Identified and classified weeds
Perez-Oritz et al. (2016)	Weed management	ML and UAVs	Integrated image processing along with machine learning and UAVs for an innovative approach to weed management
Ampatzidis & Partel (2019)	Plant breeding	DCNN, multispectral imaging, and UAVs	Evaluated phenotypic traits in citrus crops
Torero (2021)	Crop harvesting	Robotics	Decreased the need for labor
Van Henten et al. (2002)	Crop harvesting	Robotics and computer vision system	Accurately detected ripeness of cucumbers
Torero (2021)	Crop price prediction	ML	Conducted market prediction and crop forecasting for wheat, maize, rice, and soybeans
Zhao et al. (2009)	Soil quality	ANN and DEM	Forecasted soil texture
Athani et al. (2017)	Soil water monitoring	IoT along with Arduino sensors	Substantially reduced manufacturing and maintenance expenses
Valdes-Vela et al. (2015)	Irrigation	Fuzzy logic	Estimated stem water potential in plants

Source: Chamara et al. (2020); Liu et al. (2023); Torero (2021); Namkhah et al. (2023).

Note: ANN: artificial neural network; DCNN: deep convolutional neural network; DEM: digital elevation model; GHG: greenhouse gas; GIS: geographic information system; IoT: Internet of Things; ML: machine learning; UAVs: unmanned aerial vehicles.

10.10 AI IN FOOD DISTRIBUTION AND CONSUMPTION

The focus of food distribution and consumption lies in providing consumers with safe, high-quality food (Ben Ayed & Hanana, 2021, as cited in Namkhah et al., 2023).

Post-harvest quality control

Post-harvest storage degrades agricultural goods through loss of weight, color, visual appearance, nutrient content, flavor, and other aspects. Environmental factors including temperature, relative humidity, air composition, and light exposure degrade harvested food, as can biological factors like respiration, transpiration, ethylene synthesis, and post-harvest diseases. AI regulates biological and environmental elements to ensure food safety and quality (Chamara et al., 2020).

ML algorithms assist in activities such as management of stocks, storage, transportation, and consumer data analytics, aiming to reduce damage and maintain quality of food (Ben Ayed & Hanana, 2021, as cited in Namkhah et al., 2023). AI optimizes supply chain management by tracking food and testing it for quality assurance at each stage (Namkhah et al., 2023).

Emphasizing the significance of food safety, various methods, including image processing (IP), are employed to categorize and identify the quality of food and its products. IP leverages technologies such as ultrasound, near-infrared spectroscopy, X-ray, and scanners to examine the shape, size, and texture of the food product (Kumar et al., 2021, as cited in Namkhah et al., 2023). This method can also be extended to packaging of products for identifying imperfections and grading quality. Applying AI in the field of sustainable food systems has led to notable progress in quality control and food grading sections of the food industry (Namkhah et al., 2023).

Babawuro et al. (2015) introduced a temperature control method for post-harvest storage of fresh cassava roots. They utilized a fuzzy logic controller to regulate storage temperature, employing two inputs and one output. The two inputs involved an error in temperature and rate of change in error, while the output included a change in fan speed.

Liu and Hu (2017) integrated algorithms like classification regression trees, neural networks, and Bayesian networks to predict and monitor the deterioration of perishable food during transportation. Ensuring access to food is increasingly vital during pandemics like COVID-19. Therefore, it is crucial to safely distribute food and essential supplies to all people during difficult times like this. Sharma et al. (2020) have introduced a robotic drive-through system designed to achieve this goal, and another study has monitored food deliveries by utilizing IoT devices.

Amin et al. (2021) employed ML to create models utilizing data obtained from US census tracts, enabling precise prediction of access to nutritious food. The model accurately recognizes food swamps and food deserts with a 72% prediction accuracy. Food deserts have been described as regions lacking adequate spatial and socio-economic access to nutritious food. Fuzzy-based models perform more effectively in addressing real-time uncertainties like proper storage and transportation of perishable foods.

Industries address the challenge of insect infestations by implementing non-destructive, cutting-edge AI techniques. Surface characteristics of fruits and vegetables have been identified by employing visible light sensors operating at wavelength ranging from 380 to 750 nm. Pearson et al. (2001), Blasco et al. (2009), López-García et al. (2010), and Blasco et al. (2016) have utilized this approach, coupled with ML techniques, to identify infestation by insects, like insect damage in pistachios, thrips in citrus fruits, scale insects in citrus fruits, and Mediterranean fruit flies in citrus fruits, respectively.

The hyper spectral imaging system can help identify internal damage caused by insect infestations without destroying the sample. Ma et al. (2014), Liu et al. (2016), and Rady et al. (2016) have applied this concept, combined with ML techniques, to identify pests such as pod borers in soybeans, fruit flies in jujube fruits, and codling moths in apples, respectively.

Drying serves as the principal means of preserving food, extending the shelf life of food by reducing the amount of moisture present. However, optimal conditions for drying must be achieved to ensure the desired shelf life of food products. Controlling these conditions manually can be challenging and, at times, impractical. AI-based techniques offer a viable solution for automating these conditions.

Food processing transforms fresh foods into edible products, extending their shelf life, enhancing safety, and preserving nutritional quality. Contamination during food processing, often caused by human handling, can significantly impact food security. AI-powered robotics can offer solutions that address labor needs in food processing activities, thereby enhancing food hygiene (Chamara et al., 2020).

Sorting and grading of food

The majority of fruits and vegetables often suffer from brown spots and bruises due to mechanical stress during post-harvest handling. Sorting fruits and vegetables after harvest is essential to meet quality standards, given that consumers are increasingly attentive to the quality and safety of food. Using AI, the process of sorting can be accelerated and made more trustworthy, with less labor required (Chamara et al., 2020).

Food grading is an essential procedure for assessing the quality and safety of food products, which depends on predetermined standards covering characteristics like shape, size, color, texture, flavor, absence of imperfections, and freshness (Namkhah et al., 2023). Manual grading is prone to inconsistency, time consumption, and contamination risks. Hence, automated grading surpasses manual grading in efficiency and accuracy (Chamara et al., 2020). AI techniques, including robotics, computer vision, and ML, have automated and optimized the process of food grading. By inspecting, classifying, and sorting food products in real time, AI can minimize errors made by humans, lower labor costs, reduce waste, and simultaneously enhance productivity, profitability, and customer satisfaction (Namkhah et al., 2023). ML algorithms can accurately distinguish genuine fruits and vegetables by assessing physical (shape, size, color) and biological attributes of each item. This may help identify the product type and adherence to specific criteria (Javaid et al., 2023). Larada et al. (2018) developed an ML-based fruit classification system for bananas, categorizing them into four classes: extra class, class 1, class 2, and class 3. An accuracy of 97% was achieved while excluding the reject class. Consequently, AI holds significant promise for effective implementation in the handling of food after harvest and the food processing industry to safeguard food security.

The acidity level of pomegranates dictates their suitability for various consumer preferences. In light of this, Fashi et al. (2020) devised a model to classify pomegranates depending on their pH levels, employing the following AI algorithms: ANN, ANFIS, and response surface methodology (RSM). The ANFIS model yielded the most favorable outcomes (Chamara et al., 2020). Sofu et al. (2016) and Valdez (2020) in apples, Ireri et al. (2019) in tomatoes, Al Ohali (2011) in date fruit, and Przybylak et al. (2020) in potatoes have devised approaches using computer vision, DL methods, and IP techniques to identify nutritious fruits and vegetables and distinguish them from the ones with imperfections. Buyers constantly anticipate fresh agricultural products with superior nutritive and sensory qualities (Chamara et al. 2020).

Table 10.3 summarizes the role of AI applications in food distribution and consumption as discussed previously.

TABLE 10.3
AI in Food Distribution and Consumption

Study	Domain	Technique	Application
Babawuro et al. (2015)	Post-harvest quality control	Fuzzy logic	Used an intelligent temperature control method for post-harvest storage of fresh cassava roots
Liu & Hu (2017)	Post-harvest quality control	ANN, classification regression tree, and Bayesian network	Predicted and monitored the deterioration of perishable food during transportation
Sharma et al. (2020)	Post-harvest quality control	Robotics	Efficient food distribution
Pearson et al. (2001); Blasco et al. (2009); López-García et al. (2010); Blasco et al. (2016)	Post-harvest quality control	ML with visible light sensors	Detected insect infestations
Ma et al. (2014); Liu et al. (2016); Rady et al. (2016)	Post-harvest quality control	Hyper spectral imaging and ML	Detected concealed internal damage caused by insect infestations without the need for sample destruction

(continued)

TABLE 10.3 (Continued)
AI in Food Distribution and Consumption

Study	Domain	Technique	Application
Amin et al. (2021)	Decision-making	ML	Identified food swamps and food deserts with 72% prediction accuracy
Larada. et al. (2018)	Sorting and grading of food	ML	Classified bananas into four classes
Fashi et al. (2020)	Sorting and grading of food	ANFIS, ANN, and RSM	Classified pomegranates based on pH levels
Sofu et al. (2016); Valdez (2020); Ireri et al. (2019); Al Ohali (2011); Przybylak et al. (2020)	Sorting and grading of food	Computer vision, DL, and IP	Distinguished healthy fruits and vegetables from defective ones

Source: Chamara et al. (2020).

Note: ANFIS: adaptive neuro-fuzzy inference system; ANN: artificial neural network; DL: deep learning; IP: image processing; ML: machine learning; RSM: response surface methodology.

10.11 AI IN FOOD WASTE MANAGEMENT

Despite the increasing global hunger, food waste and losses remain extensive and inconsistent. On average, individuals discard 120 kg of food annually. While 828 million individuals experienced hunger in 2021, post-harvest food loss along the supply chain was estimated to be 13.2% globally, failing to meet the goal of significantly decreasing the food losses after harvest by 2030. Moreover, an extra 17% of food was wasted at household, food service, and retail levels (The Sustainable Development Goals Report, 2023).

Minimizing food wastage, which encompasses both food loss and food waste, presents a clear avenue to enhance food security without escalating the impact of production on environment. Food loss entails a decline in edible food mass occurring during every stage of the food supply chain, from production to processing, whereas food waste pertains to losses at the consumer and retail levels. Addressing food loss and food waste represents a significant possibility to alleviate production demands, considering that out of 1.6 billion tonnes of food wasted along the supply chain, 1.3 billion tonnes is edible (Gustavsson et al., 2011; Institution of Mechanical Engineers, 2013, as cited in Cole et al., 2018).

Effective post-harvest handling practices throughout the supply chain, along with robust infrastructure and logistics support, may help alleviate the loss of fresh produce (Cole et al., 2018). Improved data tracking throughout the agriculture supply chain (including storage temperatures) or implementing sensors in food items to identify pathogens or indicators of spoilage like CO_2 could enhance trust in extending use-by dates, potentially mitigating food waste (Erickson & Fausti, 2021).

Food production and consumption sustainability pose significant hurdles within the food supply and distribution networks. However, tackling these hurdles becomes feasible through the creative incorporation of AI, providing a fresh strategy to reduce food wastage at different points in the food cycle (Namkhah, Z. et al., 2023).

Faezirad et al. (2021) presented a novel food waste reduction model using ML in Tehran universities. In their investigation, the reservation mechanism used to assess food demand sometimes caused unexpected meal loss. A more accurate demand prediction technique was needed to address this issue. They integrated an ML model with the reservation system while contemplating the factors influencing the demand of the students. These factors include day of the week, consecutive holidays, food attributes (including price and name of the food), reservations classified by accommodation and academic degree, and attendance history. Academic level, living status, and dining hall involvement were also evaluated. This integrated model cut food waste by 79% (Namkhah et al., 2023).

10.12 CHALLENGES OF AI APPLICATIONS IN THE AGRICULTURE SUPPLY CHAIN

Although AI has been proven beneficial in the food supply chain, it also poses unique challenges, some of which are discussed below.

Unemployment

The adoption of AI-powered agricultural robots is largely seen as a potential threat to jobs traditionally reliant on manual labor. However, the growing notion that AI could also replace numerous white-collar positions is gaining traction, indicating that AI may pose risks of job displacement in both white- and blue-collar sectors within agriculture, as well as across various sectors of society (Sparrow et al., 2021).

AI affordability and the digital divide

Undoubtedly, farmers embracing new technologies and opportunities in digital agriculture incur certain costs. However, it is crucial to proceed with caution to prevent further widening of the digital divide within farming communities. Ensuring that all farmers can access the benefits of AI and digital agriculture necessitates accessible networks, databases, and advanced analytics algorithms. This accessibility encompasses the ability to upload and gather data from wireless sensors in the field and machinery operating there. This underscores the need for affordable broadband Internet access, not only in residential areas but also in agricultural fields (De Baerdemaeker 2023).

Ownership concentration

The integration of AI into agriculture is likely to bring about an increase in claims regarding intellectual property rights related to farming methods and food processing. Consequently, this trend may further widen the gap between wealthier and poorer enterprises.

Loss of autonomy

The emergence of AI and big data could result in a significant reduction in the autonomy of farmers, subjecting them to a network of commercial and institutional pressures dictated and enforced by machines. Additionally, AI systems are likely to increase surveillance of agricultural workers, as the data they generate will be used to track and monitor their activities.

Susceptibility to cyberattacks

Implementing AI exposes users to the risk of hacking and various cyberattacks orchestrated by malicious entities, which should be acknowledged as a potential threat in agriculture, as in other sectors. Though it may appear speculative, the prevalence of ransomware attacks is on the rise across industries, with certain incidents resulting in millions of dollars in damages (Sparrow et al., 2021).

Transparency and reliability

Expanding the use of AI technologies in agriculture hinges on the establishment of trust among farmers and consumers in the services provided. Ensuring transparency in the supply chain and the handling of data collection and utilization is paramount, and concerns about privacy, confidentiality, and data ownership may arise. Technology users, including farmers, may seek guidance on safeguarding themselves against unexpected usage, unwanted consequences, and potential physical or financial harm (De Baerdemaeker, 2023).

Data bias

The effectiveness of ML systems heavily relies on the quality of the training data, and the presence of bias within this data can result in unintended consequences. In the realm of agriculture, two types of bias are particularly notable. Initially, agricultural AI tools were expected to be marketed in Europe, the USA, and possibly China. This generates a risk of farmers in other countries adopting these AI tools based on data sourced from crops or soil in the mentioned countries, leading to significant challenges when applied locally elsewhere. Furthermore, if the data used to train agricultural AI systems fail to capture the challenges faced by small-scale landowners and people native to the region, these systems will inherently exhibit bias against traditional practices. Consequently, agricultural AI is likely to offer inadequate support to indigenous and small-scale farmers, and in some cases, may not function effectively in these contexts (Sparrow et al., 2021).

10.13 STRATEGIES TO OVERCOME THE CHALLENGES

There is a great need to address challenges to ensure digital technologies remain efficient and inclusive. Below are some strategies that can be employed to address these challenges.

- Nations need to prioritize the adoption of renewable energy sources, particularly solar energy, to power robotics in agriculture.

- Developing agriculture value chains is essential to capitalize on their benefits and generate higher-paying employment opportunities.
- Addressing illiteracy is a crucial strategy for fostering a comprehensive digital revolution, emphasizing the need to invest in human resources, by providing quality education and inclusion of women in the workforce.
- There is a need to promote a new generation of well-trained farmers, offering digital training that enables them to leverage advanced technologies for profit.
- Governments should invest in human capital and enact policies and regulations to ensure that everyone, particularly smallholders who are major food producers, can partake in the emerging digital economy.
- Establishing an environment that guarantees accessibility, adaptability, and suitability is imperative. This includes making technologies affordable for all users, ensuring that the content they provide is beneficial and that users can utilize them effectively.
- Agriculture stakeholders must prioritize cybersecurity by addressing potential threats such as management of risk (including third parties), data privacy and integration, non-repudiation, control of access, robustness, and scalability to minimize vulnerabilities and enhance protection against cyberattacks (Torero, 2021; De Baerdemaeker, 2023; Demestichas et al., 2020).

10.14 CONCLUSION

Challenges such as adverse weather, political instability, and economic issues can compromise food security, resulting in decreased well-being. Individuals face challenges in accessing sufficient nutrition due to structural factors like poverty. The food system has a role in the accessibility of nutritious food to individuals. A sustainable food system aims to meet present needs while preserving ecosystems and promoting fairness and justice throughout the supply chain. Decision-making processes and data collection are essential at each stage of the agricultural supply chain to ensure efficient distribution and utilization of food resources.

As agriculture grapples with increasing demands due to population growth, automation emerges as a critical solution, with AI playing a central role in optimizing various components, technologies, and applications. AI represents a transformative force in revolutionizing the agricultural sector. Through ML, DL, and robotics, AI systems have demonstrated remarkable capabilities in processing vast datasets, identifying patterns, and generating user-friendly outputs. In the context of global food and nutrition security, AI-powered precision agriculture emerges as a pivotal solution to address food insecurity and hunger challenges. Despite facing hurdles such as data overload, AI's potential to foster adaptability and resilience in agriculture underscores its crucial role in shaping a sustainable and resilient future for food production on a global scale.

AI empowers farmers to achieve higher yields with limited resources by enhancing resource allocation and reducing wastage, while also enabling dynamic control of environmental factors for food safety assurance. Additionally, AI-driven advancements hold promise for overcoming labor shortages, improving productivity, and mitigating environmental impact by reducing the use of pesticides and fertilizers.

Ultimately, AI's transformative potential offers significant benefits to the agricultural sector, enhancing efficiency, sustainability, and resilience in meeting global food production challenges.

AI applications, ranging from crop yield prediction to insect and disease management, offer innovative solutions to enhance productivity and address challenges in food production. Addressing food distribution and consumption is crucial for ensuring the delivery of safe, high-quality food to consumers while minimizing waste. AI may enhance the safety and quality of food by regulating environmental and biological factors during post-harvest storage and distribution. Moreover, AI technologies facilitate food waste management by improving demand prediction, optimizing waste collection routes, and reducing food waste through innovative approaches.

While AI presents numerous benefits for the food supply chain, it also brings forth challenges that must be addressed. These challenges include the potential for unemployment due to automation, concerns about the affordability of AI technology widening the digital divide, concentration of ownership leading to inequalities, exploitation, and surveillance of farmers, vulnerability to hacking and cyberattacks, and biases in AI systems. To overcome these challenges, strategies must be implemented including creation of higher-wage jobs, promotion of literacy and digital training for farmers, and enhancement of cybersecurity measures. By addressing these challenges proactively, the agricultural sector can harness the benefits of AI while mitigating its potential negative impacts, ensuring a more sustainable and inclusive digital revolution in farming.

REFERENCES

AGRIVI. (2020). Crop Diseases: The Nightmare of Every Farmer. Retrieved from https://blog.agrivi.com/post/crop-diseases-the-nightmare-of-every-farmer

Ahmed, S., de la Parra, J., Elouafi, I., German, B., Jarvis, A., Lal, V., Lartey, A., Longvah, T., Malpica, C., Vázquez-Manjarrez, N., Prenni, J., Aguilar-Salinas, C. A., Srichamnong, W., Rajasekharan, M., Shafizadeh, T., Siegel, J. B., Steiner, R., Tohme, J., & Watkins, S. (2022). Foodomics: A data-driven approach to revolutionize nutrition and sustainable diets. *Frontiers in Nutrition*, *9*. https://doi.org/10.3389/fnut.2022.874312

Al Ohali, Y. (2011). Computer vision based date fruit grading system: Design and implementation. *Journal of King Saud University – Computer and Information Sciences*, *23*(1), 29–36. https://doi.org/10.1016/j.jksuci.2010.03.003

Allen, T., & Prosperi, P. (2016). Modeling sustainable food systems. *Environmental Management*, *57*(5), 956–975. https://doi.org/10.1007/s00267-016-0664-8

Amin, M. D., Badruddoza, S., & McCluskey, J. J. (2021). Predicting access to healthful food retailers with machine learning. *Food Policy*, *99*. https://doi.org/10.1016/j.foodpol.2020.101985

Ampatzidis, Y., & Partel, V. (2019). UAV-based high throughput phenotyping in citrus utilizing multispectral imaging and artificial intelligence. *Remote Sensing*, *11*(4). https://doi.org/10.3390/rs11040410

Anandhakrishnan, T., & Jaisakthi, S. M. (2022). Deep convolutional neural networks for image based tomato leaf disease detection. *Sustainable Chemistry and Pharmacy*, *30*, 100793.

Athani, S., Tejeshwar, C. H., Patil, M. M., Patil, P., & Kulkarni, R. (2017). Soil moisture monitoring using IoT enabled arduino sensors with neural networks for improving soil management for farmers and predict seasonal rainfall for planning future harvest in

North Karnataka-India. *Proceedings of the International Conference on IoT in Social, Mobile, Analytics and Cloud, I-SMAC 2017* (pp. 43–48). https://doi.org/10.1109/I-SMAC.2017.8058385

Babawuro, A. Y., Umar, S. A., Fatai, S., Salami, M. J. E., & Sidek, S. N. (2015). Fuzzy logic based intelligent temperature controller for cassava post-harvest storage system. *International Conference on Artificial Intelligence, Electrical & Electronics Engineering (AIEE '15), Kuala Lumpur.* Abu Dhabi: EACEEE. DOI: https://doi.org/10.17758/R1515033

Barrero, O., Rojas, D., Gonzalez, C., & Perdomo, S. (2016). Weed detection in rice fields using aerial images and neural networks. *2016 21st Symposium on Signal Processing, Images and Artificial Vision, STSIVA 2016, Bucaramanga, Colombia.* New York: IEEE. https://doi.org/10.1109/STSIVA.2016.7743317

Ben Ayed, R., & Hanana, M. (2021). Artificial intelligence to improve the food and agriculture sector. In *Journal of Food Quality* (Vol. 2021). Hindawi Limited. https://doi.org/10.1155/2021/5584754

Bestelmeyer, B. T., Marcillo, G., McCord, S. E., Mirsky, S., Moglen, G., Neven, L. G., Peters, D., Sohoulande, C., & Wakie, T. (2020). Scaling up agricultural research with artificial intelligence. *IT Professional*, *22*(3), 33–38. https://doi.org/10.1109/MITP.2020.2986062

Blasco, J., Aleixos, N., Gómez-Sanchis, J., & Moltó, E. (2009). Recognition and classification of external skin damage in citrus fruits using multispectral data and morphological features. *Biosystems Engineering*, *103*(2), 137–145.

Blasco, J., Cubero, S., & Moltó, E. (2016). Quality evaluation of citrus fruits. In Da-W. Sun (Ed.), *Computer Vision Technology for Food Quality Evaluation* (2nd ed.). San Diego: Academic Press.

Bradshaw, C. J. A., & Brook, B. W. (2014). *Human population reduction is not a quick fix for environmental problems.* Proc. Natl. Acad. Sci. (PNAS) U.S.A. 111, 6610–16615. https://doi.org/10.1073/pnas.1410465111

Capone, R., El Bilali, H., Debs, P., Cardone, G., & Driouech, N. (2014). Food system sustainability and food security: Connecting the dots. *Journal of Food Security*, *2*(1), 13–22. https://doi.org/10.12691/jfs-2-1-2

Chamara, R. M. S. R., Senevirathne, S. M. P., Samarasinghe, S. A. I. L. N., Premasiri, M. W. R. C., Sandaruwani, K. H. C., Dissanayake, D. M. N. N., De Silva, S. H. N. P., Ariyaratne, W. M. T. P., & Marambe, B. (2020). Role of artificial intelligence in achieving global food security: A promising technology for future. *Sri Lanka Journal of Food and Agriculture*, *6*(2), 43–70. https://doi.org/10.4038/sljfa.v6i2.88

ChandraKarmokar, B., Samawat Ullah, M., Kibria Siddiquee, Md., & Md. Rokibul Alam, K. (2015). Tea leaf diseases recognition using neural network ensemble. *International Journal of Computer Applications*, *114*(17), 27–30. https://doi.org/10.5120/20071-1993

Cole, M. B., Augustin, M. A., Robertson, M. J., & Manners, J. M. (2018). The science of food security. *NPJ Science of Food*, *2*(1). https://doi.org/10.1038/s41538-018-0021-9

De Baerdemaeker, J., & European Parliament. Directorate-General for Parliamentary Research Services. (2023). *Artificial Intelligence in the Agri-Food Sector: Applications, Risks and Impacts.* Brussels: EPRS.

Demestichas, K., Peppes, N., & Alexakis, T. (2020). Survey on security threats in agricultural iot and smart farming. In *Sensors (Switzerland)* (Vol. 20, Issue 22, pp. 1–17). MDPI AG. https://doi.org/10.3390/s20226458

Devereux, S. (2000). *Food Insecurity in Ethiopia.* www.researchgate.net/publication/50200941

Eddy, P., Smith, A., Hill, B., Peddle, D., Coburn, C., & Blackshaw, R. (2008). Hybrid segmentation– Artificial neural network classification of high resolution hyperspectral imagery for site-specific herbicide management in agriculture. *Photogrammetric Engineering & Remote Sensing*, *74*, 1249–1257.

Ehrlich, P. R., & Harte, J. (2015). Food security requires a new revolution. *International Journal of Environmental Studies*, *72*(6), 908–920. https://doi.org/10.1080/00207233.2015.1067468

El Bilali, H., Bassole, I. H. N., Dambo, L., & Berjan, S. (2020). Climate change and food security. *Agriculture and Forestry*, *66*(3), 197–210. https://doi.org/10.17707/AgricultForest.66.3.16

Ericksen, P. J. (2008). Conceptualizing food systems for global environmental change research. *Global Environmental Change*, *18*(1), 234–245.

Erickson, B., & Fausti, S. W. (2021). The role of precision agriculture in food security. *Agronomy Journal*, *113*(6), 4455–4462. https://doi.org/10.1002/agj2.20919

Faezirad, M., Pooya, A., Naji-Azimi, Z., & Amir Haeri, M. (2021). Preventing food waste in subsidy-based university dining systems: An artificial neural network-aided model under uncertainty. *Waste Management and Research*, *39*(8), 1027–1038. https://doi.org/10.1177/0734242X211017974

FAO. (2008). *Climate Change and Food Security: A Framework Document*. Rome, Italy: Food and Agriculture Organization.

FAO, IFAD, UNICEF, WFP & WHO. (2019). *The State of Food Security and Nutrition in the World 2019: Safeguarding Against Economic Slowdowns and Downturns*. Rome: FAO.

Fashi, M., Naderloo, L., & Javadikia, H. (2020). Pomegranate grading based on pH using image processing and artificial intelligence. *Journal of Food Measurement and Characterization*, *14*(6), 3112–3121.

FSIN and Global Network Against Food Crises. (2024). GRFC 2024. Rome. www.fsinplatform.org/grfc2024

Gunaratne, M. S., Radin Firdaus, R. B., & Rathnasooriya, S. I. (2021). Climate change and food security in Sri Lanka: Towards food sovereignty. *Humanities and Social Sciences Communications*, *8*(1). https://doi.org/10.1057/s41599-021-00917-4

Gustavsson, J., Cederberg, C. & Sonesson, U. (2011). *Global Food Losses and Food Waste — Study conducted for the International Congress*. Rome: FAO.

Hua, Y., Zhang, N., Yuan, X., Quan, L., Yang, J., Nagasaka, K., & Zhou, X.-G. (2019). Recent advances in intelligent automated fruit harvesting robots. *The Open Agriculture Journal*, *13*(1), 101–106. https://doi.org/10.2174/1874331501913010101

Institution of Mechanical Engineers. (2013). Global Food, Waste Not Want Not. London: IME. https://catalogue.unccd.int/1482_IME-Global-Food-Report.pdf

International Society of Precision Agriculture (ISPA). (2021). *Precision ag Definition*. Monticello, IL: ISPA. www.ispag.org/about/definition

IPCC. (2012). Summary for policymakers. In Field, C.B., V. Barros, T.F. Stocker, D. Qin, D.J. Dokken, K.L. Ebi, M.D. Mastrandrea, K.J. Mach, G.-K. Plattner, S.K. Allen, M. Tignor, & P.M. Midgley (eds.), *Managing the Risks of Extreme Events and Disasters to Advance Climate Change Adaptation. A Special Report of Working Groups I and II of the Intergovernmental Panel on Climate Change*. Cambridge: Cambridge University Press.

Ireri, D., Belal, E., Okinda, C., Makange, N., & Ji, C. (2019). A computer vision system for defect discrimination and grading in tomatoes using machine learning and image processing. *Artificial Intelligence in Agriculture*, *2*, 28–37.

Javaid, M., Haleem, A., Khan, I. H., & Suman, R. (2023). Understanding the potential applications of Artificial Intelligence in Agriculture Sector. *Advanced Agrochem*, *2*(1), 15–30. https://doi.org/10.1016/j.aac.2022.10.001

Jordan, M. I., & Mitchell, T. M. (2015). Machine learning: Trends, perspectives, and prospects. *Science*, *349*, 255–260.

Jorgensen, S., Xu, L., & Costanza, R. (Eds.). (2016). *Handbook of Ecological Indicators for Assessment of Ecosystem Health*. Boca Raton: CRC Press/ Taylor & Francis.

Kumar, I., Rawat, J., Mohd, N., & Husain, S. (2021). Opportunities of artificial intelligence and machine learning in the food industry. *Journal of Food Quality*, 2021. https://doi.org/10.1155/2021/4535567

Kuwornu, J., Mensah-Bonsu, A., & Ibrahim H. (2011). Analysis of foodstuff price volatility in Ghana: Implications for food security. *Journal: European Journal of Business and Management*. www.researchgate.net/publication/228838064

Lakshmi, V., & Corbett, J. (2020). How artificial intelligence improves agricultural productivity and sustainability: A global thematic analysis. In Proceedings of the 53rd Hawaii International Conference on System Sciences. HICSS Conference Office, *Wailea, HI, USA*. (pp. 5202–5211). Hawaii.

Larada, J. I., Pojas, G. J., & Ferrer, L. V. V. (2018). Postharvest classification of banana (Musa acuminata) using tier-based machine learning. *Postharvest Biology and Technology*, *145*, 93–100.

Lecun, Y., Bengio, Y., & Hinton, G. (2015). Deep learning. In *Nature* (Vol. 521, Issue 7553, pp. 436–444). Nature Publishing Group. https://doi.org/10.1038/nature14539

Liu, G., He, J., Wang, S., Luo, Y., Wang, W., Wu, L., & He, X. (2016). Application of near-infrared hyperspectral imaging for detection of external insect infestations on jujube fruit. *International Journal of Food Properties*. 19(1): 41–52.

Liu, T., & Hu, A. (2017). Model of combined transport of perishable foodstuffs and safety inspection based on data mining. *Food and Nutrition Sciences*, *08*(07), 760–777. https://doi.org/10.4236/fns.2017.87054

Liu, Z., Wang, S., Zhang, Y., Feng, Y., Liu, J., & Zhu, H. (2023). Artificial intelligence in food safety: A decade review and bibliometric analysis. In *Foods* (Vol. 12, Issue 6). MDPI. https://doi.org/10.3390/foods12061242

López-García, F., Andreu-García, G., Blasco, J., Aleixos, N., & Valiente, J. M. (2010). Automatic detection of skin defects in citrus fruits using a multivariate image analysis approach. *Computers and Electronics in Agriculture*, *71*(2), 189–197. https://doi.org/10.1016/j.compag.2010.02.001

Ma Y., Huang M., Yang B., & Zhu Q. (2014). Automatic threshold method and optimal wavelength selection for insect-damaged vegetable soybean detection using hyperspectral images. *Computers and Electronics in Agriculture*, *106*, 102–110.

Mohamed, A. A. (2017). Food security situation in Ethiopia: A review study. *International Journal of Health Economics and Policy*, *2*(3), 86–96. https://doi.org/10.11648/j.hep.20170203.11

Nabavi-Pelesaraei, A., Abdi, R., & Rafiee, S. (2016). Neural network modeling of energy use and greenhouse gas emissions of watermelon production systems. *Journal of the Saudi Society of Agricultural Sciences*, *15*(1), 38–47. https://doi.org/10.1016/j.jssas.2014.05.001

Namkhah, Z., Fatemi, S. F., Mansoori, A., Nosratabadi, S., Ghayour-Mobarhan, M., & Sobhani, S. R. (2023). Advancing sustainability in the food and nutrition system: a review of artificial intelligence applications. In *Frontiers in Nutrition* (Vol. 10). Frontiers Media SA. https://doi.org/10.3389/fnut.2023.1295241

de Oliveira, R. C., & de Silva, R. D. S. E. (2023). Artificial intelligence in agriculture: Benefits, challenges, and trends. In *Applied Sciences (Switzerland)* (Vol. 13, Issue 13). Multidisciplinary Digital Publishing Institute (MDPI). https://doi.org/10.3390/app13137405

Owino, L., & Söffker, D. (2022). How much is enough in watering plants? State-of-the-art in irrigation control: Advances, challenges, and opportunities with respect to precision irrigation. *Frontiers in Control Engineering*, *3*. https://doi.org/10.3389/fcteg.2022.982463

Pawlak, K., & Kołodziejczak, M. (2020). The role of agriculture in ensuring food security in developing countries: Considerations in the context of the problem of sustainable food production. *Sustainability (Switzerland)*, *12*(13). https://doi.org/10.3390/su12135488

Pearson, T. C., Doster, M. A., & Michailides, T. J. (2001). Automated detection of pistachio defects by machine vision. *Applied Engineering in Agriculture, 17*(5), 729–732.

Peixoto, M. S., Barros, L. C., Bassanezi, R. C., & Fernandes, O. A. (2015). An approach via fuzzy systems for dynamics and control of the soybean aphid. In X. Luo, A.A. Almohammedi, S. Guan, & D. Pamucar (eds.), *Proceedings of the 2015 Conference of the International Fuzzy Systems Association and the European Society for Fuzzy Logic and Technology* (pp. 1295–1301). Atlantis press. https://doi.org/10.2991/ifsa-eusflat-15.2015.183

Perez-Ortiz, M., Gutierrez, P. A., Pena, J. M., Torres-Sanchez, J., Lopez-Granados, F., & Hervas-Martinez, C. (2016). Machine learning paradigms for weed mapping via unmanned aerial vehicles. *2016 IEEE Symposium Series on Computational Intelligence, SSCI 2016*. https://doi.org/10.1109/SSCI.2016.7849987

Pham, T. N., Tran, L. Van, & Dao, S. V. T. (2020). Early disease classification of mango leaves using feed-forward neural network and hybrid metaheuristic feature selection. *IEEE Access*, *8*, 189960–189973. https://doi.org/10.1109/ACCESS.2020.3031914

Policy Brief Changing Policy Concepts of Food Security. (2006). www.foodsecinfoaction.org/

Przybylak, A., Kozłowski, R., Osuch, E., Osuch, A., Rybacki, P., & Przygodziński, P. (2020). Quality evaluation of potato tubers using neural image analysis method. *Agriculture (Switzerland)*, *10*(4). https://doi.org/10.3390/agriculture10040112

Rady, A., Ekramirad, N., Rady, A., Adedeji, A., Alimardani, R., Bessin, R., & Strang, J. (2016). *Hyperspectral Imaging for Detection of Codling Moth Infestation and Prediction of Quality in GoldRush Apples Hyperspectral Imaging for Detection of Codling Moth Infestation and Prediction of Quality in Gold-Rush Apples*. www.researchgate.net/publication/305650954

Russell, S. J., & Norvig P. (2016). *Artificial Intelligence: A Modern Approach*. Harlow, England: Pearson Education Ltd.

Saiz-Rubio, V., & Rovira-Más, F. (2020). From smart farming towards agriculture 5.0: A review on crop data management. In *Agronomy* (Vol. 10, Issue 2). MDPI. https://doi.org/10.3390/agronomy10020207

Sarker, I. H. (2021). Machine learning: Algorithms, real-world applications and research directions. *SN Computer Science*, *2*, 160.

Sarku, R., Clemen, U. A., & Clemen, T. (2023). The application of artificial intelligence models for food security: A review. In *Agriculture (Switzerland)* (Vol. 13, Issue 10). Multidisciplinary Digital Publishing Institute (MDPI). https://doi.org/10.3390/agriculture13102037

Sharma, A., Zanotti, P., & Musunur, L. P. (2020). Drive through robotics: Robotic automation for last mile distribution of food and essentials during pandemics. *IEEE Access 8*, 127190–127219.

Sofu, M. M., Er, O., Kayacan, M. C., & Cetişli, B. (2016). Design of an automatic apple sorting system using machine vision. *Computers and Electronics in Agriculture*, *127*, 395–405. https://doi.org/10.1016/j.compag.2016.06.030

Soori, M., Arezoo, B., & Dastres, R. (2023). Artificial intelligence, machine learning and deep learning in advanced robotics, a review. In *Cognitive Robotics* (Vol. 3, pp. 54–70). KeAi Communications Co. https://doi.org/10.1016/j.cogr.2023.04.001

Sparrow, R., Howard, M., & Degeling, C. (2021). Managing the risks of artificial intelligence in agriculture. *NJAS: Impact in Agricultural and Life Sciences*, *93*(1), 172–196. https://doi.org/10.1080/27685241.2021.2008777

Story, M., Hamm, M. W., & Wallinga, D. (2009). Food systems and public health: Linkages to achieve healthier diets and healthier communities. *Journal of Hunger and Environmental Nutrition*, *4*(3–4), 219–224. https://doi.org/10.1080/19320240903351463

The State of Food Security and Nutrition in the World 2022. (2022). *In The State of Food Security and Nutrition in the World 2022*. Rome: FAO. https://doi.org/10.4060/cc0639en

The Sustainable Development Goals Report 2023. (2023).

Torero, M. (2021). Robotics and AI in food security and innovation: Why they matter and how to harness their power. In von Braun, J., Archer, M. S., Reichberg, G. M., & Sorondo, M. S. (Eds.), *Robotics, AI and Humanity*. (pp. 102–107). https://doi.org/10.1007/978-3-030-54173-6

Valdes-Vela, M., Abrisqueta, I., Conejero, W., Vera J., & Ruiz-Sánchez, M. C. (2015). Soft computing applied to stem water potential estimation: A fuzzy rulebased approach. *Computers and Electronics in Agriculture*, *115*, 150–160.

Valdez, P. L. (2020). Apple defect detection using deep learning-based object detection for better postharvest handling. *Paper presented at the ICLR 2020 Workshop on Computer Vision for Agriculture (CV4A). 12 May, 2020.*

Van Henten, E. J., Hemming, J., Van Tuijl, B. A. J., Kornet, J. G., Meuleman, J., Bontsema, J., & Van Os, E. A. (2002). An autonomous robot for harvesting cucumbers in greenhouses. *Autonomous Robots*, *13*(3), 241–258. https://doi.org/10.1023/A:1020568125418

Zhao, Z., Chow, T. L., Rees, H. W., Yang, Q., Xing, Z., & Meng, F. R. (2009). Predict soil texture distributions using an artificial neural network model. *Computers and Electronics in Agriculture*, *65*, 36–48.

Zhou, L., Zhang, C., Liu, F., Qiu, Z., & He, Y. (2019). Application of deep learning in food: A review. *Comprehensive Reviews in Food Science Food Safety*, *18*, 1793–1811.

Index

Note: Figures are indicated by *italics*. Tables are indicated by **bold**.

For Product Safety Concerns and Information please contact our EU representative GPSR@taylorandfrancis.com
Taylor & Francis Verlag GmbH, Kaufingerstraße 24, 80331 München, Germany

www.ingramcontent.com/pod-product-compliance
Lightning Source LLC
LaVergne TN
LVHW011122300926
849160LV00008B/477

* 9 7 8 1 0 3 2 7 8 2 9 6 6 *